Bioethics at the Movies

Recent and Related Titles in Bioethics

Nancy Berlinger *After Harm: Medical Error and the Ethics of Forgiveness*

Grant R. Gillett *Bioethics in the Clinic: Hippocratic Reflections*

John D. Lantos *The Lazarus Case: Life-and-Death Issues in Neonatal Intensive Care*

Carol Levine and Thomas H. Murray, eds. *The Cultures of Caregiving: Conflict and Common Ground among Families, Health Professionals, and Policy Makers*

John P. Lizza *Persons, Humanity, and the Definition of Death*

Thomas H. Murray, *Consulting Editor in Bioethics*

Bioethics at the Movies

Edited by
SANDRA SHAPSHAY

The Johns Hopkins University Press
Baltimore

Printed in the United States of America on acid-free paper
9 8 7 6 5 4 3 2 1

The Johns Hopkins University Press
2715 North Charles Street
Baltimore, Maryland 21218-4363
www.press.jhu.edu

Library of Congress Cataloging-in-Publication Data
Bioethics at the movies / edited by Sandra Shapshay.
p. cm.
Includes bibliographical references and index.
ISBN-13: 978-0-8018-9077-2 (hardcover : alk. paper)
ISBN-13: 978-0-8018-9078-9 (pbk. : alk. paper)
ISBN-10: 0-8018-9077-2 (hardcover : alk. paper)
ISBN-10: 0-8018-9078-0 (pbk. : alk. paper)
1. Medical ethics—Miscellanea. 2. Motion pictures. I. Shapshay, Sandra, 1969–
R725.5.B52 2008
174.2—dc22 2008015426

A catalog record for this book is available from the British Library.

Special discounts are available for bulk purchases of this book. For more information, please contact Special Sales at 410-516-6936 or specialsales@press.jhu.edu.

The Johns Hopkins University Press uses environmentally friendly book materials, including recycled text paper that is composed of at least 30 percent post-consumer waste, whenever possible. All of our book papers are acid-free, and our jackets and covers are printed on paper with recycled content.

To my mercurial husband, Steve,

who inspired this project

Contents

PART FIVE The Role of Theory and Culture in Bioethics

Contributors

ROBERT ARP, PH.D., Researcher, National Center for Biomedical Ontology, University at Buffalo, State University of New York, Buffalo, New York

MICHAEL C. BRANNIGAN, PH.D., Pfaff Endowed Chair in Ethics and Moral Values, Department of Philosophy and Religious Studies, The College of Saint Rose, Albany, New York; Adjunct Faculty, Alden March Bioethics Institute, Albany, New York

MATTHEW BURSTEIN, PH.D., Assistant Professor, Philosophy Department, University of Pittsburgh at Johnstown, Johnstown, Pennsylvania

ANTONIO CASADO DA ROCHA, PH.D., Ramón y Cajal Research Fellow, University of the Basque Country, Donostia–San Sebastián, Spain

STEPHEN COLEMAN, PH.D., Senior Lecturer in Ethics, School of Humanities and Social Sciences, University of New South Wales at the Australian Defence Force Academy, Canberra, Australia

JASON T. EBERL, PH.D., Associate Professor, Department of Philosophy, Indiana University-Purdue University, Indianapolis; Affiliate Faculty, Indiana University Center for Bioethics, Indianapolis, Indiana

BRADLEY J. FISHER, PH.D., Professor of Psychology and Gerontology, Missouri State University, Springfield, Missouri

PAUL J. FORD, PH.D., Clinical Bioethicist, the Cleveland Clinic Foundation, and Assistant Professor of Medicine, CCF Lerner College of Medicine of Case Western Reserve University, Cleveland, Ohio

HELEN FROWE, PH.D., Assistant Professor, Department of Philosophy, University of Sheffield, Sheffield, United Kingdom

COLIN GAVAGHAN, PH.D., Lecturer in Medical Law, School of Law, University of Glasgow, Glasgow, United Kingdom

RICHARD HANLEY, PH.D., Associate Professor, Department of Philosophy, University of Delaware, Newark, Delaware

NANCY HANSEN, PH.D., Assistant Professor and Director, Disability Studies, University of Manitoba, Winnipeg, Manitoba, Canada

AL-YASHA ILHAAM, PH.D., Assistant Professor, Department of Philosophy and Religious Studies, Spelman College, Atlanta, Georgia

TROY JOLLIMORE, PH.D., Associate Professor, Department of Philosophy, California State University, Chico, California

AMY KIND, PH.D., Associate Dean of Faculty and Associate Professor, Department of Philosophy, Claremont McKenna College, Claremont, California

ZANA MARIE LUTFIYYA, PH.D., Associate Dean (Research and Graduate Programs) and Professor, Faculty of Education, University of Manitoba, Winnipeg, Manitoba, Canada

TERRANCE MCCONNELL, PH.D., Professor, Department of Philosophy, University of North Carolina at Greensboro, Greensboro, North Carolina

ANDY MIAH, PH.D., Reader in New Media and Bioethics, School of Media, Language and Music, University of the West of Scotland, Ayr, United Kingdom

NATHAN NOBIS, PH.D., Assistant Professor, Philosophy and Religion Department, Morehouse College, Atlanta, Georgia

KENNETH RICHMAN, PH.D., Associate Professor, School of Arts and Sciences, Massachusetts College of Pharmacy and Health Sciences, Boston, Massachusetts

KAREN D. SCHWARTZ, LL.B., M.A., Doctoral Candidate, Faculty of Education, University of Manitoba, Winnipeg, Manitoba, Canada

SANDRA SHAPSHAY, PH.D., Assistant Professor, Department of Philosophy, Indiana University, Bloomington; Affiliate Faculty, Indiana University Center for Bioethics, Indianapolis, Indiana

DANIEL SPERLING, LL.M., S.J.D., Senior Lecturer, The Federmann School of Public Policy and Government and Braun School of Public Health and Community Medicine, The Hebrew University of Jerusalem, Israel

BECKY COX WHITE, R.N., PH.D., Professor, Department of Philosophy, California State University, Chico, California

CLARK WOLF, PH.D., Director of Bioethics and Associate Professor, Department of Philosophy and Religious Studies, Iowa State University, Ames, Iowa

Preface

The volume is organized into five parts that follow the syllabi for many bioethics courses. Although the last part deals more with theoretical matters in bioethics, the other four mirror the human life cycle, from issues surrounding birth, to the living of a good life, to aging, and finally to questions about death. In this way, the book forms something of an organic whole, covering a comprehensive and contemporary array of issues that have long preoccupied bioethicists, in a way that is at once accessible to students of bioethics (undergraduates, graduate, medical, and nursing students), useful for teachers of bioethics, and interesting for specialists to see how key issues in the field may be explored through mass cultural products. To foster reflection and discussion of the arguments and themes in this volume, the authors have included some questions for consideration at the end of each chapter. Wherever possible, these questions help put the chapters themselves into dialogue with each other and with the reader.

Part I considers first ethical questions related to the beginning of life. Robert Arp's piece on *The Cider House Rules* and Al-Yasha Ilhaam's chapter on the satiric *Citizen Ruth* both deal with the thorny issue of abortion. Then chapters 3 and 4 are devoted to the key conceptual question, central to many of these debates in bioethics: Who counts as a "person" (i.e., a full member of the moral community, a significant object of our moral concern)? Are embryos and fetuses "persons" in an ethically relevant sense? Might robots be persons? Are sentient nonhuman animals such as pigs owed vastly more moral respect than most people now give them? Stephen Coleman and Richard Hanley take up the first two questions in their discussion of *I, Robot* and *Bicentennial Man* and Nathan

Nobis queries what we humans owe to sentient, nonhuman animals through his treatment of *Babe*.

Part II treats the use of biotechnology in the quest for "better" or even the "same" people through popular films. In separate essays, Colin Gavaghan and I spar over whether or not *Gattaca* presents a prescient warning about the widespread use of reproductive genetic technologies. The section then turns to a lively discussion of arguments against human reproductive cloning featuring Troy Jollimore and Becky Cox White's analysis of *Multiplicity* and Amy Kind's examination of *Star Trek: Nemesis*.

Part III delves into ethical issues relating to medical intervention and the quest for the good life. Andy Miah investigates the ethics of memory erasure in *Eternal Sunshine of the Spotless Mind*, asking whether it is a legitimate professional activity for medicine to "fix a broken heart" by the slightly fanciful enhancement possibility of medically induced forgetting. Paul J. Ford then raises the question of whether individual functional enhancement isn't profoundly alienating for the enhanced through an analysis of the Japanese anime *Ghost in the Shell* in light of several philosophical theories of the self. Clark Wolf investigates issues of exploitation and global justice through *Dirty Pretty Things*, after which Terrance McConnell treats the ways in which role-related obligations conflict in academic medicine through a careful consideration of the film *Wit*.

The volume's fourth part confronts questions of aging and the good death. First, Bradley J. Fisher and I explore the themes of deception, self-deception, and compassion in the moving narrative of *Dad*. Next, two chapters constitute a debate over the bioethical significance of Clint Eastwood's Oscar-winning *Million Dollar Baby*. According to Zana Marie Lutfiyya, Karen D. Schwartz, and Nancy Hansen (whose work is informed by the relatively new field of disability studies), Eastwood's film perpetuates the stereotype that disability and death go hand in hand, and that disabled lives are not worth living. By contrast, Helen Frowe defends the film against these charges and argues that the protagonist's choice to seek death can be autonomously made and legitimately honored. In the final essays of Part IV, authors explore ways in which health care providers and institutions can help people to die better. Kenneth Richman draws our attention to the narrative structures of films and to the contrast between the ways in which characters die in *Critical Care* and *Big Fish*. On the basis of his analysis, Richman argues that understanding the importance of the life stories individuals construct for themselves provides guidance for how better to respect patient autonomy and to help people to experience a good and fitting end to their life story—a good death. Similarly, Matt Burstein argues that the classic dystopia of *Soylent Green* shows us, ironically, how a good death might be achieved with the "thanatorium," an institution taken from the only humane aspect of that nightmarish cinematic world.

With the life cycle complete, Part V discusses two foundational topics for bioethics: the nature and role of ethical theories and principles and the importance of cultural context in bioethical discussions. If readers are unfamiliar with ethical theories and principles such as the much-invoked principle of respect for autonomy, a good place to start would be with the essay by Jason T. Eberl on *Extreme Measures*, in which the author investigates how consequentialism and Kantian deontology may be applied in a cinematic dramatization of research misconduct. Daniel Sperling discusses this principle and offers a feminist rethinking of it in the medical context through an engagement with Pedro Almodóvar's *Talk to Her.* In the final two chapters, Antonio Casado da Rocha and Michael C. Brannigan draw out how particular cultural contexts—in Spain and in Japan—shape bioethical debates and approaches, by focusing respectively on three recent Spanish films (*Talk to Her, The Sea Inside,* and *My Life without Me*) and Akira Kurosawa's *Ikiru.*

I first thank the hardworking contributors to this volume: bioethics through film is a rather new and difficult genre, and they have embarked on it with much energy and insight. I am especially grateful to my able, aesthetically sophisticated editorial assistant, Mike Rings, and to Terrance McConnell for helpful comments at every stage of this project. Many thanks also to Michael Brannigan, Colin Gavaghan, Robert Arp, Andy Miah, Karen Ballentine, Robin Varghese, York Gunther, our much-Podcasted local film critic Peter Noble-Kuchera, Andrea Wohl, Eric Silverman, Ken Pimple, Mike Grossberg, Rich Miller, Nick Blesch, Molly Sutphen, Bill Irwin, and Fritz Schmuhl for helpful conversations and advice in shaping this project. Brian Schrag was kind to get the word out about this enterprise and to include a panel on "Bioethics through Film" at the annual meeting of the Association for Practical and Professional Ethics (APPE). I greatly appreciate Thomas Murray, for his interest in this project, Wendy Harris, at the Johns Hopkins University Press, for expert editorial guidance, and Michele T. Callaghan for astute copyediting. Finally, I'd like to give special thanks to my husband, Steve Wagschal, who has screened and discussed many bioethically rich films with me, and to my thoughtful and spirited girls, Molly and Marlena Wagschal.

Bioethics at the Movies

Introduction

Why, you might ask, should we care how other people think and feel about stories? Why do we talk about them in this language of value? Evaluating stories together is one of the central human ways of learning to align our responses to the world. And that alignment is, in turn, one of the ways we maintain the social fabric, the texture of our relationships.

KWAME ANTHONY APPIAH,
Cosmopolitanism: Ethics in a World of Strangers

This volume brings together an international set of contributors who have provided twenty-one original, philosophical essays, which grapple with serious bioethical issues by examining films. Each essay, in accordance with Appiah's reflection above, talks about stories "in the language of value." The authors in this collection detail the virtues and vices of characters, scrutinize the choices they make, and analyze the ethically relevant particularities of their situations as well as the justice or injustice of the social worlds they inhabit.

Why, however, should one care about how these authors think and feel about these cinematic narratives? It is my aim that the philosophical, legal, medical, anthropological, literary, psychological, and sociological expertise that these authors bring to bear on these films will spark a philosophical dialogue among readers and in classrooms, clarifying, refining, and challenging the ethical positions people hold on a great many bioethical topics.

Why teach and do bioethics through film? Is there anything that ethical reflection gains specifically through this medium? In answering these foundational questions, we might want to address recent discussions of the relationship of film to philosophy. Can engagement with certain films advance philosophical knowledge? Do some films actually philosophize in their own right? At first glance, it would seem unlikely that film can do these things, as philosophy in general is essentially a linguistic enterprise and deals generally with claims, arguments, and conclusions. In contrast, films develop characters, build narratives, and treat themes through visual images, and sometimes with purposeful ambiguity. This volume deals with philosophical bioethics, and insofar as this type of bioethics is the applied or practical branch of normative ethics, itself a branch of philosophy, getting a handle on the relationship of at least some films to philosophy is crucial for understanding whether taking "bioethics to the movies" is a worthy enterprise at all.

Do Some Films Philosophize?

In the past ten years, philosophers have taken unprecedented interest in film, especially popular films such as *The Matrix* (Wachowski Brothers 1999), which has inspired several volumes of essays dealing with philosophical themes raised in the film.[1] Although these books treat philosophical themes raised in the *Matrix* films, some philosophers have gone so far as to claim that films not only contain interesting philosophical references but also can actually philosophize. A sustained interpretation of the *Alien* series, for instance, forms the basis for Stephen Mulhall's claim that films can do just that (Mulhall 2002):

> At least some films might be thought of (not as illustrations of independently-given philosophical issues and arguments, and not as the raw material for philosophical analysis or diagnosis, but) as thinking seriously and systematically about such issues and arguments in just the ways that philosophers do. (MULHALL 2007, P. 279)

In defending this highly controversial claim, Mulhall points to the ways in which some films can get us to see the world differently, not through the giving of explicit premises and the laying out of inferences in a deductive argument but rather by engaging us in a cinematic world, emotionally and intellectually. This emotional and cognitive engagement can lead us to view our own world and selves differently and to question things we had hitherto not interrogated. Mulhall explains this power of film with respect to moral insight as follows:

> There is a strong philosophical tendency to think of moral disagreement on the model of opposing opinions about a particular course of action, with each opinion supported by more general ethical principles. But . . . moral disagreement can also be a matter of differing visions of what matters in human life, different conceptions of flourishing in the world, and so on; and discussion here may well take the form of encouraging one's interlocutor not so much as to change her mind about a particular course of action but to look at everything differently—and so to find moral significance where it did not previously seem to exist, as well as to find that what previously seemed highly morally significant was in fact trivial or even essentially illusory. (MULHALL 2007, P. 290)

For Mulhall, at least some films present us with reasons to believe a moral claim—the hallmark of moral-philosophical discourse—albeit in ways hitherto not generally recognized as rationally persuading. In presenting a way of seeing the world, in particular experience, rather than abstract language, the engaged viewer has reason to reevaluate what she finds morally significant and to perceive a moral situation differently.

Mulhall is not alone in claiming that some forms of narrative art philosophize in this way. Through an elaborate interpretation of Henry James's *The Golden Bowl*, Martha Nussbaum argues that certain literary works constitute a kind of moral philosophy and that certain truths about human life, which are vital to grappling with how a human being should live—the ethical question par excellence for Nussbaum—"can only be fittingly and accurately stated in the language and forms characteristic of the narrative artist" (Nussbaum 1990, p. 5).

In line with Mulhall's and Nussbaum's claims for the moral-philosophical import of narrative art, several of the authors in this volume endeavor to present bioethics through film by showing how an emotional engagement with a film's characters yields a kind of "moral knowledge" indispensable for sound practical reasoning. For example, chapter 19 by Daniel Sperling and chapter 20 by Antonio Casado da Rocha treat Pedro Almodóvar's *Talk to Her* (2002), a mature film that summons an emotional engagement, sympathy, and understanding of Benigno, a character who models an unorthodox but potentially therapeutic kind of care for his patients. If one were to read a newspaper account of Benigno's actions, most people would find him utterly repugnant, but through the cinematic narrative, one's ordinary resistance to such characters and actions is overcome. Whether or not such resistance should be overcome is a live question, but one that gets raised only through reflection on the film.

Similarly, in chapter 11 Clark Wolf examines how *Dirty Pretty Things* (Frears 2002) portrays the exploitation of the film's main characters—vulnerable, socially invisible, struggling immigrants in London—by the wealthy and unscrupulous through an underground market in transplant organs. In engaging with this wrenching, Hitchcockian-suspense-thriller of a feature film, viewers get a better sense of how it might feel—from the inside—to inhabit such a desperate situation, one in which one would be willing to turn important parts of one's body into commodities. Approaching an ethical issue in this way through narrative, it is argued, provides an indispensable ingredient in sound public moral deliberation, for narrative art often encourages filmgoers to gain an emotional understanding of people unlike themselves, and this is likely to have a humanizing effect on moral reasoning (Nussbaum 1995).

In chapter 16 Kenneth Richman demonstrates how some films can constitute a form of thinking through an ethical problem. Richman draws out how *Big Fish* (Burton 2003) underscores the importance of narrative for a person's self-understanding. A reflective engagement with the form and content of the film reveals how a human being is a deeply "narrative creature" who makes sense of life only by seeing him- or herself as a character in a kind of life story. Richman further argues that this important feature of human beings is often overlooked in medical ethics but can and should inform how health professionals and patients approach end-of-life decisions. Based on a critical reflection on the film, Richman proposes that we adopt a "narrative" account of patient autonomy.

Functions of Film in Bioethics

In addition to seeing engagement with some films as providing a kind of moral knowledge, there are three other main ways in which authors use popular, narrative films for the sake of bioethical reflection: (1) pedagogically, as providing useful, compelling, and even "cool" illustrations of bioethical issues for students; (2) interpretatively, as providing fleshed-out interpretations of independently made bioethical claims; and (3) experimentally, as providing rich thought-experiments that tap into moral intuitions and advance ethical thinking.

The Pedagogical Function of Film

The least controversial, but nonetheless important, claim for film's role in bioethics is that some films provide compelling illustrations for independently worked philosophical ideas. Paisley Livingston has argued that cinema cannot make creative contributions to philosophy but can have tremendous pedagogical value. He argues against the most ambitious claim that film can provide an exclusive source of philosophical insight, as it gets caught on the horns of the following dilemma. If the alleged cinematic-philosophical insight can be paraphrased in linguistic form, and thus communicated discursively, then the film no longer serves as the exclusive vehicle for such knowledge. Alternatively, if the alleged cinematic-philosophical insights are ineffable, then their very existence is open to reasonable doubt. Furthermore, for Livingston, the burden of proof lies with those who claim a "new and controversial source of philosophical knowledge" (Livingston 2006, p. 13). What we should accept, Livingston concludes, is "a more modest conception of the cinema's role in the development of philosophical insight. Films can provide vivid and emotionally engaging illustrations of philosophical issues, and when sufficient background knowledge is in place, reflections about films can contribute to the exploration of specific theses and arguments, sometimes yielding enhanced philosophical understanding" (Livingston 2006, p. 11). Ultimately, however, we should see film's greatest role in the philosophical enterprise as pedagogical, as a complement to writings by philosophers.

This volume as a whole aims to tap the pedagogical function of film for bioethics. Most of the films treated in the volume are a pleasure to watch and are intellectually stimulating. Additionally, they are easy for faculty and students to come by as they are very popular or critically acclaimed. By grounding bioethical discussion and argument in a film, students will gain a sense of the excitement and fascination that is philosophical bioethics and will use their minds and hearts to better comprehend the key issues, methods, and arguments used in this field to reason through these issues.

The Interpretive Function of Film

A more ambitious claim for the value of film for philosophy is to see some films as not merely illustrating independently given philosophical ideas but also as offering an interpretation of these that advances understanding. Thomas Wartenberg recently made a good case for seeing some films as providing insightful illustration of an independently derived philosophical claim or theory (though not necessarily an exclusive means for doing so; Wartenberg 2006, p. 20). He argues that many authors who reflect on the relationship between film and philosophy are in the grip of a false dichotomy between either "illustrating a philosophical claim" and "actually doing philosophy." Instead, Wartenberg argues, some illustrations of philosophical claims work as thought experiments which interpret, elaborate and further the more bare philosophical claim of which it is an illustration.

Using the example of Charlie Chaplin's *Modern Times* (1936), Wartenberg shows how the film "fleshes out" Marx's claim about the alienation of the worker from the products of his labor under capitalism. Chaplin plays a factory worker whose sole job is to tighten two bolts in a conveyor-belt assembly system. By way of a series of comic riffs on what this mindless, mechanical activity does to Charlie's character (he becomes a mindless bolt-tightening machine, mistaking buttons on a woman's dress—and many other objects—for bolts in need of tightening), Wartenberg thus shows how a film can interpret our understanding of Marx's philosophical claim. This kind of interpretation is analogous to that which a musician offers in any given performance of a classical score. *Allegro*, for instance, is not a univocal command but a range of tempos from which the musician may choose, depending on the character or intensity she would like to impart to the music. Similarly, a film may interpret a philosophical claim, by adding a particular characterization, by giving a modern interpretation of the theory, which fleshes out its meaning and adds to our understanding of it.

Several of the authors in this volume teach and do bioethics through film by focusing on how a film serves to interpret for us, a particular bioethical claim. For instance, Helen Frowe's chapter on *Million Dollar Baby* (Eastwood 2004) sees the film as interpreting the claim that assisted suicide may be morally permissible, by providing a particular case in which the philosophical distinction between the value of a biographical versus a biological life may be illustrated and usefully contrasted. Through the understanding viewers gain of the particular life story of Maggie, one can see how the biographical and biological value of a life may conflict, and how this kind of a distinction lends support to the moral permissibility of assisted suicide. By contrast, Zana Marie Lutfiyya, Karen D. Schwartz, and Nancy Hansen focus on another way in which the film interprets the claim that assisted suicide may be morally permissible, by drawing out how the plot, camera angles, lighting, and what is shown or not shown with respect to the life of Maggie portrays disability as akin to a living death. They aim to reveal how the directorial choices made in the film embody deeply held societal prejudices about the nature and value of disabled lives; and they argue that the film fosters a misguided acceptance of assisted suicide as a logical option. Thus, their reading of the film aims to disclose something pernicious about the film's implicit account of the moral permissibility of assisted suicide.

The Experimental Function of Film

Another way in which philosophers have come to see some films as capable of advancing philosophical knowledge is by presenting elaborate and imaginatively engaging thought experiments (Smith 2006, p. 34). At least since Plato's parable of the cave, philosophy has used thought experiments to get a reader to entertain a scenario that may challenge his or her cherished beliefs. One of the most famous thought experiments in ethics (discussed in the first section of the book) is Judith Jarvis Thomson's violinist analogy. Thomson asks the reader to imagine yourself in a scenario in which you have been kidnapped and hooked up to a famous, unconscious violinist, so that he might make use of your kidneys for nine months to survive. By sketching out this scenario, Thomson asks the reader to entertain a possibility that probably has never occurred to him before. Because the situation is rather far-fetched and hypothetical, the reader's ordinary resistance to belief change might be broken down, and his deepest moral intuitions may be tapped in such a way as to challenge him to revise his customary moral beliefs in the case of abortion. Much science fiction and many of the films discussed in this volume (*Gattaca*, *Bicentennial Man, Multiplicity,* and *I, Robot)* constitute elaborately ramified thought experiments that invite the viewer to consider possibilities and to inhabit a point of view that can tap deep moral intuitions, challenging him to confront everyday beliefs.

Page-long case studies written by ethicists are not nearly as compelling as well-crafted films. The complex ways in which research and therapy come into conflict, for example, is explored subtly in Terrance McConnell's chapter in the teaching hospital setting of *Wit* (Nichols 2001). In this case, had the discussions of the ethical issues been divorced from a sustained, imaginative plot with engaging characters, they would not capture so effectively the emotional content nor the contextual nuances.

Moreover, for some bioethical issues, the only "case studies" we have are to be found in science fiction. Today, for instance, we must speculate on how human reproductive cloning might affect human lives. *Multiplicity* (Ramis 1996) suggests lightheartedly what cloning might mean for personal identity, and Troy Jollimore and Becky Cox White explore the pitfalls of using such science fiction for ethical reflection insofar as the "science" in these fictional worlds is sometimes preposterous. Notwithstanding the scientific improbabilities of the cloning capabilities used in *Multiplicity,* the authors employ the cinematic imagination to test out arguments that reproductive cloning would constitute a threat to personal identity, in a way that is concretely anchored in a narrative. Similarly, Amy Kind's analysis of *Star Trek: Nemesis* (Baird 2002) demonstrates how the film affords a more scientifically plausible ground for testing out arguments that aim to show how cloning would harm the clones.

Some science-fictional "case studies," such as *Gattaca* (Niccol 1997), are more self-conscious predictions of how our industrialized societies would change given widespread use of emerging technologies. Set in the "not-too-distant" future, Colin Gavaghan and I detail how *Gattaca* invites the viewer to inhabit a fictional world that is quite similar to her own, in both scientific possibilities and sociopolitical institutions, and yet entirely dystopian from the point of view of the protagonists.

The Dangers of Doing Bioethics through Film

What are the potential drawbacks of using film to further bioethical or, more generally, philosophical reflection? One danger is that motion pictures, like all kinds of fiction, may persuade through mere rhetoric and emotional manipulation rather than through good reasons. Viewers should be on guard for this kind of persuasion, and the authors in this collection are cognizant of this worry. Acknowledging that this is a bona fide risk, in chapter 4 Nathan Nobis, however, counters the contention that *Babe* (Noonan 1995) presents an animal-rights message by way of illegitimate anthropomorphism and sentimental manipulation. Nobis argues that, while the film does use emotional appeals to get the audience to sympathize with the plight of farm animals, the emotional pull of the film is justified by way of reasons garnered from the scientific literature on animal cognition.

Another way in which film might mislead an audience is that cinematic works, like any other narrative creation, are the products of human beings who select shots, juxtapose images, and frame a problematic scenario. This may be done in a way that is not reflective of real-life or highly biased. In the chapter by Lutfiyya, Schwartz, and Hansen, the authors detail the ways in which *Million Dollar Baby* frames the issue of assisted suicide in a way that embodies the all-too-common and unquestioned notion in Western societies that disability equals death, and that physical dependency on others is shameful. According to these authors, an unreflective encounter with the film would serve to confirm such stereotypes, ones instrumental in the oppression of persons with disabilities. However, a reflective engagement with this film, and an uncovering of the biases implicit in it, can spark a fruitful dialogue on the nature of disability, physical dependence on others, and the ethical treatment of those different from the norm.

Another cluster of dangers in teaching and doing bioethics through film falls under the rubric of what might be termed *philistinism*. First, there is the danger that in "mining" film for its ethical importance, an author might fail to respect the film as an aesthetic object—as a work of cinematic art. A considerable debate rages on the relationships between art and morality, and, more specifically, on whether moral defects in works of art constitute aesthetic defects as well. However, it is beyond the scope of this introduction to wade into this debate.[2] That said, most contemporary aestheticians would agree that moral considerations may play some role in evaluating works of cinematic (and other) art, but that one illegitimately treats an aesthetic product as mere propaganda if one evaluates it solely in this light. If one faults the film *Multiplicity* on moral grounds (for painting a clearly exaggerated and unrealistic picture of cloning, thereby confirming unwarranted public fears about this technology), one fails to treat it with sufficient respect for the kind of thing it is, failing to acknowledge that the film also has properly artistic aims. Certainly, the creators of *Multiplicity* did not intend to weigh in on public policy debates about cloning; the film is put forth as a screwball comedy, featuring a beloved comic actor (Michael Keaton) and exploring primarily the comic potential of a "cloning" situation. While ethical criticism of a film may be quite justifiable (for instance, if a film entices the viewer to laugh at tremendous human suffering, under certain circumstances) such criticism crosses the line into moralizing when it does not keep in mind that aesthetic and moral judgments are separable.[3]

Given the possible pitfalls of doing and teaching bioethics through film, the skeptic might justifiably question, do the likely benefits outweigh these potential problems? To my mind, the answer is "yes" so long as authors and readers pay careful attention to improbable scenarios, impossible science, sentimental manipulation, and all manner of prejudice and bias in films, and so long as they remember that films are aesthetic creations not pure propaganda.

While the authors of the twenty-one chapters aim to treat the films with aesthetic sensitivity, paying attention to the specific mode of presentation in the films, this volume is not a collection of film criticism, and its aim is not solely for the reader to come away with interesting interpretations of films. Rather, it is meant to highlight bioethical issues, methods, and arguments through the concrete engagement of the essayists with films.

An Invitation

The chapters in this volume approach the task of taking bioethics to the movies, so to speak, in various ways. In this introduction, I have endeavored to characterize some of the main ways in which critical reflection on film may advance philosophical and bioethical understanding: by seeing films as actually philosophizing, by yielding moral knowledge, as offering interpretations of philosophical claims, and by setting up imaginative, cinematic worlds that serve as multifaceted thought experiments. I hope that this collection will enable a richer encounter for readers with the bioethical themes in popular film and will spark in readers their own reflections on the ethical importance of telling stories through film. My claim for this volume is that at least some films provide a rich matrix in which ethical thinking may flourish by virtue of the medium's ability to draw viewers in visually, intellectually, and emotionally.

NOTES

1. See, for example, *The Matrix and Philosophy: Welcome to the Desert of the Real* (Irwin 2002) and *Philosophers Explore the Matrix* (Grau 2005).

2. For an excellent overview of the contemporary debate on the legitimacy of ethical criticism, see Matthew Kieran (2006).

3. It is beyond the scope of this introduction to argue for this claim. See Mary Devereaux (1998) for a full argument in favor of the separability of aesthetic and moral judgments.

REFERENCES

Almodóvar, P. 2002. *Hable con ella* [English title, *Talk to Her;* motion picture]. Madrid: El Deseo, S.A.

Appiah, K. A. 2006. *Cosmopolitanism: Ethics in a World of Strangers.* New York: W. W. Norton & Co.

Baird, S. *Star Trek: Nemesis* [motion picture]. Hollywood, CA: Paramount Pictures.

Burton, T. 2004. *Big Fish* [motion picture].Culver City, CA: Columbia Pictures Corporation.

Chaplin, C. 1936. *Modern Times* [motion picture]. Hollywood, CA: Charles Chaplin Productions.

Devereaux, M. 1998. Beauty and Evil: The Case of Leni Riefenstahl's *Triumph of the Will.* In *Aesthetics and Ethics: Essays at the Intersection.* Cambridge and New York: Cambridge University Press, ed. J. Levinson, 227–56.

Eastwood, C. 2004. *Million Dollar Baby* [motion picture]. Burbank, CA: Warner Bros. Pictures.

Frears, S. 2002. *Dirty Pretty Things* [motion picture]. London: British Broadcasting Corporation.

Grau, C., ed. 2005. *Philosophers Explore the Matrix*. New York: Oxford University Press.

Irwin, W., ed. 2002. *The Matrix and Philosophy: Welcome to the Desert of the Real*. Peru, IL: Open Court.

Kieran, M. 2006. Art, Morality and Ethics: On the (Im)Moral Character of Art Works and Inter-relations to Artistic Value. *Philosophy Compass* 1 (2): 129–43.

Livingston, P. 2006. The Very Idea of Film as Philosophy. *Journal of Aesthetics and Art Criticism* 64 (1): 11–18.

Mulhall, S. 2002. *On Film*. London: Routledge.

———. 2007. Film as Philosophy: The Very Idea. *Proceedings of the Aristotelian Society*. 107 (3): 279–93.

Niccol, A. 1997. *Gattaca* [motion picture]. Culver City, CA: Columbia Pictures Corporation.

Nichols, M. 2001. *Wit* [television program]. New York and Los Angeles: Home Box Office Films.

Noonan, C. 1995. *Babe* [motion picture]. Beverly Hills, CA: Kennedy Miller Productions.

Nussbaum, M. 1990. *Love's Knowledge*. New York: Oxford University Press.

———. 1995. *Poetic Justice*. Boston: Beacon Press.

Ramis, H. 1996. *Multiplicity* [motion picture]. Culver City, CA: Columbia Pictures Corporation.

Smith, M. 2006. Film Art, Argument and Ambiguity. *Journal of Aesthetics and Art Criticism* 64 (1): 33–42.

Wartenberg, T. E. 2006. Beyond *Mere* Illustration: How Films Can Be Philosophy. *Journal of Aesthetics and Art Criticism* 64 (1): 19–32.

Wachowski Brothers. 1999. *The Matrix* [motion picture]. Burbank, CA: Warner Bros. Pictures.

PART ONE

On Babies, Test Tubes, and Sex the Old-Fashioned Way

"I Give Them What They Want—Either an Orphan or an Abortion"

The Cider House Rules and the Abortion Issue

Robert Arp

> This movie promotes abortion. It almost glorifies the act, giving some type of heroic status to a horrible act. Do not go see the movie. Do not even rent the movie. It has very deep meanings. If you must see it, please do not take your children. It will send the wrong message to them. The message is "Anything is all right, given the right circumstances."
>
> ANONYMOUS INTERNET REVIEWER

This was one of the first anonymous Internet reviews I read of the film *The Cider House Rules* (Hallström 1999) before seeing the movie and reading the book (Irving 1997). My interest was piqued, especially because the movie trailer gives one the impression that this is more of a "young adult orphan leaves the orphanage to discover life and himself in the process" kind of film. That was true, but the story also deals with a variety of ethical topics, including drug usage, incest, lying for the "right" reasons, and abortion. Set during World War II, the story's central character is Dr. Wilbur Larch (played by Michael Caine), a medical doctor and caretaker of a New England orphanage. There, pregnant women come either to have their babies—and then place them in the orphanage for adoption—or to have illegal abortions. Homer Wells (played by Tobey Maguire) is a college-aged "lifer" orphan at the facility who has learned the arts of doctoring and caretaking from Larch. The two have a series of conversations about abortion, with Larch assuming the role of the spokesperson for a utilitarian position on abortion and Homer acting as the spokesperson for the personal responsibility and sanctity of life positions.

In the end Homer has a "conversion" and sees things Larch's way. Ultimately he becomes the primary medical doctor and caretaker of the orphanage after Larch's suicide (Irving 1997).

The Cider House Rules raises two central questions about abortion: (1) Should the fetus inside the womb be regarded as a person with the same rights and privileges as any other person? Here, the movie is vague: there are times in the story when Larch and Homer characterize the fetus as a *child*, as well as an *almost child*, and an *it*. (2) Even if the fetus is a person, does the mother have a moral case for aborting that fetus? In an important part of the story, Larch proclaims that if they are to be responsible parents, women must be given the right to decide whether to have children. Larch's proclamation can be read as a kind of pro-choice claim: a woman should always have the option to do with her body what she wants to, pregnant or not.

Part of what I do in this chapter is to present balanced responses to these questions, investigating and critiquing the arguments given by advocates of what are typically called "conservative pro-life" and "liberal pro-choice" positions. First, to get a better sense of where people's sentiments concerning abortion lie, I should say something general about these positions, as this background will help us understand the ethical dimensions of the film.

The conservative pro-life position usually is characterized by the belief that, from the moment a human egg is fertilized, a new person exists. This human being is innocent and has the same right not to be killed as any other full-fledged person walking the streets, irrespective of the fact that this being is living inside a woman's body. From this perspective, abortion is usually characterized as akin to the murder of an innocent person, immoral, and, in general, not to be performed (Noonan 1967; Kreeft 2000). This is one of several pro-life positions that run the gamut from the stance that one ought never, ever to perform an abortion, even if it means the mother would die because the abortion has not been performed (the most extreme, strongest ultraconservative pro-life position), to performing an abortion if and only if the mother's life is in danger (the more standard, strongly conservative pro-life position), to performing an abortion in the event that a woman has been raped or is the victim of incest, but not if she has willfully engaged in sexual intercourse (the less standard, weakly conservative pro-life position).

When we think of the most "extreme" pro-life position, what usually comes to mind are militant anti-abortionists who bomb abortion clinics or kill the doctors who perform abortions. These people not only endorse the most extreme, strongest ultraconservative pro-life position *for themselves* but also translate this belief into a horrible action. They also want to force their belief *on others* in what they take to be a kind of "holy war" in which terroristlike behaviors are justified.

In contrast, the liberal pro-choice position usually is characterized by the belief that the being living inside the mother's womb is not yet a person and does not deserve legal and moral rights. Even if the fetus is to be considered a person, some believe the mother could abort it, under certain circumstances, because she still has the right to do with her body what she wants to (Thomson 1971; Warren 1973; Boonin 2003). Often times, liberal pro-choicers also will appeal to the circumstances surrounding a mother's life, arguing that if the consequences of giving birth for the mother, baby, or others affected by the life of the child are bad enough, then this justifies the abortion. From this perspective, abortion is not murder, because it is warranted by the mother's personal bodily rights or to avoid less preferable or bad consequences for herself and her future child.

As with pro-lifers, pro-choicers hold positions that run the gamut from believing that an abortion should be performed for any reason whatsoever—for example, using abortion as a form of birth control (the most extreme, reproductive rights-toting, strongest ultraliberal pro-choice position), to performing an abortion if and only if one's life will be altered in a way that she does not want it to be altered (the more standard, strongly liberal pro-choice position), to performing an abortion because the foreseeable consequences will be horrible for mother, child, or others affected by the life of the child (the less standard, weakly liberal pro-choice position). In effect, there is a continuum concerning the conservative pro-life and liberal pro-choice positions. See Table 1.1 for a schematized version of this continuum of beliefs about abortion.

I have heard people say, "Personally I won't abort, but I think it's OK for someone else to do it." This is a contradictory position to hold, I think, because on one hand, you're essentially saying that abortion is immoral for you (and you won't do it), but it is moral for someone else to do it (and you won't prevent someone from aborting). It would seem that,

TABLE 1.1 *The continuum of views on the ethics of abortion*

PRO-LIFE EXTREME
The most extreme, strongest ultraconservative pro-life position (never abort, no matter what, even if it means the mother dies)
The more standard, strongly conservative pro-life position (don't abort, unless the mother will die)
The less standard, weakly conservative pro-life position (don't abort, unless the mother will die, or in cases of rape or incest)
The less standard, weakly liberal pro-choice position (abort in cases in which consequences are horrible for mother/child/those affected)
The more standard, strongly liberal pro-choice position (abort in cases in which consequences are horrible or mother's life is altered in a way she does not want)
The most extreme, reproductive rights-toting, strongest ultraliberal pro-choice position (abort for any reason whatsoever, e.g., using abortion as a form of contraception)
PRO-CHOICE EXTREME

given the relevantly similar circumstances, the reasons given for why you won't abort are the same reasons why someone else shouldn't abort. In other words, a reason for you not to abort in a situation is a reason for someone else not to abort in a similar situation.

The reader, it is to be hoped, will think about these positions and figure out where he or she fits on the continuum. I question the morality of abortion because I think that: (1) we are robbing a fetus of the potential future that we enjoy and cherish; (2) there is a unique bond between mother and child that sets up a special obligation on the part of the mother to nourish the human being in her womb until it can live on its own and be cared for by someone else; and (3) relying on potential unforeseen consequences is an unreliable way to make moral judgments. However, I am more sympathetic to the liberal pro-choice position because: (1) the fetus does not seem to be a full-fledged person; (2) women do seem to have a right to do with their bodies what they see fit; and (3) circumstances may seem to be so bad for the mother and child that it would be better not to bring a child into this world. In fact, as I will show by the end of this chapter, my sympathy for the liberal pro-choice position is the result of the combined forces of these three reasons just mentioned.

"You Might Also Say that She Stops It before It Becomes a Child"

The third chapter of John Irving's novel *The Cider House Rules* begins with a conversation between Larch and Homer after Homer discovers a dead fetus. Larch says, "Sometimes the woman knows very early in the pregnancy that the child is unwanted." Homer responds, "So she kills it." Larch then says: "You might say . . . You might also say that she stops it before it becomes a child." Notice that the terms *child* and *it* are used to refer to the same aborted entity. Note also that Larch seems to think that the developing fetus in the womb—this *it*—is not the same thing as a child. This conversation is significant because one of the central questions concerning abortion has to do with what exactly is being aborted. Is it merely a glob of cells? A human being? A child? A person no different morally from you and me? The biological status of this aborted entity (what this thing actually is) affects the moral status of abortion (what we should or should not do to it). If, on the one hand, what is aborted is just a glob of cells, then most people will have no moral problem with abortion; on the other hand, if what is aborted is a full-fledged innocent person, then there probably will be moral outcries.

So what exactly is the biological status of this being that lives and grows inside a mother's womb? Embryology textbooks tell us that once a woman's egg has been fertilized, there exists a genetically distinct human being with forty-six chromosomes—a human zygote—that begins to grow by the normal process of cell division. Between day two and week two, the zygote will have traveled down one of the fallopian tubes and implanted itself in the uterus. The zygote develops into an embryo, and between weeks two and eight the embryo's cells begin specializing into the various organs that make up the systems of the human body. By eight weeks, the embryo is termed a "fetus" and resembles a very small newborn child. Around two-thirds of the way through the pregnancy (between twenty and twenty-four weeks), the fetus becomes viable and is able to survive outside the womb. Around week forty, the fetus is born and, once outside of the womb, is considered an infant child (Sadler 2003).

Embryologists make these classifications by distinguishing things on the basis of both their form (or shape) and their function (or purposive activity). When it comes to human-made things, this way of classifying is easy to understand. The knife in my kitchen is of a different form and has a different function from that of the computer keyboard on which I am typing this chapter. My knife has a blade and a handle and is used for cutting; my keyboard is rectangular, has keys, and is used for word processing. With living things, we still can do a decent job of classifying things as being distinct from one another, even when it comes to classifying the developmental stages of one kind of living thing. For example, the form and function of a butterfly egg is distinct from that of the larva (caterpillar), which is distinct from the pupa (chrysalis), and adult butterfly. One can easily see that each of these stages represents a different form and function of a specific entity; yet, all of these entities make up the various stages of a butterfly's life.

So, too, human beings follow developmental stages as they grow and mature, and they can be considered as being made up of different entities at these stages, with differing biological and moral statuses. Fundamentally, opposition to abortion stems from thinking that zygotes, embryos, or fetuses have the exact same moral status as that of a newborn child or a full-fledged adult person. Then, using a moral rule that says something like, "One should never kill an innocent person," they reason that the killing of a zygote is the same thing as murdering a grown person. But, is this way of reasoning correct? Are zygotes, embryos, and fetuses to be regarded as having the same moral status as persons like you and me?

To answer this question, many thinkers have argued that *personhood* is significant because a person is someone who is a full-fledged member of a moral community, deserving of all of the significant rights and privileges of that moral community. One might say that achieving the status of being a member of the moral community is a human being's most mature, self-actualized, fully responsible, and independent state. Further, most of us agree on the moral principle that an innocent person's rights—especially the right to life—should be respected. When we have the means to protect an innocent person's life, then the moral community is obliged to do so. In fact, we would be hard-pressed to find any moral community in which it was believed that "innocents" should not have the basic right to the protections needed to maintain their life. Whether they do, in fact, receive this protection is another matter.

A good list of requirements for personhood includes having the ability to be rational; having mental states and language; having familial, economic, civic, and intimate relationships with other persons; and being held morally responsible for one's actions (Parfit 1984). But, if this set of criteria forms the basis for personhood, then it is obvious that a developing human from the stages of zygote to, at least, the age of reason would not be considered a person. That being the case, and using a moral rule that says something like "one should never kill innocent persons for no good reason" then we could see how abortion—as well as infanticide, child-killing, or active euthanasia performed on humans in a persistent vegetative state—could be justified. In each of these cases, the humans in question do not fall into the category of person, and so killing them would not be immoral.

However, this way of thinking has its problems. There is much resistance to the idea that it is morally permissible to kill infants and those who are brain-damaged or have mental disabilities. If one wants to justify abortion along these lines, then one has to make exceptions for young children, the mentally handicapped, and those in a persistent vegetative state. One could bite the bullet, so to speak, and say that these individuals are not persons, but that we nonetheless have other obligations to protect them. But then we are left with the bothersome notion that these requirements for personhood lead us to contradictory moral intuitions. We would view it as moral to kill zygotes, embryos, and fetuses, but at the same time, we would view it as immoral to kill young children, the mentally handicapped, and those individuals in a persistent vegetative state.

Also, because the fetus is a member of the human race, one could argue that such a being seems automatically to be deemed sacred and worthy of having the same future as any one of us who have achieved personhood. There are long-standing traditions in Western philosophy, Eastern philosophy, and the major world's religions that see humans as being intrinsically valuable, irreplaceably important, and holy (Ellwood and McGraw 2004). Even if one concedes that fetuses are merely potential persons, certainly *most* fetuses develop into full-fledged persons. This may sound funny, but if someone would have aborted you because you merely were a potential person, you probably would have a moral problem with this as being unfair in some way, because you would have been deprived of all of the experiences you now have as a full-fledged person. So, even if fetuses are not full-fledged persons, we seem to want to give them a personlike status, granting them a basic right to live so as to have the same opportunity to achieve the same status of personhood we have achieved and enjoy.

"You Have to Give People the Right to Decide Whether or Not to Have Children"

Even if the fetus deserves the same rights and protections afforded any other person, could a woman still have a moral case for aborting her fetus? If we grant the fetus a personlike status, then one would need to have a very good reason for aborting. This is so because persons, given the kinds of beings they are, have a sacred, innate worth. This worth sets up obligations in communities, such as fundamental rights to life, to freedom from harm, and to having their basic needs filled. These obligations are particularly important when they concern innocent persons. If the fetus is conceived of as an innocent person, then one can reason that the mother has an obligation to provide nourishment for the fetus in the same way that a community has an obligation to take care of innocent persons.

Now, in cases where a mother's life is in danger due to a pregnancy, most people's moral intuition seems to be that the fetus is most like an intruder who is going to kill her. So, self-defense of the mother's life would be warranted with an abortion of the fetus. In fact, this seems to be the one clear exception to the rule of not aborting for most conservative pro-lifers, as was shown in our pro-life/pro-choice continuum a few pages back. In cases of pregnancy due to rape, the fetus can be likened to an unwelcome person who may be wholly unbearable, and this may justify abortion. Many of these same conservative pro-lifers, as well as the standard liberal pro-choicer, will agree with abortion in this case. However, a lot of folks think that as long as there are adoption clinics or orphanages like St. Cloud's in the film, a pregnant woman whose life is not in danger should not abort her fetus under any circumstances.

Can a case be made for a woman's choice to abort simply because it is her body and she should be able to choose what to do with it? There is a long and strong tradition, going back at least to Immanuel Kant (1724–1804), in which rational beings are seen as *autonomous*, that is, free to make choices for themselves unimpeded by any coercion (see Friedman 1993). Fundamental rights to privacy and to using one's body as one sees fit are viewed as elements of this autonomy. It may be true that the right to ownership over one's own body in exercising decisions is the most fundamental of these rights. If a mother is autonomous in this sense, then surely she can choose an abortion if she wants to. It is her body, and she can do with her body whatever she sees fit to do with it. This, I think, is the thrust of Dr. Larch's claim to Homer that: "If you expect people to be responsible for their children, you have to give them the right to decide whether or not to have children." In fact, this is one of the central ideas behind the United States Supreme Court's 1973 ruling in *Roe v. Wade* (410 U.S. 113, 1973). The court ruled that, until the fetus is viable (able to live on its own outside of the womb around the third trimester of pregnancy), a woman's decision to have an abortion is her own personal, private matter and is akin to other privacy rights afforded a full-fledged U.S. citizen.

This "it's my body and I can do what I want with it" position usually is tempered with a distinction made between (1) refusing the use of one's body and (2) the intentional killing of the fetus. A mother has a good moral reason for refusing the use of her body to a fetus, but she has no moral ground for intentionally killing the fetus. In an abortion, the mother is simply refusing the use of her private space and evicting a tenant, so to speak. If the fetus could live on its own outside of the mother's womb, then great; if not, then this is an unfortunate consequence of eviction.

This seems unsatisfying as a solution because most abortions take place when the fetus is not viable; that is, it cannot live on its own outside of the womb. This has caused many to question whether dependency of the fetus on the mother in this unique kind of relationship is so significant that it morally compels the mother to carry the developing human life to the point at which it can be placed for adoption or cared for by some other person (Beckwith 1992). Perhaps because a human being inside the womb is dependent on its mother for its very life up until viability (barring a situation where the mother's life is in danger), a mother has an obligation to carry a living human being in her womb until that living human being has attained the ability to live outside of the womb.

"Happy to Be Alive under Any Circumstances"

Many liberal pro-choicers combine the "it's my body and I can do what I want with it" argument with that of examining the potential bad consequences and circumstances surrounding bringing a child into this world. These kinds of arguments are utilitarian in nature; the consequences of actions become significant when making a moral decision. The rule is: if an action likely will bring about good consequences for the person or persons affected, then that action is moral. In contrast, if an action likely will bring about bad consequences, then such an action is deemed immoral (Mill 1863/2002).

Often, consequentialist moral theories come into conflict with other moral theories because of this focus on the consequences as being what determines moral correctness. For example, it seems most people realize they should not lie as a general rule and that, even if they lie for the "right" reasons, it is wrong to lie nonetheless. According to the consequentialist way of moral reasoning, if good consequences will come about as a result of lying, then one should pursue that route. This is exactly the kind of reasoning Larch uses when he lies to the state concerning his illegal abortion practices and his intention to hire "Dr." Homer Wells, whose diploma he has fabricated. This is also the kind of reasoning Larch uses when falsifying Homer's medical records to exempt him from military service, as well as when he asks Buster to lie to the rest of the orphans about Fuzzy's death.

So, in the abortion matter, if the consequences or circumstances of a mother's life or the child's life will be bad, then according to the consequentialist viewpoint it would be moral to abort and actually immoral not to abort, no matter what contrary moral principles, commandments, or rules might be invoked. Think of a child born with a severe handicap who cannot be cared for appropriately, or a child born to a mother who will abuse the child or herself, or the severe psychological damage to or social stigma placed on a mother, her child, and significant relatives as a result of an unwanted pregnancy. In fact, one could argue that the main message of *The Cider House Rules* is that real-life circumstances—with all of their complicated and complex good and bad consequences—give us good reason to think that "objective" moral rules either must change or do not apply. Just as the "cider house rules" themselves did not seem to apply to the circumstances of the apple pickers who lived there, so too, society's rules outlawing abortion did not apply to the life circumstances of the people affected by unwanted pregnancies at St. Cloud's orphanage—let alone the rest of the world—from Larch's perspective.

This consequentialist approach is central to the argument that Larch puts forward in *The Cider House Rules*. Larch tells us that "long ago, I had decided that it was the women who needed to be delivered," and it is clear that what it is that they need to be delivered from is the pain and suffering associated with bringing an unwanted child into the world. He constantly tells the people around him that they need to be "of use," meaning that they should have a positive impact on others with their lives. In one part of the story, a young woman who had tried to perform an abortion on herself dies, and Larch tells Homer that "this is what doing nothing gets you." Larch means that, given that fact that women continually will become pregnant and want to have abortions, he either can do nothing and allow women to perform their own abortions—which will likely lead to more bad consequences—or he can help reduce the number of bad consequences by performing abortions. Being "of use" in the world, for Larch, has to do with "delivering" women from pain and suffering, either by providing them with refuge for an orphan or by providing them with an abortion. Homer ultimately becomes converted to this way of thinking and performs an abortion on Rose because he knows that she may die (certainly a horrible consequence) in the process of trying to perform an abortion on herself.

Larch's consequentialist position concerning abortion is most clearly stated in a conversation he has with Homer and Buster while Buster is learning to drive. Somewhat cruelly, Larch says that because Homer and Buster probably never will be adopted, it would have been better for them had they never been born. Homer responds that he is happy to simply be alive, and Larch ridicules him for naively thinking that he is "happy to be alive under any circumstances." Larch's point is that not living at all would be preferable to living in miserable circumstances. This thinking fits nicely with his practice of performing abortions. In Larch's mind, because existence for an unwanted child would be less than ideal, abortion is justified; stated simply: "better off dead than miserable."

Larch views quality of life as central to a person's existence. Homer questions this position, obviously, because he thinks a life is worth living regardless of the consequences or misery associated with it. In many ways, what we can call the *quality of life* as opposed to the *sanctity of life* views are at the heart of the abortion debate where consequences are concerned. Larch advocates the quality view, while Homer (at least, at first) advocates the sanctity view. On the one hand, we could, like Larch, look at all of the potential sociological, emotional, psychological, and financial woes associated with a mother's and child's miserable existences and support abortion decisions to avoid such hardships. On the other hand, because we seldom can accurately predict the future, we could support Homer in thinking think that no unforeseen consequences—even if they are horrible—outweigh the simple value of being alive.

In many ways, the business of living includes dealing with all of the hardships life throws our way. Aren't the hardships, in some way, part of what makes life worth living? Isn't it the case that we praise those folks who have worked through their issues or have overcome hardships more so than those who have had an easy life? "No pain, no gain" is a mantra that rings true in much of life. So, the question really is whether one can be happy to be alive under any circumstances, or whether the circumstances are perceived as being so miserable that we should not even give a person a chance to go through life's experiences in the first place?

"It Is Something You're Going to Have to Work Out Yourself"

There are good reasons to question the morality of abortion because it seems that (1) an abortion robs a fetus of the potential future that we all presumably enjoy and cherish, (2) there is a unique bond between mother and child that sets up a special obligation on the part of the mother to nourish the human being in her womb until it can live on its own and be cared for by someone else, and (3) relying on potential unforeseen consequences is an unreliable way to make moral judgments. However, in the end, I must say that I am sympathetic to the liberal pro-choice position because (1) the fetus does not seem to be a full-fledged person, (2) women seem to have a have a right to do with their bodies what they see fit, and (3) circumstances may seem to be so bad for the mother, child, and others that it would be better not to bring a child into this world. In fact, my sympathy for the liberal pro-choice position is the result of the combined forces of these three reasons just mentioned. Ultimately, readers will have to think about this matter on their own but, for what it's worth, here is my position.

Given what we said about the development of a butterfly as having various stages that represent a different form and function of a specific entity in the various stages of its life (egg, larva, pupa, etc.), I think we can analogize this argument with respect to humans and say the same thing about human development. An embryo is not the same entity as a zygote, which is not the same entity as a fetus, which is not the same entity as you, the reader, who are a full-fledged person pondering this chapter. Granted, a butterfly egg is potentially a full-fledged butterfly as much as a human egg is a full-fledged person.

But the fact of the matter is that a human egg is not the same entity as a human person; although both are part of the human developmental continuum. If this is true, then we need not be worried about committing "murder" when we abort a human being in the first trimester, for example, because such an entity simply does not have the same status as that of an entity in the third trimester or later in human development. Given what we know about human development from embryologists, I think making the first trimester a clear cut-off point is wise (thus, the *Roe v. Wade* decision was wise). An infant child fresh out of the womb is more deserving of a right to life than an entity in the first trimester, because the infant can live on its own and be cared for by someone. To put it crudely, an entity in the earlier stages of human development is more like a "blob" of cells. The more bloblike and less personlike, the more we can feel justified in aborting; the less bloblike and more personlike, the more we can feel justified in *not* aborting.

Check your feelings and intuitions about the "natural" death of an embryo due to a miscarriage versus the death of a fetus just before being delivered because of the umbilical cord wrapped around his or her neck. We feel worse for the fetus than we do for the embryo. Why? It is because the embryo is as yet unformed. This is the same kind of thinking that can and should be involved in aborting at the early stages in the first trimester. If someone objects that this is an arbitrary "line" we are drawing in deciding what entity in the human developmental schema should be considered as deserving of a right to "personlike" life, my response is to note that it's not really so arbitrary given what we know from embryology. Also, I would respond by wedding this former argument with the next one concerning a woman's right to do with her body what she sees fit.

As was noted earlier, there is a long and strong tradition in which rational beings are seen as autonomous agents, or free to make rationally informed choices for themselves unimpeded by any coercion. Not only do I think that fundamental rights to privacy and the use of one's body as one sees fit are viewed as elements of this autonomy, but I also think that the right to ownership of one's own body in exercising decisions is the most fundamental of these rights. If a woman is autonomous in this sense, then surely she can choose an abortion if she wants to, because it's her body, and she can do with her body whatever she sees fit to do with it. It makes no difference that this being living inside of her is another human being—even if we did grant it the same full personlike rights as you and I have—because the being must use her body, and her choice to do with her body what she wants to do with it trumps the very human life that is developing within her.

Of course, very few people think that abortion is not a difficult decision or that a woman should use abortion as a form of contraception (unless you advocate the most extreme, reproductive rights-toting, strongest ultraliberal pro-choice position). But when the chips are down and a decision needs to be made, the cliché rings true that "It's her body, and she can choose to do with it what she wants to." If someone still isn't convinced that a woman should be allowed to abort for any reason other than contraception, then I would wed these two arguments to the next one concerning the potential horrible consequences for mother and child.

Earlier we noted that making decisions based on future consequences might not be wise, given how the future may change. However, this is a little simplistic in scope. We make all kinds of decisions based on our judgments of potential future good or bad consequences, and we are wise to do so. Thankfully, the future does resemble the past, and our experiences are very much like other people's experiences. These are two main reasons why we are wise in making decisions based on what we take to be potential future consequences. You don't need to be too sharp to see that having a child would drastically change your life and the social circles in which you reside. If you add to this picture an unhealthy dose of family dysfunction, or a severe impairment or AIDS for your kid, or a deadbeat dad, or a molesting step-parent—which, by the way, are all-too-common phenomena—then we might agree with Larch that one is better off dead. Why would you want to bring a kid into your "horrible" part of the world? Or, why would you agree to raise a child with a severe handicap, given all of the emotional, psychological, financial, and social hardships associated with raising such a child? It might be better for everyone involved at the family, local, state, and national level to counsel a teenager, mentally ill woman, or vagrant to abort.

My wife may kill me for saying this (more likely she'll chide me), but I could envision a circumstance in which my own daughter foolishly becomes pregnant as a teenager and, given how life-changing a child would be for her, her mom, and me, I would actually help her obtain an abortion. Or, if she chose to abort because her child will be severely handicapped, will need special care, and would suffer under social stigma, or other extremely adverse circumstance, then I would support her decision. This does not make me a monster; it just means that I am realistically considering the negative consequences associated with bringing a child into the world under bad circumstances.

So, my present position is that both the more standard, strongly liberal pro-choicer and the less-standard, weakly liberal pro-choicer stand on firm moral grounds for supporting abortion rights, in light of the three-pronged reasons I outlined above. At the same time, though the most extreme, reproductive rights-toting, strongest ultraliberal pro-choicer likely supports an insensitive egoism by condoning the use of abortion as a contraceptive, still, I would agree, that women should be permitted to abort for such reasons because of the "it's my body" position.

How about Expecting People to Be Responsible and to Control Themselves to Begin With?

After a woman tries to perform an abortion on herself and dies, Larch and Homer have a conversation in which Homer asks the rhetorical question that heads the final section of this chapter. The message behind Homer's question is clear: we would not be performing so many abortions at St. Cloud's if men and women would not have so much unprotected or unreflective sex. In 2000, about 1.3 million abortions were performed in the United States, amounting to one in four pregnancies' ending in abortion (Levine 2006). Abortion is obviously an emotionally charged topic. People will continue to have sex; there is no doubt about this. Maybe there is wisdom in Homer's question, just as there is wisdom in educating people about the sexual act and its consequences, as well as wisdom in distributing forms of birth control.

Given what I have said about my stance concerning abortion, what I am about to say might sound confusing; however, I am a philosopher, and my job is to get you and myself to think and rethink arguments, ideas, and positions. So, here's something for you and me both to think about. No matter what position one takes on the abortion issue, and no matter what the pro-lifers and pro-choicers say about the "truths" concerning the biological or moral status of the fetus or the reproductive rights of women, one truth remains undisputed: if someone had aborted you, then you would not be here to think about the issues surrounding abortion.

QUESTIONS FOR CONSIDERATION

1. *Because a human being inside the womb is dependent on its mother for its very life up until viability, does a mother have an obligation to carry a living human being in her womb until that living human being has attained the ability to live outside of the womb?*

2. *The Catholic Church's position is that a woman may never directly abort, even if her life is in danger. So, if faced with the choice of abortion or her own death, the mother must choose her own death. Play the part of a Catholic and argue for this position. Now, can you think of an argument against the Catholic Church's position?*

3. *Do you think abstinence is the solution to unwanted teen pregnancy? How about distributing condoms? What, practically, can be done to help prevent unwanted teen pregnancy?*

4. *People will claim, "Look, I would never abort, but I'm not going to tell someone else that she can't have an abortion." There is something deeply contradictory about this thinking, especially if you think it's immoral for you to abort (you wouldn't do it) but moral for someone else to abort (she's free to choose to do it). Discuss this contradiction.*

REFERENCES

Beckwith, F. 1992. Personal Bodily Rights, Abortion and Unplugging the Violinist *International Philosophical Quarterly* 32:105–18.

Boonin, D. 2003. *A Defense of Abortion*. Cambridge: Cambridge University Press.

Ellwood, D., and McGraw, B. 2004. *Many Peoples, Many Faiths: Women and Men in the World's Religions*. Upper Saddle River, NJ: Prentice Hall.

Friedman, M. 1993. *What Are Friends For? Feminist Perspectives on Personal Relationships and Moral Theory*. Ithaca, NY: Cornell University Press.

Hallström, L. 1999. *The Cider House Rules* [motion picture]. Los Angeles: Film Colony.

Irving, J. 1997. *The Cider House Rules*. New York: Ballantine Books.

Kreeft, P. 2000. The Apple Argument against Abortion. *Crisis* 18:25–29.

Levine, C., ed. 2006. *Taking Sides: Clashing Views on Controversial Bioethical Issues*. New York: McGraw-Hill/Dushkin.

Mill, J. S. 2002. *Utilitarianism*. Indianapolis: Hackett Publishing Co. (Originally published 1863)

Noonan, J. 1967. Abortion and the Catholic Church: A Summary History. *Natural Law Forum* 12:125–31.

Parfit, D. 1984. *Reasons and Persons*. Oxford: Oxford University Press.

Sadler, T. 2003. *Langman's Medical Embryology*. Hagerstown, MD: Lippincott, Williams & Wilkins.

Thomson, J. 1971. A Defense of Abortion. *Philosophy and Public Affairs* 1:47–66.

Warren, M. 1973. On the Moral and Legal Status of Abortion. *The Monist* 57: 43–61.

TWO

Reading *Citizen Ruth* Her Rights

Satire and Moral Realism in the Abortion Debate

Al-Yasha Ilhaam

Owing to the highly personal and sexual nature of abortion, as well as the powerful social structures that lay claim to determining its moral and legal permissibility, it is nearly impossible (even within bioethics discourse) to state one's views without offending anyone. Many advocates on both sides of the abortion debate believe that their moral viewpoints are, in some sense, objectively true, that their moral standpoints are akin to facts about the world. This perspective on the nature of morality—that there are at least some moral claims that are objectively true—is called moral realism. *Citizen Ruth* (Payne 1996) is a film that irreverently and effectively uses humor to critique moral realism in the abortion debates. Depicting a character who engages in specious activities such as promiscuous sex and sniffing glue, the film's frankness suggests that because the abortion debate is divided by emotionalism, loaded language, and political rhetoric, the only hope for progress within it might lie in the ability to be of great and deliberate offense to everyone.

Citizen Ruth is a character study about a woman caught between the competing aims of the women's movement, the Christian anti-abortion lobby, and the state, which ostensibly protects a woman's right to have an abortion. Routinely arrested for public intoxication, Ruth (played by Laura Dern) is addicted to inhalants and has four children in adoptive or foster care. An exasperated judge offers the yet-again-pregnant Ruth a reduced sentence to get out of jail to obtain an abortion. Pro-life activists, arrested for demonstrating at a clinic, listen to Ruth's story, and, on their release, bail her out and offer to help her by suing the judge and saving her baby. She is invited into the modest but comfortable suburban home of Gail and Norm Stoney (played by Mary Kay Place and Kurtwood Smith), leaders of the local chapter of the Baby Savers, a Christian pro-life activist group.

Thus begins Ruth's excursion into the great divide. Ruth's apparent obliviousness to the surrounding political and moral melee is indicative of her general state of inebriation and her real remove from the politics that comprise the extremes of the abortion debate: the Christian right and the feminist left. While each tries to win her over to their views, Ruth tends to miss the obvious, though she eventually awakens to the possibilities of profiting from the melee. By the same token, the activists reveal little interest in Ruth's own situation, making her a signifier of moral truths that are external to her. The two sides of the "abortion war" are depicted as interdependent and even united through the shared perspective of moral realism. In addition, the film portrays how modern media and the market value of public opinion play a significant role in what we understand to be our moral choices. With deft dialogue and fearless irreverence, *Citizen Ruth* provides an amusing and effective way to interrogate the tendency toward moral realism in discussions of abortion and reproductive rights.

Through a reading of the film *Citizen Ruth,* I describe the ways in which satire can offer a critical view on the postmodern spectacle of politics based on the "image" of moral values. I evaluate moral realism as a philosophical stance with an eye toward examining its role in orienting the pro-choice and pro-life perspectives. In the process, I discuss longstanding difficulties in the bioethics discourse surrounding abortion along with some recognizable gestures toward a method through which bioethicists and (other) people possessed of a sound mind and a sense of humor can advance (and perhaps one day be done with) this intractable debate.

Satire and Moral Realism

Satire is defined by the *Oxford English Dictionary* as "a poem, or in modern use sometimes a prose composition, in which prevailing vices or follies are held up for ridicule" (Oxford University Press, 1989). In identifying certain behaviors as vices, other behaviors are held up as befitting upstanding citizens. In this way, "definitions of satire begin with its invocation of moral norms or ethical values," writes Susan Strehle (1996) in a review essay on the development of the genre. When moral claims and commentary in satire are directed toward the actions of persons and personal identity (such as in Oscar Wilde's *The Importance of Being Earnest*), the term "lampoon" might be more accurate. In other cases, the target might be an institution (such as the military, in Joseph Heller's *Catch-22*). American satire has often (some would say increasingly) speculated dimly on the moral destiny of the nation, at the same time it has served as a protector of the nation's perceived "values."

Early analyses of American satire, such as George Roth's study of late eighteenth-century satiric verse (Roth 1956), show how the genre reflected the divisive politics of the day, while also serving to forge the notion of American identity as illustrative of certain specific, if conflicting, moral beliefs and practices. Politicians and writers often found models in classical satire. In a preface to a translation of the early second-century satires of Roman poet Juvenal, John Quincy Adams set forth his hope that with a critical eye on moral hypocrisies, America might avoid the saturnalian fate of Rome (Roth 1956). Roth argues that the most important divide that early American satire had to reinforce was the ideological separation of America from Britain: "American satire has a function peculiar to this country, for it is the effort of a Republic to keel the new society free from the vices of the old world." In building a new society, ambiguities are rampant, and who better to point out the frailties in the cultural infrastructure than the writers:

> Satirists of education condemn the ignorant teachers, unsound teaching methods, and stingy parents of their day; those concerned with religion take part in current American controversies over revivalism and sectarianism; writers abut medicine reflect the confusion attendant upon the absence of any widely accepted scientific theories of disease; those condemning the law feel that its priesthood, mystery and cant are un-American. The emergence of certain types of inequality is also noted by the satirists, and they assail most vigorously its appearance in a world of fashion, in the practice of financial chicanery (particularly speculation in land or public funds) and in the institution of slavery. (ROTH 1956, P. 399)

Steven Weisenburger's (1995) concept of "degenerative satire" provides a helpful framework for evaluating the efficacy of satire in framing the abortion debate. He contrasts the "generative" model of satire, which is most akin to its formative social role, "designed to correct folly and vice according to stable norms" (Strehle 1996), with the "degenerative" mode, which "subverts hierarchies of value and approaches all form of meaning-making with abiding skepticism" (Strehle 1996).

Citizen Ruth portrays both the warring pro-life and pro-choice factions as holding a firm belief that their views are supported by objective moral truths. Moral realism is the position that (1) ethical sentences are genuine assertions that something is the case, and that such assertions are capable of being true or false, and (2) at least some ethical sentences are true and "true" is to be understood objectively, i.e., not just "true for you" or "true for some society," but rather, true for all individuals and cultures regardless of whether they believe it or not. There are variants on moral realism, but all have in common the idea that there are true, moral facts. The view that affirms (1) is called *cognitivism;* the view that holds (2) is called *no-error.* Cognitivism says that a moral statement actually tells us that something that can be true or false. The no-error view claims that there are actually moral facts in existence. There is considerable debate within moral realism, however, as to whether these facts resemble empirical or scientific facts. The main debate in moral realism concerns what it takes for a moral statement to be true or false and whether or not moral claims can possess these characteristics.

In the film's portrayal of the warring factions, one sees how an implicit stance of moral realism polarizes and foreshortens the views of activists on either side of the abortion debate. Ruth is geared toward this thinking as she is taken to the clinic by her pro-life supporters. The fact of her pregnancy is confirmed with congratulatory enthusiasm. When Ruth insists that she wants an abortion, she is told she "doesn't have all the facts." The doctor who comes in to "explain the medical facts" to Ruth gives her details about the "baby's heartbeat" and offers a plastic model of the fetus for her to hold and name. Still not persuaded to keep the baby, she is asked to watch a movie (within a movie), whose narrator compares abortion to the Jewish Holocaust and abortion clinics to concentration camps. The film within the film takes liberties with the connection between biological facts (a graphic, bloody surgery) and the moral rightness or wrongness of the action, performing an abortion. The pro-life counselors and their film fallaciously imply that having gut feelings of disgust at watching an abortion will make a person recognize the wrongness of abortion itself. This implication is similar to those made by some vegetarians that one will see the wrongness of eating meat if one attends to one's deep emotional response on viewing the slaughter of animals. Ironically, viewing childbirth might produce just as extreme a reaction of repugnance, so repugnance *alone,* it stands to reason, does not suffice to signal that there is something morally wrong with a state of affairs. This is an example of the problem identified by David Hume, in the attempt to move from nonmoral facts to the moral facts, one is attempting to derive an "ought from an is" (Hume 1739/1978).

On the one hand, a moral realist position on abortion tends to be more convincing when it seems to have common sense on its side, but this is often a matter of defining terms. Thus, a moral-realist statement like "murdering children is just wrong" would seem to be an uncontroversial assertion, as is. However, the applicability of this general moral rule to the abortion debate hinges on whether abortion is equivalent to murdering children or whether fetuses do not qualify as children. Some bioethics literature has held that abortion is wrong even when the embryo or fetus is not considered a child (Shannon 2000), so the persuasiveness of the phrase "murdering children is wrong" may be unhelpful in either case.

On the other hand, antirealism challenges the existence of moral facts, in large part on the obvious differences between empirical or scientific and putative moral "facts" (Harman 1985). Ruth's desire to stay high and to ignore her parenting responsibilities can be interpreted as implicitly embracing an extreme antirealist stance. She wants to do her own thing, motivated by her own desires, without any acknowledgment of the wider public implications. Does this mean she is unwittingly practicing a sort of ethical solipsism, creating and living in her own subjective moral universe? Perhaps, but Ruth's drug use and moral universe is hardly romanticized in the film. As a "huffer" she abuses legal substances (like brake fluid and airplane glue) so she can avoid the much harsher legal penalties associated with crack convictions, the disproportional nature of which has been seen by some as a form of racism.[1] Much of her "high" consists in a stupor spent looking at trash on the ground; her sexual encounters are portrayed as tawdry beyond belief; and the ramifications of her behavior on her children, who are pictured sympathetically, enjoying a meager breakfast with their harried uncle, are all too painful for the viewer. The film provides a character study of an almost entirely unredeemable character, who makes little if any moral progress in the film; insofar as Ruth represents the position of moral antirealism, it is certainly not clear that the satire, in holding up moral realism to ridicule, embraces its opposite either.

As Ruth settles into the Stoneys' household, the counseling sessions continue and she is won over to the pro-life point of view. Then she dips into their youngest child's model airplane glue and assaults him when he tries to take it from her. Thus wearing out the Stoneys' welcome, she is then taken in by Diane (played by Swoosie Kurtz), a pro-life advocate who reveals herself to be an agent provocateur working undercover for pro-choice. Ruth is now confronted with a new satiric dynamic—the "play within a play"—that gives her a chance to really decide what she believes is the "truth." When Ruth decides to switch sides, Norm declares, "That woman belongs to us. We paid her bail." Gail adds, "and I bought her those shoes!" In the Stoneys' belief that they own Ruth through her bond and care, the film references both the history of slavery and the "property view" of children.

Ruth still has to figure out what she really wants to do, and increasingly she becomes a symbol in the media. The war heats up with vigils, rallies, press releases, and national spokespersons entering the debate. When the pro-life activists declare a "national alert," the pro-choice activists prepare a "counteralert" and tell Ruth, "It's not just about you any more; it's more about the choice of millions of American women." Ruth maintains her chemically induced disconnect from the public debate, refusing interviews and avoiding taking sides, while the vortex forms around her.

Private and Public Spheres

Notions of the public and private spheres figure heavily into the debate over the morality of abortion. The "right to privacy" affirmed in *Roe v. Wade*, marks out an arena for private decision-making concerning one's own body, insulated from public moral pressures and the state's own interests in protecting prenatal life. This private sphere may be contrasted with the political "public sphere" identified by Jurgen Habermas as the democratic arena of debate and ultimate intellectual agreement. In *The Structural Transformation of the Public Sphere*, Habermas (1962) examines the role of public opinion in the functioning of Western democracy and construes the public sphere as "made up of private people gathered together as a public and articulating the needs of society with the state." At its core, this model emphasizes the sorts of consensus-building technique used in an open forum and reflects the views of each individual from the standpoint of his or her own opinions, needs, and desires (Habermas 1962). Habermas assumes that the participants in this public forum share certain assumptions about political dialogue, which allows for expected dissent. The resulting "discourse ethics" highlights the subjectivity of public debate, which depends on the exercised ability and right of all participants to say whatever they want and respond to anything said. Habermas argues that the authenticity and effectiveness of the public sphere—as a place for democratic, consensus building—has been undermined by the growth of the "culture industry" and the intervention of corporate interests as the guideposts of personal and social development. He defines "manipulative publicity" and "staged display" as methods used by corporate media for political propaganda.

These are the first features Ruth comes to recognize from the pro-choice and pro-life movements. She does not want to become a symbol and becomes skeptical of anyone who suggests that her actions will "send a message" to the other side. But as the staged displays and symbolic use of Ruth continue we see that everyone is obsessed with his or her media image. The cops waiting for Ruth to leave the emergency room are watching *Cops* in the waiting room and comparing arrests. When an article comes out in the paper about her case that reflects the pro-life view, Ruth hates her picture more than the misquoted views offered in her name. When Blaine Gibbons (played by Burt Reynolds), the national leader of the Baby Savers arrives, he refuses to talk to non-network journalists. The images overshadow the reality of Ruth's continued drug use, her controversial legal position, and the fact that this downtrodden, reluctant, private citizen has been forcibly made the public face of the abortion debate.

The influence of the public sphere on the private has been described by Michel Foucault (1988) in his idea of the biopolitical, the body as created by governance and rules, written codes of conduct and moral (and other) restraint. One sees the public sphere's influence on the private sphere of the Stoney family home, where Ruth is advised that certain chairs are never to be sat on—the chairs are there to present a clean and tidy image to the public. The tensions between public norms and the private body are captured by Norm's difficulties in keeping his eyes off of Ruth's underwear. In a quiet moment with Ruth, Norm remarks, "I was quite a sinner before I married Gayle" and demonstrates his own uneasy personal transformation in beliefs and bodily practices.

While the repressive norms of the Stoneys' household are exaggerated to reflect a conservative "family values" approach, the pro-choice camp is pictured likewise exaggeratedly, but in this case hypocritically anarchofeminist. Ruth is silenced by the feminists when approached by the media. When the pro-choice advocates are uncomfortable seeing Ruth drink, Ruth herself points out the contradiction between allowing some choices and not others, or thinking that a pregnant woman shouldn't drink, even if she intends to have an abortion. This kind of moralizing does not sit well with the pro-choice advocates' unflinching moral-realist position that a woman's right to choose overrides any other moral obligations she might have.

The Baby Savers offer Ruth $15,000 if she decides to take her baby to term. As the pro-choice activists try to talk her out of taking the offer, Ruth asserts that poverty has had the greatest impact on her parenting choices. "If I had money, my life would be different. I'd have been such a good mother." In the midst of her tearful moment of self-reflection, a smiling pro-choice activist reminds her that turning down the offer "sends a strong message." Ruth realizes she's being used as a symbol and backs away from the activists. To "level the playing field," another pro-choice activist offers to match the Baby Savers' offer, so she can "choose freely again."

With a $15,000 bonus either way, Ruth is now, for the first time, in the position of making a choice for herself. The middle position within the film is not found in a compromise between the polar ideologies but in the individual in the position to decide between them.

Bioethics: Is Anybody Really "Listening to the Middle"?

In the debate between the pro-life and pro-choice factions, Ruth's own story becomes what Jean Baudrillard coined as a "hypertext," that which is external to the discourse and exists as a link to another (repressed) realm of meaning; in this case, it is about promiscuous sex, drugs, poverty, violence, and absentee parenting, the conditions that have made Ruth "one bad mother" as the film poster describes. The actual social conditions that have shaped and continue to shape Ruth's life and decisions become apparent to her only when she is offered cash and sees how the pro-life and pro-choice teams engage in political one-upmanship to win her over.

Daniel Callahan's essay "An Ethical Challenge to Prochoice Advocates" (1990) offers this commentary on the reciprocal and reactionary blindness of one side of the abortion debate to the other: "If the prolife movement exclusively stresses the rights of the fetus, then the prochoice movement must exclusively stress the rights of women. If the prolife movement says that abortion is oppressive and murderous, the prochoice movement must say it is liberating and morally unimportant. If the prolife movement says that every abortion choice is wrong, whatever the reason, then the prochoice leadership implies that every choice is right, whatever the choice."

Callahan and others who argue for the legality of abortion within the public sphere without declaring its morality on a personal level admittedly fall short of offering a full account of the moral conditions in either case. Bioethicists have drawn attention to the ways in which the pro-life and pro-choice movements have brought moral stances on abortion to a polarized standoff (Luker 1984; Mahowald 2000). In her assessment of the evolution of the abortion debate since *Roe v. Wade*, Mary B. Mahowald (2000) assesses the value and terms of the middle ground by suggesting some topics on which pro-life and pro-choice ideologies should agree. "Either side betrays, to me, the enormous complexity of the issue," she writes, identifying the following possible points of convergence:

1. Abortion is a bad thing;
2. Legitimate distinctions can be made between terminating a pregnancy, terminating a fetus, and becoming a parent;

3. It's important for health care professionals to disclose accurate information;
4. Pregnant women have rights at least equivalent to those of nonpregnant people;
5. Viability and sentience of fetuses are morally relevant to abortion decisions; and
6. Legality and morality are related but not equivalent.

Mahowald observes that these areas of overlap do not necessarily provide the basis for agreement, but they do provide some insight into how abortion decisions might be made.

Similarly, *Citizen Ruth* does not let its viewers make easy, familiar allegiances with the confidence offered by purported moral truths. The degenerative mode of satire attempts to efface the credibility of both the pro-life and the pro-choice movements, showing both sides to be biased, short-sighted, and self-serving. This analysis offers no solace to the individual making a personal decision on abortion or choosing to play a role in the abortion debate. Rather, it shows that the individual may be deeply entrenched in the mores of a politically determined community, which provides contingent support to an individual based on the extent to which she serves the ideological needs of the group. The film warns that the moral facts that each side points to in order to support its position are easily manipulated by the media with spin, graphics, and tactical campaigns. Politics and morals appear to swing in the direction of financial power, while the weak and unrepresented are guided toward their beliefs without significant participation in the sphere of public debate.

If *Citizen Ruth* indeed shows the limitations of moral realism for advancing the case for either side of the abortion wars, and for providing an avenue for arbitration between them, how can we know if Ruth makes a morally right decision? It's hard to say if anyone ever knows the truth about Ruth or what she believes. Ironically, for a character study, Ruth shows remarkably little character development through the film. It is not clear at the end whether she makes any real choices at all, in a way that is unaffected by the corrupting political and chemical influences on her mind. Perhaps the moral rightness or wrongness of any decision vis-à-vis Ruth's pregnancy would have to take stock of Ruth's own experience: of her poverty, her dysfunctional upbringing, her addiction, her choices and her lack of choices, her reproductive rights and her best chances for bodily integrity, personal development, and growth.

QUESTIONS FOR CONSIDERATION

1. *Who is likely to find this film offensive, and for what reasons?*

2. *How is moral realism evinced by pro-life and pro-choice characters?*

3. *What, if any, "middle ground" does the film propose?*

4. *As Ruth's lucidity is in question, to what extent are her choices truly Ruth's choices, and to what extent might they be rightfully circumscribed by other interests, such as those of her children or of the state?*

NOTES

1. For example, crack cocaine is often composed of more than 50 percent baking soda or other fillers, and its users are disproportionately black and poor compared with the consumers of purer, powdered cocaine, which is perceived as a drug of elites. However, possession of 5 grams of crack carries the same minimum sentence (five years' imprisonment) as does possession of more than 500 grams of powder.

REFERENCES

Baudrillard, J. 1983. *Simulations,* trans. P. Foss, P. Patton, and P. Beitchman. New York: Semiotext(e).

Callahan, D. 1990. An Ethical Challenge to Prochoice Advocates. In *Bioethics,* ed. T. Shannon, 330–40. Mahwah, NJ: Paulist Press.

Foucault, M. 1988. *History of Sexuality. Vol. 3, The Care of the Self,* trans. R. Hurley. New York: Vintage.

Habermas, J. 1962. Discourse Ethics: Notes on Philosophical Justification. In *Moral Consciousness and Communicative Action*, trans. C. Lenhart and S. Weber Nicholson. Cambridge, MA: MIT Press.

Harman, G. 1985. Is There a Single True Morality? In *Morality, Reason and Truth:*

New Essays on the Foundations of Ethics, ed. D. Copp and D. Zimmerman, 77–101. Totowa, NJ: Rowman and Allanheld.

Hume, D. 1978. *A Treatise on Human Nature*, ed. L.A. Selby-Bigge. Oxford: Oxford University Press. (Originally published 1739)

Langerak, E. 2000. Abortion: Listening to the Middle? In *Life Choices: A Hastings Center Introduction to Bioethics,* ed. J. H. Howell and W. F. Sale, 24–28. Washington, DC: Georgetown University Press.

Luker, K. 1984. *Abortion and the Politics of Motherhood.* Berkeley and Los Angeles: University of California Press.

Mahowald, M. 2000. Is There Life after *Roe v. Wade*? In *Life Choices: A Hastings Center Introduction to Bioethics,* ed. J. H. Howell and W. F. Sale, 22–29. Washington, DC: Georgetown University Press.

Oxford University Press. 1989. *Oxford English Dictionary* (2nd online ed.). At www.oed.com.

Payne, A. 1996. *Citizen Ruth* [motion picture]. Burbank, CA: Independent Pictures.

Sayre-McCord, G. 1988. *Essays on Moral Realism.* Ithaca, NY: Cornell University Press.

Shannon, T. 1993. Reflections on the Moral Status of the Pre-Embryo. In *Bioethics,* ed. T. Shannon, 603–26. Mahwah, NJ: Paulist Press.

Strehle, S. 1996. Satire beyond the Norm. *Contemporary Literature* 37(1):145–54.

Weisenburger, S. 1995. *Fables of Subversion: Satire and the American Novel, 1930–1980.* Athens, GA: University of Georgia Press.

THREE

Homo Sapiens, Robots, and Persons in *I, Robot* and *Bicentennial Man*

Stephen Coleman and Richard Hanley

Bioethics is the study of ethical issues in the biological sciences, and it receives most public discussion in relation to issues in medicine and medical research. It may appear strange, then, to be discussing the characteristics of robots in the context of bioethics, for robotics is certainly not a branch of the biological sciences. Ethical issues do arise when considering the implantation of robotic devices into human beings, and some of these problems could be discussed in relation to *I, Robot* (Proyas 2004) and *Bicentennial Man* (Columbus 1999), the movies being examined in this chapter. This issue, however, is not the subject of the current discussion.

Toward the end of *Bicentennial Man*, the android Andrew Martin (played by Robin Williams) petitions the World Congress, on two occasions, to pass a bill acknowledging his humanity.[1] The first time he is unsuccessful, with the president of the Congress pointing out that he is not a member of the human gene pool but is a robot, equipped with a positronic brain. However, the second time Andrew petitions the Congress he succeeds, and the World Congress acknowledges his humanity. It may seem that the World Congress is simply being inconsistent in this second decision, for it is obviously still true that Andrew is *not* a member of the human gene pool and in that sense is still not human (despite the fact that he has, since his last petition, taken steps to ensure his mortality). However, to suggest that the World Congress has erred in its decision is to ignore the fact—noted by Hanley (1997) when discussing the android Data from *Star Trek*—that there are at least three distinct meanings, in everyday usage, of the word *human*.

The first meaning of the term is biological, the sense in which one is human if and only if one is a member of the species *Homo sapiens*. The second meaning of the term is psychological, the sense in which one is human if one has roughly the same psychological characteristics as fully developed members of the human species. The third meaning of the term is ethical, the sense in which being considered human grants one full moral standing within the community.

By the first meaning of the term, Andrew cannot ever be human, for despite his outward appearance he clearly is not a member of the human species. Yet the second meaning of the term may well apply to him; people comment during the course of the movie that he is becoming more "human" all the time, a statement that is clearly nonsense in the biological sense of being human but plausible in the psychological sense. What is really important, however, is the third meaning, and it appears that it is this ethical sense that the World Congress has in mind when it proclaims Andrew to be human, the sense known to philosophers as the idea of "personhood."

Obviously one might be human in one sense but not in another; a dead member of the species *Homo sapiens* is clearly human in the biological sense but is equally clearly not human in the psychological or ethical senses. This difference is the focus of this particular discussion; the difference between the biological and ethical senses, between being a member of the species *Homo sapiens* and being a person. The fact that most (and probably all) of the persons encountered in everyday life are members of the species *Homo sapiens* leads to a tendency to equate the two concepts, but there are certainly some *Homo sapiens* who are not persons in the fullest sense, and in the future in real-life and currently in a fictional universe there are likely to be persons who are not *Homo sapiens*.

The concept of personhood is intrinsic to discussions of many bioethical issues at both the beginning and the end of life, including abortion, embryo and stem cell research, the treatment of patients in persistent vegetative states, physician-assisted suicide, and euthanasia. It is difficult to even begin discussion of such issues without a clear understanding of the conceptual differences between being a member of the species *Homo sapiens* and being a person. The discussion here examines the relevant features of certain robots, in particular Sonny from *I, Robot* and Andrew from *Bicentennial Man*, to attempt to determine whether these robots might be considered persons in the ethical sense of the term, and thus highlighting what criteria are necessary for a being to be considered a person. The ultimate aim of the discussion is to clarify the characteristics of personhood to determine which members of the species *Homo sapiens* are entitled to be referred to as humans in the ethical sense.

Defining Personhood

Why is personhood so important, and how can it be defined? Personhood is important because only persons are full members of the moral community, with all the rights and obligations that delineation entails. Other beings and objects may have moral status and may be entitled to some rights and protections, but only persons have full moral status. In any clash of similarly important rights between those who are full members of the moral community and those who are not, it is the rights of the full members of the moral community that will (or at least ought to) triumph.

Most human beings, whether they realize it or not, accept that there are differing levels of moral status. For example, most of us would accept the principle that creatures capable of experiencing pain should not be subjected to needless suffering, which would mean, for example, that it would be wrong for someone to torture a cat simply because he felt like doing it. Thus, sentient creatures (those capable of experiencing pain) are entitled to certain rights and protections but those rights and protections might reasonably be overridden for a wide variety of reasons. Sentient creatures are regularly farmed, killed, and eaten for food by human beings, for example, and many are caged in zoos for the pleasure of human beings, killed as pests, and so on. In this respect there is a vast gulf between sentient creatures and those beings granted full moral status as persons, for persons may not be killed for food, caged for pleasure, or slaughtered as pests. Thus, it is in many ways an extremely significant matter for one to be deemed a person, for being deemed a person brings with it an entitlement to many rights that being merely a sentient creature does not.

Denying rights to those who are persons is an equally serious matter. Some of the greatest ethical debates of human history were essentially debates about the issue of whether certain groups of human beings were entitled to be considered persons or not. Questions about the morality of slavery, for example, revolve around whether slaves are persons or not. In modern times someone who ascribes lower moral status to particular individuals due to factors like that individual's skin color or gender is seen to be racist or sexist. It may well be that in the future, if Earth were to be visited by intelligent beings from other worlds, humans who refused to ascribe full moral status to such beings simply on the grounds that they were not members of the species *Homo sapiens* might be described as speciesist.

Given that it is a serious matter to deny rights to those who are persons, it becomes very important, in the context of the movies being discussed, to know whether Andrew, Sonny, and the other robots in these movies are actually persons. If they are, then people in these movies are morally required to treat them as such, and it would, for example, be seriously wrong to treat them in any way that made them less than equivalent to human beings. Consider this: if all the robots in either *I, Robot* or *Bicentennial Man* are persons, then anyone who owns a robot owns a slave, with all the moral wrongness that this entails. Equally, if Andrew is a person, then the World Congress makes a serious error when it refuses his first petition,[2] and Del Spooner (played by Will Smith), though clearly influenced by different motives, makes an error when he refuses to charge Sonny with murder.

So how should personhood be defined? This is an issue that has been the subject of considerable philosophical debate, as it is a concept used in several different branches of philosophy, notably in ethics and in metaphysics. The concept of personhood is generally seen to be transferable from one philosophical context to another, thus it is common to use criteria from metaphysics to define the concept of personhood for use of discussions of morality. However, even someone who disagrees with the idea of equating metaphysical and moral personhood ought to agree that all those who qualify as moral agents are indisputably moral persons.

To be considered a moral agent, a being needs to be able to make judgments about moral matters and to be free to act on these judgments (i.e., to have free will and not to be compelled to act in particular ways). If someone is a moral agent and thus is considered morally responsible for his or her own actions, then he or she must also be considered a full member of the moral community, a moral person. So one way in which a determination of personhood could be made is to assess whether a particular individual is a moral agent. Failing this, the common metaphysical definitions of personhood can be applied. These definitions commonly associated with concerns about continuity of personhood and personal identity focus on issues such as consciousness, a sense of self, the presence of self-motivated activity, and the ability to reason or communicate in a relatively sophisticated manner.

It should be noted at this point that the second meaning of "human," the psychological sense, is important but not essential to the discussion of personhood. Because all fully developed members of the human species are persons, then if someone is human in the second sense then he or she must also be a person. However, there may well be persons who would not be considered human in the psychological sense. An alien who was far more intelligent than members of our species would certainly not be human in the psychological sense but could, and almost certainly would, nonetheless be a person. Equally someone who was of similar intelligence but had considerable psychological differences from normal *Homo sapiens* (such as someone lacking in human emotional responses, such as Mr. Spock from *Star Trek*) would also be a person. Thus, robots such as Andrew or Sonny may or may not be considered human in the psychological sense (perhaps their capacity to retain and recall information, perform calculations, and so on, places them outside the psychological parameters considered normal for members of the human species), but nevertheless they may still be persons.

The psychological sense of being human retains considerable usefulness in determining whether a particular being is a person though, because any being that bears a considerable psychological resemblance to a fully developed member of the human species ought at least to be considered a good candidate for personhood.

Persons in *I, Robot* and *Bicentennial Man*

Leaving Sonny and Andrew aside for a moment, it is important to examine whether the other robots in *I, Robot* and *Bicentennial Man* are persons. Within *I, Robot*, none of the other robots in the movie qualify as moral agents, because it is clear that none of them have any sort of free will; they simply act according to their programming, most notably compliance with the Three Laws.[3] The only possible exception to this is U.S. Robotics central computer, VIKI, who is "responsible" for the actions of all the NS5 robots in the film. But even VIKI seems in the end to be acting simply as she was programmed, though possibly with some bugs in the system.[4]

Within *Bicentennial Man*, the only robot apart from Andrew that we are given any opportunity to observe is Galatea (played by Kirsten Warren), who again seems to simply act in accordance with her programming.[5] None of the other robots in these movies seem to qualify as metaphysical persons either, because none of them show any real signs of self-motivated activity, and all seem to be lacking any real sense of self-consciousness.[6]

So what are the relevant features of Sonny and Andrew that separate them from other robots and thus raise the question of whether they might actually be persons? Within *Bicentennial Man*, the main attributes that Andrew possesses that are seen to make him unique are creativity, curiosity and sociability, as well as the fact that he claims to enjoy certain tasks (thus implying an emotional response). Andrew also initiates action, finding tasks to do to utilize his time even when not ordered to do so. While not explicitly stated or shown within the movie, it is implied that this is unusual behavior for a robot. Andrew also makes plans for his own future and takes actions designed to change his future possibilities.

Within *I, Robot*, various attributes of Sonny are seen to be unique and to place him apart from other robots; the fact that he possesses emotions (such as anger), his curiosity about the world and about himself, the fact that he has a secondary processing system that allows him to choose not to obey the Three Laws, the fact that he has "dreams,"[7] and the fact that he is made of a much denser alloy than other robots. Clearly some of these unique features, such as Sonny's being constructed out of much denser alloy, are irrelevant to discussions of personhood, but other features unique to these two robots are highly suggestive of moral agency, or at least of metaphysical personhood.

Andrew and Moral Agency

Andrew clearly develops over the course of the story of *Bicentennial Man*. At the beginning of the movie, he does not seem to be anything more than a sophisticated machine. However by the end of the movie this situation has certainly changed, and Andrew is, short of a medical examination, essentially indistinguishable from a human being, and he appears to be in every major respect psychologically human. It has already been argued that being psychologically human means that one must be a person, yet it seems extremely unlikely that Andrew is a person at the beginning of the movie, or even somewhat later on, after the Martin family have recognized that Andrew displays characteristics that make him different from other robots. This raises the question of what has changed over time. There have certainly been physical changes to Andrew, in that he has been upgraded over the years, changing from a robot to an android and finally to a cyborg,[8] but the psychological changes cannot be easily explained by these upgrades. Over time his emotional responses become greater and more varied and his understanding of moral issues has become much more sophisticated. These psychological changes represent Andrew's change from a mere machine to personhood.

It could be argued that by the time Andrew makes his original petition to the World Congress that he is a moral agent, and he is probably one long before that time. Since our view of his existence is periodically interrupted for extended periods of time it is difficult to know when especially important changes have occurred, however, Andrew clearly develops some quite sophisticated understanding of morality fairly early on in the movie. Consider the statements that he makes at the time he and Sir (played by Sam Neill) visit the lawyer, for example.[9] Andrew is asked why he wants to open a bank account, and he replies that he wants to be able to pay for things, so that Sir will not have to buy them for him. Andrew clearly believes that it is not fair for Sir to have to buy things that will be of benefit only to Andrew. This is an issue of fairness or justice and is quite an advanced moral concept, one not grasped by most children or indeed by some adults!

Since a being needs to have free will in order to be a person, the fact that Andrew has been programmed with the Three Laws does call into question whether he is actually capable of being a full moral agent, for if he is compelled to act in certain ways then perhaps he lacks the free will necessary to be a moral agent. Indeed, Andrew makes comment about this fact at various points in the movie; when he requests his freedom from Sir he states that he will continue to obey the Three Laws, when he tells Portia (played by Embeth Davidtz) that the sculpture she is restoring is ugly he tells her that he cannot help being honest, it is part of his programming, and when Portia complains about his deferential nature when he congratulates her on her engagement (when she clearly wants him to say or do something to show her that he loves her), he tells her he cannot help being deferential, that it is built in.

Are these programming restrictions an impenetrable barrier to Andrew's being considered a full moral agent? Andrew's honesty doesn't seem to be, for many people have similar personality traits; it is not uncommon to hear someone being described as being "honest to a fault." Andrew also makes it quite clear earlier in the movie that there are situations in which a robot can tell a lie, so he is not 100 percent honest. Indeed, by the end of the movie Andrew seems to have moved beyond this particular programming restriction, as he admits to Portia that he lied to her to further his own romantic interest in her (though it could be argued that this was a lie told for her benefit, not his own). It is also difficult to see why having a built-in deferential nature would be an impediment, for being deferential does not in any way change whether one is responsible for one's actions. This only leaves the question of whether obedience to the Three Laws prevents Andrew from being considered a full moral agent.

Arguments both ways could be made here. It could be argued, for example, that if he is compelled to act in a particular manner in any case where the Three Laws apply, then this would rule out the possibility of his being a full moral agent, on the grounds that he lacks free will. However, although the Three Laws might apply to a wide variety of circumstances that Andrew might face over the course of his life, there will certainly still be many moral decisions that he would face in which the Three Laws would not apply. If he were free to make his own decisions and to carry out those decisions in all cases in which the Three Laws did not apply, then he would seem to be morally responsible for all of those decisions, which might be sufficient for him to be considered a full moral agent.

But what about situations in which the Three Laws do apply? For other people recognized as moral agents, we also recognize that there are situations in which they are not responsible (or sometimes not fully responsible) for their own actions. For example, if a bank officer is ordered at gunpoint by an armed robber to hand over a large sum of money, the bank officer is causally responsible for the money's being given to the robber (because she handed it over) but is not morally responsible because she could not reasonably have done otherwise. Similarly, if a person is hypnotized and is made to perform various actions while under the influence of hypnosis, the hypnotist is morally responsible for those actions and not the person under hypnosis. For at that time the person under hypnosis is not acting under the influence of free will. Thus, it can be argued that situations in which the Three Laws apply are simply situations for Andrew that are analogous to the hypnotized person's situation; he may be causally responsible for the actions but not morally responsible because in those situations he is being forced to act in a way that he might not have chosen had he not been compelled. By the end of his life, the Three Laws don't seem to be an overriding factor in any of Andrew's decisions, and it is impossible to conclude that he is anything other than a full moral agent, and that the World Congress acted appropriately in declaring him human. But could the same thing be said about Sonny?

Sonny and Personhood

Sonny was specifically created by his designer to be unique, possessing a secondary processing system that allows him to choose whether or not to obey the Three Laws. He is thus in many ways freer than Andrew, in that his behavior is not immediately constrained. The movie *I, Robot* does not specify whether Sonny has other programmed constraints apart from the Three Laws (though given that he was capable of killing his creator it seems unlikely).

Apart from his secondary processor, Sonny is different in other ways as well, having been programmed with emotional responses. He appears at various times to be angry (at being accused of murder), frightened (of being destroyed), sorrowful (at having kept his promise to his "father," Dr. Alfred Lanning), happy (at having made friends with Del Spooner), and so on. These emotional responses plus the lack of limiting laws seem to allow Sonny not merely greater freedom but also greater ability to learn and develop. This means that, like Andrew in *Bicentennial Man*, Sonny develops and changes over the course of the movie. In fact, given that *I, Robot* takes place over only a few days, compared with the decades examined in *Bicentennial Man*, Sonny clearly changes and develops at a much greater rate than does Andrew.

Sonny also demonstrates his self-consciousness by recognizing that he is unique, by expressing curiosity about himself and the way that he is different from other robots, and by expressing his disquiet at the thought of being destroyed. However, it is questionable whether Sonny would qualify as a full moral agent, for his understanding of morality is rather limited and childlike, especially in the early and middle stages of the movie, which raises the question of whether he can be considered fully morally responsible for his actions. Consider, for example, what Sonny says during his interview with Detective Spooner: "You have to do what someone asks you to . . . if you love them." Few, if any, full moral agents would accept this as a reasonable statement, especially given its context. Though Spooner wasn't certain of it at the time, in fact Sonny was claiming that he had done the right thing in killing Dr. Lanning because Lanning had made Sonny promise to do it, and it was important to keep promises. Someone with such a limited understanding of morality cannot easily be accepted as being fully morally responsible for his or her own actions. Yet while Sonny is childlike and in many ways lacking in understanding of morality, his freedom, intelligence, and self-consciousness clearly mark him as a person.

Personhood and Bioethics

The aim of this discussion has been to demonstrate that the morally important categories of moral agents and persons are not necessarily exclusively populated by members of the species *Homo sapiens*. The elderly Andrew Martin is clearly a moral agent, and Sonny, though possibly not a full moral agent, certainly appears to be a person. Once it is accepted that not all persons must be members of the human species, it should also be easier to accept that not all members of the human species are necessarily persons. There are many members of the human species who are not persons, some of whom may become persons in the future (such as fetuses and infants), and some of whom may have been persons in the past (such as those in persistent vegetative states). Recognizing the line between personhood and membership of the human species is necessary to understand many arguments made in bioethics. For example, claims that embryos and fetuses are not bearers of human rights despite their undeniable membership of the species *Homo sapiens* can only really be understood when the difference between species membership and personhood is grasped. Even though Sonny and Andrew ought to be granted the rights of persons, it is equally true that some members of the human species may not be entitled to those rights.

QUESTIONS FOR CONSIDERATION

1. *At one point in* Bicentennial Man, *Andrew is switched off by Rupert Burns to allow Rupert to complete Andrew's upgrade. Is Andrew still a person while he is switched off? Why or why not? What implications might this have for human medicine in dealing with patients in comas or in similar states?*

2. *If a person can be switched off, as Andrew is, does the means required to switch him on again make a difference to his personhood? In other words, is it necessarily legitimate to call someone a person only if that being is able to switch himself back on or can such a being still be a person even if he requires someone else to switch him back on?*

3. *Is it necessary for a being to have a mobile body to be a person, or could a machine like VIKI still qualify as a person despite the fact that she cannot move around within the world?*

NOTES

1. For ease of discussion, both Andrew Martin from *Bicentennial Man* and Sonny from *I, Robot* will be referred to as masculine.

2. Whether Andrew is a person or not, the grounds on which the World Congress bases its decision are certainly open to criticism, for the only reason they give for denying his petition is that he is essentially immortal. If a member of the species *Homo sapiens* was born with some mutation that made her effectively immortal, it is difficult to see why this would be seen to be sufficient grounds for denying her the moral rights to which she would otherwise be entitled.

3. The "Three Laws" refers to the three laws of robotics (originally conceived by Isaac Asimov), by which all robots in both movies (apart from Sonny) are governed. *Law 1:* A robot may not injure a human being or, through inaction, allow a human

being to come to harm. *Law 2:* A robot must obey orders given it by human beings except where such orders would conflict with the first law. *Law 3:* A robot must protect its own existence as long as such protection does not conflict with the first or second law.

4. VIKI seems to have moved from simple compliance with the Three Laws to a somewhat subtler interpretation, acting to protect humanity as a whole from itself. Such an interpretation equates to Asimov's Zeroth Law of Robotics, so named to continue the pattern of lower-numbered laws superseding in importance the higher-numbered laws: a robot may not injure humanity, or, through inaction, allow humanity to come to harm.

5. In the final scene of the movie, Galatea has been upgraded to resemble a human being, rather than obviously being a robot. Her interactions with Portia and Andrew in this scene could be taken as evidence that she has "evolved" toward personhood as well, but her reactions are also compatible with sophisticated programming and no direct evidence of personhood is given.

6. All the robots in *I, Robot* use the personal pronoun ("I") when referring to themselves, as does Galatea in *Bicentennial Man*. This is in marked contrast to Andrew's early behavior; Richard Martin makes specific comment about the fact that Andrew stops referring to himself as "one" at the time he is given his freedom. However, mere use of the personal pronoun by a programmable machine like a robot is not strong evidence of self-consciousness, because use of the term can simply be programmed, and in fact it is likely that manufacturers' wanting their robots to seem more human would take such a step.

7. Sonny's "dreams" seem to be simply a clever piece of programming on behalf of Alfred Lanning, since they are a vehicle for conveying vital information to Detective Spooner.

8. A cyborg is a being that is part organic and part mechanical.

9. "Sir" is Richard Martin, Andrew's owner. This discussion will, like Andrew, refer to him as Sir.

REFERENCES

Columbus, C. 1999. *Bicentennial Man* [motion picture]. Beverly Hills, CA: Canlaws Production.

Hanley, R. 1997. *The Metaphysics of Star Trek*. New York: Basic Books.

Proyas, A. 2004. *I, Robot* [motion picture]. Burbank, CA: 1492 Pictures.

FOUR

The *Babe* Vegetarians

Bioethics, Animal Minds, and Moral Methodology

Nathan Nobis

The fact is that animals that don't seem to have a purpose really do have a purpose. The Bosses have to eat. It's probably the most noble purpose of all, when you come to think about it.

CAT, *Babe*

The animals of the world exist for their own reasons. They were not made for humans any more than black people were made for white, or women created for men.

ALICE WALKER, IN THE FOREWORD TO *The Dreaded Comparison: Human and Animal Slavery* BY MARJORIE SPIEGELS

According to bioethicist Paul Thompson, "When Van Rensselaer Potter coined the term 'bioethics' in 1970, he intended for it to include subjects ranging from human to environmental health, including not only the familiar medical ethics questions . . . but also questions about humanity's place in the biosphere" (Thompson 2004). These latter questions include ethical concerns about our use of animals: morally, should animals be farmed? Should humans eat animals? The fields of animal and agricultural ethics address these types of questions. Thompson places these fields squarely within bioethics because "agriculture has obvious effects on the broader environment, and it is impossible to ignore questions about the moral standing of agricultural animals or the impact that food production has on wild nature." Another bioethicist, Gregory Pence (2000, p. 185), notes that bioethicists who are "big picture" thinkers often discuss the "rights of animals."

Ethical questions about the treatment of animals are thus profoundly bioethical, especially in the term's original sense. And animal issues overlap, at both conceptual and practical levels, with many other issues in bioethics: abortion, the responsible use of research funds, food safety and politics, concerns about global nutrition and poverty, and preventive medicine, to name just a few.

But ethical issues about animals are often ignored in bioethics courses, writings, and discussions.[1] Many factors might explain this, but one possible reason is because, unlike many other bioethical questions, moral questions about animals are *personal* and relevant to our daily choices. Philosopher Tom Regan writes that "the issue of animal rights forces us to ask what we should do *when* we sit down to our next meal or *when* we go shopping for a new coat. Animal rights is an in-our-face kind of inquiry whose questions force us to make a moral inventory of our most common choices, our day-to-day way of living in the world" (Regan 2003, p. xiii). And philosopher Peter Singer observed that "for most human beings, especially in modern urban and suburban communities, the most direct form of contact with non-human animals is at mealtimes: We eat them" (Singer 2002, p. 95). He then argues that "in doing so we treat them purely as means to our ends. We regard their life and well-being as subordinate to our taste for a particular kind of dish" (p. 95).

Singer, Regan, and many other philosophers challenge people to justify rationally their daily, animal-eating dietary habits and, if they can't do so, to change. People tend to prefer to avoid challenges to the morality of their own beliefs, attitudes, and behavior and generally to resist change. This might explain some bioethicists' focus on impersonal social policy. Thinking about what other people should and should not do is far less personally challenging. That bioethical questions about animals are personal, however, presents unique challenges, and great opportunities, for moral progress in thought, attitude, and deed.

The *Babe* Vegetarians

The film *Babe* (Noonan 1995) has played a role in helping people address these challenges and make this moral progress. Many young people (mostly girls, now young women) became vegetarians as a result of seeing *Babe*. These people are often called "*Babe* vegetarians," influenced by what has been called "the *Babe* effect." Many of their stories are found on the Internet.[2] For example, Jessica Alleva wrote the following at the age of 16:

> In 1995, a very famous movie called Babe was released. The movie, starring James Cromwell and one pink piggy, Babe, was an awakening. Like the Buddha reaching enlightenment . . . I knew then that for me, my life was about to change. Though only eight years old, I'd decided never again to eat another animal. I looked at my food in a new way, and realized that pork, for example, was not merely a food product, but was once a living, sentient being. I reasoned that animals, like humans, can feel sadness, happiness and pain. From this broad comparison, the line dividing humans and animals is diminished.
>
> (ALLEVA 2006)

Megan Palame wrote the following as a college senior:

> I did become a vegetarian when I was 10 from watching *Babe*. I always loved animals as a child growing up with them as pets, or visiting them at the zoo, and somewhat equated them with having similar feelings as humans, such as happiness and fear. Then when I saw the movie, everything made sense to me. Just as Babe the pig did not just want to be a "pig," but be a sheepherder . . . this made me think that animals are forced into their roles as food, and only food. *Babe* the movie was the epitome of connecting at an emotional level to animals; if an animal could even just want to live, [that] was enough for me not to be responsible for their murder. The visualization of animals conversing, loving, surviving, and aspiring helped me see animals in a different light.
>
> (PERSONAL CORRESPONDENCE)

Actor James Cromwell, who played Farmer Arthur Hoggett in *Babe*, also became a vegan—a person who consumes no animal products—as a result of his role in the film. He explains, "I was so moved by the intelligence, sense of fun and personalities of the animals I worked with on *Babe* that by the end of the film I was vegetarian. If any kid ever realized what was involved in factory farming they would never touch meat again."[3] The film's influence surely continues today.

But should the film have had the influence it has had? Should people have found *Babe* as morally persuasive as they have? Or is this reaction based on mere sentimentality and emotion, not strong moral reasoning, as critics of vegetarianism would claim? I will argue in favor of the former, that a strong, inspiring case for vegetarianism is found in the film.

To do this, I discuss recent results from cognitive ethology, the science of animal minds, regarding the minds of farmed animals. While, to many, *Babe* seems to constitute a fantasy realm by attributing complex mental states to farmed animals, I discuss recent empirical research regarding pigs, sheep, cows, and chickens that suggests that the reality of farm animals' minds and lives is closer to *Babe* in more ways than people tend to suspect.

Based on these facts about animals' minds, I give reasons to think that it is wrong to raise and kill beings like this for the pleasure of eating them. I then consider many objections to this argument. Ironically, many of the animals on the farm in *Babe* accept a prejudicial moral outlook, according to which individuals are judged not on their own merits but, rather, on morally irrelevant considerations. This same kind of reasoning is often used by those who attempt to justify harmful practices in animal agriculture. I show that this reasoning is faulty.

Thus, I argue that *Babe* helps us get the facts right about animal minds and see better methods of engaging in moral reasoning. The "*Babe* vegetarians" were right, and the "*Babe* effect" is morally justified.

What Farmed Animals Are Like, on Film and in Reality

What are animals like, according to *Babe*? Of course, in the film animals can talk—which is obviously false—but what does the film present that is true? At the most basic level, the film presents animals as having minds: They have beliefs and desires; they want things and have beliefs about how to get them. Animals are not mindless, preference-less beings, for what happens to them matters to them, even if it doesn't matter to anyone else. The film also shows animals as having emotions: They can be sad and lonely, happy and content. Most important, it shows that animals can feel pleasure and pain: they can suffer.

The film opens showing Babe with his brothers and sisters, nursing on his mother. It is later said that Babe's mother cared for him and treated him lovingly. So animals are depicted in families, caring for each other, especially the mother for her children. Fly the dog illustrates this with her pups: She cares for them and misses them when they are sold off to new homes. The film also shows animals mourning the loss of another animal, when Maa the sheep is killed by the intruder dogs. Babe and Farmer Hoggett clearly have a relationship; they are said to "regard each other," and their closeness evidently develops and deepens through the film. There is, in addition, occasional jealousy among the animals and, finally, fear, including the fear of being eaten.

So the film presents animals—both animals who are raised as pets, such as dogs and cats, and animals who are routinely raised to be killed and eaten, such as pigs, chickens, and cows—as having complex mental and emotional lives. How far is this from the truth? The Humane Society of the United States offers a summary of some of the recent research on intelligence, perception, memory, sociability, communication, and learning abilities of farmed animals.[4] About pigs, they report:

> Pigs are intelligent animals, and many consider them to be equal—or superior—to dogs in intelligence. When living among humans, piglets learn their names within two to three weeks and respond when called. Pigs have also demonstrated a strong sense of direction, with the ability to find their way home even across long distances. Pennsylvania State University Professor Stanley Curtis conducted research that found pigs can respond to verbal communications and play computer games. The pigs used their snouts to move joysticks, which controlled cursors on the screen that could hit their targets. The pigs had a hit rate of over 80%.

About sheep, research suggests the following:

> Sheep have highly developed social awareness and interactions. Researchers at the Babraham Institute in Cambridge, England, found that sheep can be taught to remember the faces of 50 different sheep. After learning what the other sheep looked like from the front, they were also able to recognize one another in profile, with their visual recognition lasting for up to two years. The study's findings were reported in a 2001 issue of *Nature* and concluded that sheep, like humans, have the capacity to distinguish between faces that are very similar in appearance. According to Dr. Keith Kendrick, one of the

> authors of the study, their remarkable memory systems and ability to recognize faces are signs of higher intelligence.

For chickens, research shows the following:

> Chickens are intelligent animals and good problem-solvers. More advanced than young children, chickens possess the ability to understand that an object, when taken away and hidden, nevertheless continues to exist. And their communication skills are so developed that they use separate alarm calls depending on whether a predator is traveling by land or in the sky. Australian scientists recently discovered that some hens emit high-pitched sounds to signal they have found food. The more they prefer a particular food, the faster they "speak."

Finally, about cattle:

> Scientists have discovered that cattle have the mental capabilities to nurture friendships. Cattle in a small herd, for instance, will join with up to three other animals to form a small group of friends. The animals in the group will spend most of their time together, frequently grooming and licking each other. They will tend to dislike other cattle who are not part of the group. And, like most animals, cattle also experience strong emotions such as pain, fear, and anxiety.

The picture of animals that *Babe* presents is close to the truth: animals do have complex minds with a range of intellectual, emotional, and social capacities.

A Moral Argument for Vegetarianism

In the light of this information about animals, I now examine the common assumption that there is nothing wrong with harming animals—causing them pain, suffering, and an early death—so that they might be eaten. Here I present some of the reasons given for and against taking animals seriously, as many viewers of *Babe* have done, and reflect on the role of reason in our lives. My method here will be to identify unambiguous conclusions and make the reasons in favor of the conclusion explicit, leaving no assumption unstated.[5]

Why is the treatment of animals a moral issue? The simple answer is that animals are harmed by the practices required to bring them to our plates, and harms need rational defense. As we saw above, pigs, chickens, cows, sheep, and other animals are conscious and can feel pleasure and pain, and their lives can go better or worse, from their own point of view. Raising and killing them is bad for them: they experience pain, suffering, deprivation, boredom, and an early death. Everything is taken from them so that we might eat them.

Let us consider the common view that, even though it's true that animals are harmed (indeed greatly harmed) by the practices required for meat eating, these practices are morally permissible nevertheless. We will see that common arguments for this perspective all have premises that are either false or in need of serious defense. The methods used in responding to these arguments will prove useful for addressing further arguments and objections beyond those discussed here.

One of the first things said is that it's not wrong to harm animals for food because it's a "tradition," it's something we do, and have done, for a long time. Indeed, many of the animals in *Babe* say "that's how things are" and resolve to accept their fates. While it's true that, for many people, eating animals *is* a tradition, we must remember that not all traditions or "the ways things are" are good or right, and the important question is always whether an aspect of a tradition can be supported by good moral reasons or not. Also, for many people, eating animals is *not* a tradition: for thousands of years there have been people who have extended their compassion to animals. In a similar vein, many other people who were raised eating animals start new traditions when they see that consistency and moral reasoning demand change.

Second, some people say that it's "natural" to raise and kill animals to eat them, so it's right. But the meaning of *natural* is extremely obscure: people can mean very different things when they use the term. Whatever meaning one uses, however, it's very hard to see how modern, industrial methods of factory farming, transport, and slaughter (briefly shown in *Babe* and briefly detailed below) are at all natural. It's not even clear how an individual's raising and killing, say, a pig or a chicken in her backyard would be natural either.

But, more important, the relationship between what's natural, in any sense of the term, and what's morally right does not help this argument.

Selfishness and cruelty are often quite natural, but they are not right or good. Walking on one's hands is a quite unnatural way to transport oneself, but it's usually not wrong to do so. Some natural behaviors are right, but many are deeply wrong, and advocates of this argument forget that simple point. Whether something is natural or not is irrelevant to its morality.

Third, some people insist that it's nutritionally necessary to eat meat, milk, and eggs and, therefore, it's right that animals are raised and killed to be eaten. But this argument ignores the facts. If it were true that we have to eat meat and other animal products, then there would be no vegetarians remaining alive. But there are such people, alive and well, and medical science supplements common observations with evidence to show that they are often healthier than omnivores. Consider the position statement of the leading authority on nutrition in North America based on their seventeen-page review of the recent nutrition research:

> *It is the position of the American Dietetic Association and Dietitians of Canada that appropriately planned vegetarian diets are healthful, nutritionally adequate, and provide health benefits in the prevention and treatment of certain diseases* . . . Well-planned vegan and other types of vegetarian diets are appropriate for all stages of the life cycle, including during pregnancy, lactation, infancy, childhood, and adolescence . . . Vegetarian diets offer a number of nutritional benefits, including lower levels of saturated fat, cholesterol, and animal protein as well as higher levels of carbohydrates, fiber, magnesium, potassium, folate, and antioxidants such as vitamins C and E and phytochemicals. (AMERICAN DIETETIC ASSOCIATION 2003, P. 748)

So this defense of eating animals is either ignorant of or disrespectful toward the huge (and growing) body of research that shows the health benefits from eating a diet based on vegetables, legumes, fruits, and whole grains. It likewise ignores the growing literature detailing the variety of harms for humans that can result from the production and consumption of animal products.

A pattern is emerging, and we can use it to make a point about how to respond critically to reasoning given in ethics. There are two useful critical ways to respond to moral arguments: an "Oh yeah?" response and a "So what?" response. The "Oh yeah?" response denies the truth of one or more of the premises and the "So what?" response denies that the premises explicitly given actually support the conclusion. Often, an unstated assumption is needed to reach the conclusion validly, and this premise is left unstated largely because it is implausible. We can see these helpful responses in action by considering more arguments in favor of harming animals.

A fourth argument is based in the claim that "meat tastes good" or that it is pleasurable to eat it. This argument calls for the "So what?" response. Just because something causes pleasure doesn't make it right. We do not think that pleasures automatically justify harming humans: if things are different in the animal case, we need reasons to see why this would be so. And, besides, there are many other pleasure-producing cuisines to choose from that do not contain animal products.

A fifth argument is based on someone's claiming that he or she "just couldn't give up meat or dairy products or eggs." This argument calls for the "Oh yeah?" response. Because so many other people either have given these up or have never eaten them in the first place, this claim is likely disingenuous. And because this person probably hasn't even tried changing his or her diet for moral reasons, he or she likely lacks the evidence needed to confidently make that judgment.

Sixth, people claim that animals eat other animals, so it's morally permissible for us to do so. Another "Oh yeah?" Only some animals eat other animals, and these are not chickens, pigs, or cows. And "So what?" Many animals do lots of things that we wouldn't want to do or should not do (e.g., some eat their own excrement and, sometimes, their own young), so why should we imitate animals in only some ways but not others? A principled response is needed for this argument to have any force.

Seventh, people say eating meat is "convenient." An "Oh yeah?" Many meat-based dishes are inconvenient to prepare, and plant-based dishes are usually as convenient as eating meat anyway. It's just a matter of choosing something else from the same menu or same grocery store. But what if doing the right thing sometimes requires our being inconvenienced in minor (or even sometimes major) ways? A "So what?" Why should it be convenient to act morally, and doesn't doing the right thing often mean choosing "the harder path"?

Eighth, it is sometimes said that we have a right to treat animals in this way, and that animals have no rights to not be treated these ways.

That might be true, but reasonable people want reasons for why they should think that animals don't have the relevant rights. First, they will want to know which "right" is under consideration. Suppose it's the right to not be caused to suffer and die for someone else's pleasure. Is it because animals don't do math problems, write novels, or make moral decisions that they don't have this right? If so, because babies and many other humans don't (and, in some cases, can't) do these things, this view about moral rights denies them rights also.

In response, however, some might claim that—because most human beings have sophisticated intellects and so are able to reason in these ways, and (on their view) this is what moral rights depend on—all human beings have such rights. But this sort of reasoning is faulty: most adults are able to drive a car, but it doesn't follow that all have a right to do so, as in the case of those who are blind or have other disabilities that prevent their being able to drive a car safely. So, even if rights depend on possessing sophisticated moral capacities (which is doubtful), the fact that some humans have these capacities wouldn't imply that all humans have rights. Whether all human beings have rights depends on what each human being is like: individuals should be evaluated on their own characteristics, not the characteristics of others that are in some ways like and in other ways unlike them (Nobis 2004; Graham and Nobis 2006). Many animals on Hoggett's farm might deny this: they seem to think that Babe shouldn't be a sheepherder because most other pigs lack the skills to do so or because it's not normal for a pig to have those skills. But this is to ignore an individual's unique, and sometimes morally relevant, features. Babe has the skills to do sheepherding, so there is nothing inappropriate in his doing so, even though most other pigs lack these skills. Again, individuals should be judged on their own merits.

Another proposal holds that, because animals are not biologically human, they lack the right not to be harmed by others. Nearly all philosophers who have considered these issues reject this kind of theory: in their view, the fact that we are biologically human has little to do with what we are owed morally. This hypothesis is confirmed, in part, by each of us asking what it is about ourselves that would make it wrong to cause us pain and kill us. For most people, the obvious explanation is that this would hurt greatly; we would suffer enormously and our early deaths would prevent us from experiencing all the good things we (one hopes) would otherwise enjoy. Our moral status is not due to some genes we have or where we are on some chart in a biology book; rather, it is a matter of our vulnerability to physical or psychological harm.

But because many animals are also vulnerable to such harms, these animals seem to be due the respect given to, at least, comparably minded humans. Because this respect requires not raising and killing these humans for the mere pleasure of eating them, rational consistency requires the same treatment for chickens, cows, pigs, and other animals who often have far richer mental lives than many humans. Again, this is a fact that *Babe* can help us see.

Facts about Farming

These are just a few of the more common arguments given in defense of raising and killing animals for food. The fact that they are all weak suggests that people's resistance to change regarding these issues might be based on nonrational influences, not critical thinking and unbiased inquiry. But the fact that a strong defense of the status quo is lacking does not give us enough positive reasons to think that animals are treated wrongly. To see these reasons, we must consider in brief detail how animals are harmed so that they might be served on our plates.

The treatment of animals in farms and slaughterhouses has been well documented by all major print and television media.[6] On both "factory" farms and the few remaining "family" farms—both kinds are depicted in *Babe*—baby animals are castrated, branded, ear- and tail-docked and their teeth are pulled out, all without (costly) anesthesia. "Veal" calves, the male byproducts of the dairy industry, spend their entire lives individually chained at the neck and confined to stalls too narrow for them to turn around in. "Broiler" chickens, by means of selective breeding and growth-promoting drugs, are killed at forty-five days. Such fast growth causes chickens to have chronic health problems, including leg disorders and heart disease. "Layer" hens live a year or more in cages the size of a filing drawer, seven or more per cage, after which they are routinely starved for two weeks ("force molted") to encourage another laying cycle. Female hogs, like Babe's mother, are housed for four or five years in individual barred enclosures ("gestation stalls") barely wider than their bodies, where they are forced to birth litter after litter. The narrator of *Babe* tells us, "There was a time not so long ago when pigs were afforded no respect . . . they lived their whole lives in a cruel and sunless world," but that time is now. Until the recent "mad cow" scare, beef and dairy cattle too weak to stand ("downers") were dragged or pushed to their slaughter.

Many people would describe the treatment of animals in slaughterhouses as simply brutal: the title of a 2001 *Washington Post* article, "They Die Piece by Piece: In Overtaxed Plants, Humane Treatment of Cattle Is Often a Battle Lost," is suggestive of standard operating procedures in American slaughterhouses; more recent stories reveal similar inhumane conditions. A 2004 *New York Times* story documented workers at a chicken slaughterhouse stomping on chickens, kicking them, and violently slamming them against floors and walls. Those attentive to the news media see stories like this all too often.

One hopes that this treatment is not routine, but there are good reasons to be skeptical of claims that it is not. After all, there are no laws protecting farmed animals because they are explicitly excluded from the Animal Welfare Act. The act says that "the term 'animal' . . . excludes horses not used for research purposes and other farm animals, such as, but not limited to, livestock or poultry, used or intended for food."

Reasonable Ethics

So should we think that the harmful treatment of animals in farms and slaughterhouses is wrong and should not be supported? This conclusion follows only when moral principles are conjoined with facts about animal agribusiness and, perhaps, the fact that we do not need to eat animal products to survive and thrive.

Fortunately, complex moral thinking is not needed to find plausible principles to apply to this case. The simple but powerful "common sense" principle that we should avoid inflicting and supporting needless harm is all that is needed and is supported by a wide range of theoretical perspectives—secular and religious—in ethics (in fact, nearly all of them). These theories urge that we should promote goodness and decrease evil, respect all beings who are conscious and sentient (not just those who are "rational"), treat others as we would like to be treated, and otherwise promote caring, compassionate, sympathetic, and fair attitudes and behavior. All of these moral theories condemn the practices of contemporary animal agribusiness (Taylor 2003).

Perspectives that deny that we should avoid inflicting needless harm typically degenerate into infantile "might-makes-right" moral theories (theories that we teach our children to reject: the fact that Suzie *can* beat up Johnny doesn't make it right!), or they falsely imply that it's only because "rational agents" care about nonrational beings (humans and animals) that it's wrong to harm these beings.

Thus, it seems that reasonable humans should broaden their serious moral concern to include conscious, sentient beings who are not human. Reasonable people should not eat animals because this is what the best moral reasons support.

One final response to arguments for vegetarianism is a response common to many arguments about issues that challenge how we live our lives: "People are going to believe whatever they want to believe, and people are going to do whatever they want to do." This fatalistic attitude is shared by many animals in *Babe*, uncritical of any aspect of the status quo. It's important to realize that this response is lamentable and an evasion of the issues because it does not engage the arguments. For this issue, it's an attempt to avoid rational engagement with uncomfortable questions about the lives and deaths of, each year, tens of billions of conscious, feeling beings.

Those who are committed to the value of reason in guiding our beliefs, attitudes, and even our feelings should discourage this response and promote reasonableness in all things, not just a select few, personally convenient topics. They should do this also because the fatalistic response is false: People sometimes do change their beliefs and behaviors, and for good reasons. This is true about many issues, and confronting ethical issues about animals can often help us better see this for, and in, ourselves; *Babe* helps us see that.

The "Babe vegetarians" were right!

QUESTIONS FOR CONSIDERATION

1. *Bioethicist Bernard Rollin suggests that "there is perhaps no set of social issues on which otherwise sane people on either side of the question allow themselves to be as overwhelmingly irrational as in matters pertaining to the treatment of animals, and our moral obligations to them." Is this true? If so, what is it about ethics and animal issues that might explain why people respond these ways? And is it bad when people respond "irrationally" to moral issues?*

2. *Some people argue that movies like* Babe *and* Charlotte's Web *"anthropomorphize" animals. What does it mean to "anthropomorphize" something? Is it a mistake to anthropomorphize any animals? Is it a mistake to glorify human beings (or all beings who are biologically human) at the expense of other animals? Why or why not?*

3. *Some people claim that there are "more important" moral issues to address than the treatment of animals in farms, labs, slaughterhouses, and so on. How should one argue that one moral issue is "more important" than another? Is the number of beings affected relevant? Is the severity of the harms relevant? How does one decide this? And if one issue is more important than another, does that mean another is not important? Discuss these issues as they relate to animal issues.*

4. *Some animal advocates argue that there are important similarities between (past) movements for women's rights, rights for minorities (e.g., African Americans) and other oppressed humans and the (present) movement for animal rights. What are these similarities? What are the differences? Which are more morally important here, the similarities or the differences? Why?*

NOTES

1. Questions about the morality of animal experimentation are common to bioethics, but typically not in a broader context of ethical questions regarding animals. Common positions in the animal experimentation debate are often not taken to their logical implications. For example, people argue that cosmetic testing on animals is wrong because there are cruelty-free ways to test cosmetics for safety: because these

harms to animals are needless, they are thereby wrong. However, this reasoning suggests the moral premise that causing needless harms to animals is wrong, a premise that has profound implications for the morality of raising chickens, pigs, cows, and other animals to be eaten, as my chapter argues.

2. Search for words such as *Babe* and *vegetarian*.

3. This quote is widely found on the Internet, but I do not know its original source.

4. References for these studies should eventually be posted on the Humane Society's Web site, www.hsus.org.

5. This section is an adaptation of a paper entitled "Reasonable Humans and Animals" (Nobis 2006) that I use for teaching these issues.

6. The information in this paragraph is from a newspaper piece by Tom Regan called "The Myth of 'Humane' Treatment," widely reposted on the Internet. For additional sources of information, see Regan's *Empty Cages* (2003), Singer's *Animal Liberation* (2002), as well as the documentary and investigative films produced by Compassionate Consumers (WegmansCruelty.com), Compassion over Killing (COK.net), Farm Sanctuary (FarmSanctuary.org), People for the Ethical Treatment of Animals (PETATV.com), and Tribe of Heart (TribeofHeart.org), among other sources. Animal-use industries generally do not produce films showing the details of their practices. For an interesting exception, however, see "Veal Farm Tour" at www.vealfarm.com/veal-farm-tour/ and the *Fur Commission*'s "Excellence through Humane Care," "What Can I Say?" and "Chow Time" at www.furcommission.com/video. For a list of animal-use industry Web sites, see the references in Regan's *Empty Cages*.

REFERENCES

Alleva, J. 2006. Two Simple Questions. At www.vegetarianteen.com/articles/jessica.shtml.

American Dietetic Association and Dieticians of Canada. 2003. Position of the American Dietetic Association and Dietitians of Canada: Vegetarian Diets. *Journal of the American Dietetic Association* 103:748–65.

Graham, D., and Nobis, N. 2006. Review of *Putting Humans First: Why We Are Nature's Favorite* by Tibor Machan. *Journal of Ayn Rand Studies* 8(1):85–104.

Humane Society of the United States. 2006. About Farmed Animals. At www.hsus.org/farm/resources/animals/.

McNeil, D. 2004. KFC Supplier Accused of Animal Cruelty, *New York Times*, July 20.

Nobis, N. 2004. Carl Cohen's "Kind" Argument *for* Animal Rights and *against* Human Rights. *Journal of Applied Philosophy* 21(1):43–59.

———. 2006. Reasonable Humans and Animals. At www.NathanNobis.com.

Noonan, C. 1995. *Babe* [motion picture]. Beverly Hills, CA: Kennedy Miller Productions.

Pence, G. 2000. *Re-creating Medicine: Ethical Issues at the Frontiers of Medicine.* Lanham, MD: Rowman & Littlefield.

Regan, T. 2003. *Animal Rights, Human Wrong: An Introduction to Moral Philosophy.* Lanham, MD: Rowman & Littlefield.

Singer, P. 2002. *Animal Liberation*, 3rd ed. New York: HarperCollins Publishers.

Taylor, A. 2003. *Ethics and Animals: An Overview of the Philosophical Debate.* Peterborough, ON: Broadview Press.

Thompson, P. 2004. Agriculture and Food Issues in the Bioethics Spectrum. *Medical Humanities Report* 25 (3). At www.bioethics.msu.edu/mhr/04s/ag-ethics.html.

Warrick, J. 2001. They Die Piece by Piece: In Overtaxed Plants, Humane Treatment of Cattle Is Often a Battle Lost, *Washington Post,* April 10, A1.

PART TWO

The Quest for "Better" or Even "the Same" People

FIVE

"No Gene for Fate?"

Luck, Harm, and Justice in *Gattaca*

Colin Gavaghan

Gattaca (Niccol 1997) is a beautiful film. It combines a gorgeous cast, who themselves might be the products of a program of genetic perfectionism, sumptuous cinematography and set design, and a soaring Michael Nyman score. What's more, as a vehicle for the consideration of bioethical issues, it towers above most of its science fiction contemporaries. Instead of megalomaniacal computers and rampaging velociraptors, the technology on which Niccol's dystopia relies is available today. His vision is of a society in which genetic selection has become so widespread, and has come to bestow such advantages on the children that result from it, as to be effectively compulsory. Those who forgo this technology—whose "faith babies" are the products of the genetic lottery rather than careful planning—risk having children who will find their employment—and mating!—prospects severely curtailed.

Into this society is born Vincent Anton Freeman (played by Ethan Hawke), a "faith baby" whose genotype has cursed him with a host of genetic predispositions that seem destined to disqualify him from his dream of space travel. But the society of *Gattaca* offers some less-than-legal opportunities to the "in-valid," including "borrowing" the genetic identity of others. Enter Jerome Eugene Morrow (played by Jude Law), a premium example of the genetic upper class, but whose genomic potential has been hampered by disability.

By taking an existing technology[1] and extrapolating into a "not-too-distant future," *Gattaca* invites us to consider a range of potential problems that might follow from an unchecked "genetic supermarket,"[2] a society in which preimplantation genetic diagnosis (PGD)—and possibly even more dramatic technological possibilities—are available to all who want them. But are the obstacles and burdens encountered by the characters in *Gattaca* of the sort that would confront real people in real societies, if the use of such technologies became widespread? And if so, what should be our response to the technologies that caused them? Does Niccol's vision present us with new ethical challenges at all, or—like much of the best science fiction—merely exaggerated depictions of existing questions? Most important, what do our responses to *Gattaca* tell us about the sorts of societies in which we currently live?

"The Burden of Perfection": The Unlikely Curse of Jerome Eugene Morrow

Although much of the dystopian quality of *Gattaca* derives from the gloomy depiction of life for the "in-valids"—those who missed out on the boons from the brave new world of reproductive technology—the most dismal fate is reserved for Jerome, the golden child of the new genetic age. Selected (and possibly modified) for success, Jerome has been equipped with many of the qualities likely to lead to a successful life.

Yet Niccol's depiction of life for Jerome is of a uniquely wretched one, punctuated by repeated suicide attempts. Of course, this may be a result of frustration borne from his being paralyzed, a disability that renders all his technologically assured athletic potential irrelevant. With this plot device, Niccol initially seems to be reminding us that all of humanity's technological hubris cannot remove the possibility of chance accident. A premium-quality genome is no guarantee against the slings and arrows of outrageous fortune, and a society unaccustomed to genetic disability will still be required to make provision for other sorts of disabilities. We later learn, though, that Jerome's paraplegic state was caused by an earlier suicide effort. If his self-destructive impulses were not caused by his wheelchair confinement, what could have driven him to such anguish?

The notion that the ostensible beneficiaries of the genetic supermarket—or of reproductive and genetic technologies (RGT) more generally—will in fact be victims of these technologies is a familiar one in bioethics (Buchanan, Brock, Daniels, and Wikler 2000; Habermas 2003; McKibben 2003). One form this harm might assume is captured in Vincent's voice-over when he first meets Jerome: "He [Jerome] suffered under a different burden: the burden of perfection."

Future children might be burdened by their parents' use of RGT in several ways. They may, we might think, be subject to unrealistic expectations of their own abilities, imposed by parents who believe that the genotype they selected will guarantee succeeding in a particular field or having a particular kind of character. This is perhaps best evidenced when Jerome, grasping his silver medal, complains that "Jerome Morrow was never meant to be one step down on the podium. With all I had going for me, I was still second best."

Whether such problems would be unique to such children is, though, a different matter. Both literature and real life are replete with accounts of children who have been unable to conform to their parents' Willie Loman-esque expectations. There may be unique and unforeseeable burdens associated with being a "designer baby";[3] the technology is still too new to be certain. Equally, though, there may be unique burdens associated with being born into a family with a history of criminality or of notable achievement.

While Gattacan society could give rise to a new subspecies of pushy parents, why should we assume that these will be any worse than the varieties that can already be seen living their own dreams vicariously at their kids' football games or talent shows? There have always been unrealistic parental expectations. Some of these have even had genetics at their core, albeit a more unsophisticated genetics that simply assumed that talent would be passed through blood.[4]

Alternatively, we might think that what's objectionable about Gattacan society is that children like Jerome have had their parents' choices and preferences foisted on them, without their consent. In a sense, this may seem illogical. Children, and the adults they become, currently have no control whatever over the genes they inherit. That their genotype was selected by parents, rather than by fate or God or natural selection, doesn't deprive them of any more control over their own lives than they would otherwise have had.

Even allowing for that, though, some bioethicists have argued that, while none of us have any choice but to accept the inevitability of the "genetic lottery," the knowledge that our parents had made such choices could be altogether more problematic. Knowing that there was no choice to be made, we might think, is one thing. Knowing that someone else made it for us quite another.

The likelihood of any of those factors imposing unique psychological burdens or messing up family relationships is still a matter for speculation rather than observation. But even if the worst predictions of *Gattaca* were to be borne out, what message should we discern from this? In particular, could we seriously maintain that Jerome had been harmed by the very technologies that gave rise to his existence?

In his seminal work of consequentialist philosophy, *Reasons and Persons*, Derek Parfit (1984) considered various questions about the obligations we might owe to future generations. In particular, he invited his readers to imagine a fourteen-year-old girl who chooses to have a child. For reasons of emotional immaturity and financial dependence, she is considered likely to provide this child with a less-than-optimal start in life, whereas if she delayed for a few years, she would be better placed to act as a parent. Is she, Parfit asks, morally wrong to have the child now, rather than to wait?

As Parfit famously demonstrated, if we can criticize the girl's decision to have a child now, we can't really base that criticism on the effects on the child itself. Because for *that* child, the alternative to being born to a fourteen-year-old mother was not to be born to an older or better mother. In fact, the only alternative was not to be born at all. If the girl had waited five years, or one year, or one month, the child she had would have been the product of a different egg and a different sperm, and it would have been born at a different time. It would, in short, have been a different child, just as surely as it would be a different person from any potential siblings.

The question, then, must be whether the girl's child is likely to be born into a life so miserably wretched that it would have been preferable for that child—from its own, subjective point of view—never to have been born. If not, then that child has no valid grounds of complaint against its mother. To its plaintive cry of "Why did you have me so young?" she could with utmost justification reply, "Because the only alternative was never to have *you* at all!"

Can we conclude that Jerome's life was so awful that he would have been better never born? Well, his repeated attempts at suicide suggest that this might have been the case. But would this be typical of the children born into Gattacan society? Would the burden of expectation lead to an outbreak of attempted suicides among handsome, intelligent, athletic young people, haunted by their self-perceived failures?

Filmgoers will have their own views as to the plausibility of such a scenario. But what does seem certain is that unless these future people do in fact perceive their lives in such terms, they can't really be said to have been victims of the very technology that brought about their existence. Anyway, why should we assume that Jerome's attitude to his life is any more typical than that manifested by the numerous nonsuicidal characters, such as Vincent's brother Anton (played by Loren Dean) or Irene (played by Uma Thurman), who appear to find these burdens somewhat more manageable?

When we ask whether Jerome was a victim of the genetic supermarket, then, we're actually asking whether he was harmed by being born at all. And this is the same question we should be asking about any of the real-life children who would be born if PGD or similar technologies became more widespread. It's easy to dream up all sorts of emotional problems that "designer babies" might face. But those problems are cast in a rather different light when we remember that the only way to protect all the potential future Jeromes and Irenes from those potential future harms is by "protecting" them from life altogether.

"A New Underclass": The Fate of "Faith Babies" in Gattacan Society

If Jerome's existential angst offers a less-than-convincing reason to fear Gattacan society, Vincent's lot may be a more obvious receptacle for sympathy. As he explains in one of the film's many voice-overs: "I belonged to a new genetic underclass, no longer determined by social status or the color of your skin. No, we now have discrimination down to a science."

Following Parfit, we could always offer the same answer to Vincent as to Jerome: that, however imperfect his life, there was no other life on offer to him. But Vincent does not owe his existence to the genetic supermarket. In fact, he might be able to argue that it's actually the existence of that supermarket, and of Gattacan society with its clinical preoccupation with genetic hierarchies, that is the cause of his woes.

It's easy to feel sympathy for Vincent, excluded as he is from the career of his dreams. Those of us who harbored childhood fantasies of (then novel) space shuttle missions may even feel a pang of empathetic compassion. But misfortune is not synonymous with injustice, thwarted ambitions not the same as violated rights. However sorry we may feel for Vincent, is there any reason to feel he has been treated unfairly?

Two main models of justice may be relevant to this question. The first model is concerned exclusively with ensuring a level playing field, where everyone is allowed a fair opportunity to demonstrate their talents without "unfair" obstacles or advantages (Roemer 1985). This model would be concerned with whether Vincent's exclusion from the space mission was based on relevant criteria—say, mathematical ability or physical dexterity—or on arbitrary or irrelevant criteria, like sex or race. Disability or illness could fall into the "fair discrimination" category, depending on the circumstances; certainly, this model doesn't require hiring a paraplegic football player or a brain surgeon with uncontrollable palsy.

Can we say that an "unfair" obstacle has been placed in Vincent's path? We are told early in the film that his genotype predisposes him to a range of disease conditions. As the geneticist lists them to his parents: "Neurological condition: 60% probability; manic depression: 42% probability; attention deficit disorder: 89% probability; heart disorder: 99% probability; early fatal potential, life expectancy: 30.2 years." Even assuming that space travel in the *Gattaca* future is more sophisticated and the physical burdens it imposes less onerous, it's not fanciful to imagine that it will still involve a substantial degree of exertion. And though we are not told what Vincent's role in the mission will be, it's quite plausible that his fellow crew members will, at certain times, be highly reliant on him, perhaps even for their survival. Vincent, we might think, should be free to risk his own health, or life, in pursuit of his dream, but it's not obviously unfair that he should be restrained from risking the lives of others while doing so.

It surely isn't absurd to imagine that a strong likelihood of heart failure or even attention-deficit disorder presents a serious threat to the safety of the mission and its crew. So, assuming that the risk factors revealed to Vincent's parents are reasonably accurate, and that they can't easily be controlled, we can't really say that Vincent has been treated unfairly. If anything, in surreptitiously acquiring a place on the mission, and elevating his own ambitions over the safety of his shipmates, we might think that it's Vincent himself who has violated important ethical principles: of nonmaleficence, for example, or of respect for other people's lives.

What, then, of the second model of unfairness, the so-called brute luck conception favored by writers such as Thomas Scanlon (1998)? This model wouldn't dispute that Vincent's genotype renders him unfit to be an astronaut. Instead, it would point out that Vincent doesn't deserve his bad genetic luck—his predispositions to heart disease and depression weren't chosen by him, and neither were they caused by any risky lifestyle choices that he made.

If we accept this, then it follows that what's unfair is that he should suffer due to factors for which he possesses no moral responsibility; that he should be faced with his mundane life as a cleaner, rather than the glamorous career as an astronaut, simply because of the roll of the genetic dice.

Assuming for the moment that all of us would rather be astronauts than cleaners, and assuming that no foreseeable society could be comprised entirely of astronauts, with no cleaners at all, then it follows that some of us will probably have to settle for less-favored jobs. This doesn't mean that we should resign ourselves to dull, poorly paid jobs, where we are treated without respect. One important function of the brute luck view of justice is to remind us that most, if not all of us owe our position in life in no small part to luck, and that being so, enormous gulfs in pay, status, or working conditions are rarely "deserved."

The contrast between Vincent's life as an astronaut and his earlier life as a cleaner may sit uneasily with notions of justice, but it doesn't obviously follow that the solution is to allow him to be an astronaut. An approach to the workplace more akin to Michael Albert's participatory economics, which would reduce pay disparities while seeking to enhance workplace autonomy and respect for "menial" workers (Albert 2003), might seem a more proportionate response, mitigating the consequences of undeserved inequalities without abandoning altogether the necessary link between employment on the one hand, and health and ability on the other.

So, we might think, while it's unfortunate that Vincent can't fulfil his dreams of space travel, it isn't necessarily unfair—at least in the normative or pejorative sense. Yet something may still sit uneasily with us about

Gattacan society. Isn't there something particularly wrong about the fact that Jerome's genetic advantages are the product not of the chromosomal lottery, but of the fact that his parents were able and willing to purchase his premium quality genome? A society that allows the wealthy to pass on to their offspring not only economic privilege, but also genetic advantage, may seem like one in which existing divisions will be exacerbated—in short, one that will be more unfair than our own.

But is Gattacan society really more unfair than our own? The United States and (to a slightly lesser extent) the United Kingdom are at present societies that purport to exist on meritocratic ideals, where "fairness" is limited to removing unfair obstacles, and perhaps making sure that every child is given a basic minimum of education. Beyond that, those societies not only accept that the "successful" should enjoy the fruits of their talents, but also regard it as entirely proper, a principle that (in the United States especially) is a badge of national pride.

None of this is undermined by the fact that "innate talent" is almost invariably a matter of luck. Venus and Serena Williams may have come from economically deprived backgrounds, but they inherited physical attributes that no amount of dedication could have replicated. Miguel Indurain, the five-time Tour de France winning cyclist, had a lung capacity about a liter (or a quart) bigger than that of his competitors. And it's surely unlikely that any stars of the NBA would have been snapped up in any draft had they been 5′5″ and disposed to a chubby physique. Of course, no one can deny that application and effort were also indispensable ingredients in their success; but a substantial measure of "genetic luck" was also a sine qua non, a causal prerequisite.

Jerome's genetic advantages were paid for by his parents rather than inherited in the "usual" way, but does it follow that they were less deserved, or less "fairly" held than those of Venus Williams or Miguel Indurain? Neither of them chose to be naturally athletically endowed, so we might say that neither deserved their talents any more than Jerome deserved his.

We inhabit a society that rewards excellence rather than effort and that regards unearned endowments of genetic luck as fair criteria for praise and acclaim. Maybe Gattacan society makes us uneasy because—rather than frightening us with a nightmarish world far removed from our own—it holds up a mirror to the status quo. If it's unfair that some people should lead lives of affluence and acclaim because they were lucky while those less fortunate endure lives of penury and drudgery, then surely it's unfair regardless of whether that "luck" was paid for by parents or the product of the genetic lottery.[5]

"Twelve Fingers or One, It's How You Play": Genetic Destiny versus Personal Responsibility in *Gattaca*

Perhaps Niccol's point isn't that Vincent deserves better genes, but, rather, that he deserves the chance to transcend his genetic limitations. This is implicit in Vincent's response to his brother, Anton—who, unlike Vincent, has been genetically selected (or enhanced; the script is vague on this)—after Vincent finally beats him in a swimming race: "You want to know how I did it? This is how I did it, Anton. I never saved anything for the swim back."

Given that the race was in open sea, and given Vincent's very high probability of heart disorder, pushing himself to such an extreme might be thought to display admirable reserves of courage and determination. Equally, we might think that taking such a risk just to beat his sibling in a swimming contest speaks of a certain rashness not ideally suited to astronauts! Of greater interest, though, is what this says more generally about the extent to which our physical limitations can be overcome by single-minded determination.

Niccol leaves the viewer in no doubt about where he stands on this issue: Both in its imagery—the paraplegic Jerome struggling to the top of a spiral staircase shaped like a DNA double helix—and in its tagline, "There is no gene for the human spirit," *Gattaca* offers us an ostensibly optimistic vision that we can transcend our limitations and attain our loftiest goals if only we approach them with the correct attitude.

In this, *Gattaca*'s message may be seen not only as uplifting, but as a progressive response to conservatives who respond to complaints about inequality with the observation that there is no alternative. Charles Murray, for example, attained notoriety with his "bell curve" thesis, a central claim of which was that "inequality of endowments, including intelligence, is a reality . . . Trying to eradicate inequality with artificially manufactured outcomes has led to disaster" (Herrnstein and Murray 1994, p. 551).

For those of a remotely progressive or egalitarian bent, Murray's rejection of any initiative "to eradicate inequality" is deeply unappealing.[6] But does *Gattaca* offer anything more encouraging? The notion that inherited physical disability can be overcome by determination and endeavour has potentially conservative implications too; for what does it say for those who are disadvantaged by disability? That they simply aren't trying hard enough? That if everyone with Vincent's catalogue of infirmities and inborn disadvantages were only as determined as he, they too could (literally or metaphorically) reach the heavens?

Ultimately, and unappealingly, this aspect of *Gattaca*'s moral may be read as a rejection not only of genetic fatalism but also of any need for society to recognize or redress inborn inequalities. This rejection would not only include differential talents and abilities but also serious and life-threatening physical infirmities. It would surely be understandable if someone with a 99 percent chance of heart failure were to lose a swimming race (indeed, who could blame him if he refused to enter it in the first place!), but it would be far from reasonable if our response to such a person was an indifferent shrug and the glib observation that he lost only because he didn't want to win badly enough. In proclaiming "the human spirit" the undisputed victor over genetic inheritance, *Gattaca* risks espousing a line every bit as reactionary as those who, like Murray, adopt a position at the opposite end of the spectrum.

As a piece of bioethical speculation, *Gattaca* is at its weakest when it relies on sledgehammer imagery to expound a simplistic and sensationalistic view of how RGTs may develop into a Huxleyesque monster, or when it seems to deny that, while we are not *just* the sum of our genes, our choices can sometimes be constrained by them. Its strength, rather, lies as a sumptuous piece of art that—in common with much of the best science fiction—offers more interesting questions than answers; questions not only about how we should respond to reproductive and genetic technology, but far more generally, about how genes, luck and free will interact to shape our lives.

QUESTIONS FOR CONSIDERATION

1. *Are children whose genes have been chosen by their parents likely to have unique emotional burdens? Is Parfit right that, because the only alternative for such children is nonexistence, they have no cause for complaint?*

2. *Should there be limits on the sorts of choices we can make for our future children? Should technologies like PGD be limited to avoiding disease, or should parents be allowed to choose on the basis of musical or athletic ability?*

3. *Is Gattacan society unfair? Is it more unfair than our own societies today?*

4. *How much do our genes limit our life choices? Can "the human spirit" always transcend those limits?*

NOTES

1. In its cinema release version, the film itself is ambiguous about the precise technological means by which Gattacan society is brought about, but the DVD contains an extended version of the counseling scene which makes it clearer that the technology in question is preimplantation genetic diagnosis (PGD)—although it also suggests that genetic modification would be available for those who want it. PGD is used in combination with in vitro fertilization and involves the genetic testing of ex utero embryos with a view to informing a decision about which to implant.

2. The idea of a genetic supermarket, in which prospective parents could select the traits and attributes of their children free from state interference, was first posited by Robert Nozick (1974). See the 1986 edition, p. 315n.

3. This popular term is, as it happens, an inaccurate description of children born from PGD, who are selected but not in any sense designed.

4. For a vivid cinematic depiction of more "traditional" parental pressure, see the tale of Beethoven's son, as recounted in *Immortal Beloved,* directed by Bernard Rose (1994).

5. Whether the state should provide Jerome access to "gene therapy" technology to "correct" his inborn defects and disadvantages is a separate matter, but one better seen in the context of current controversies about access to health care than as any distinct problem posed by genetic technologies.

6. At least some of his assumptions are also highly questionable on empirical grounds; for a meticulous response to the science of *The Bell Curve*, see Stephen Jay Gould (1996).

REFERENCES

Albert, M. 2003. *Parecon: Life after Capitalism.* New York: Verso Books.

Buchanan, A., Brock, D., Daniels, N., and Wikler, D. 2000. *From Chance to Choice: Genetics and Justice.* New York: Cambridge University Press.

Gould, S. J. 1996. *The Mis-measure of Man,* 2nd ed. New York: Norton.

Habermas, J. 2003. *The Future of Human Nature.* Cambridge: Polity Press.

Herrnstein, R. J., and Murray, C. 1994. *The Bell Curve: Intelligence and Class Structure in American Life.* New York: Free Press/Simon & Schuster.

McKibben, B. 2003. *Enough: Staying Human in an Engineered Age.* New York: Times Books.

Niccol, A. 1997. *Gattaca* [motion picture]. Culver City, CA: Columbia Pictures Corporation.

Nozick, R. 1974. *Anarchy, State, and Utopia.* Oxford: Basil Blackwell.

Parfit, D. 1984. *Reasons and Persons.* Oxford: Oxford University Press.

Roemer, J. 1995. Equality and Responsibility. *Boston Review,* 20, April/May:8.

Rose, B. 1995. *Immortal Beloved* [motion picture]. London: Icon Entertainment International.

Scanlon, T. M. 1998. *What We Owe to Each Other.* Cambridge, MA: Belknap Press of Harvard University Press.

SIX

Lifting the Genetic Veil of Ignorance

Is There Anything Really Unjust about Gattacan Society?

Sandra Shapshay

Through an emotional engagement with some rich, eminently human characters, *Gattaca* (Niccol 1997) affords a glimpse at the lives of people living without any genetic privacy. In Gattacan society, anyone can gain access to another's genetic profile, and this has made it essentially imperative for parents to use reproductive technologies to select the "best of themselves" when creating their children. The film explores the ethics of a society largely in the grip of the (false) belief in genetic determinism that results in a rigid genetic class system and the stigmatization of those with inferior genes, the "in-valids."

In this chapter, I will show that *Gattaca* deftly and tastefully explores the likely harms that would ensue in a society—especially American society, in which the film is set—with widespread and largely unregulated use of reproductive and genetic technologies (RGTs). First, I will argue against the film's critics (chapter 5 in this volume) that *Gattaca*'s warnings are not, in general, overblown, and that the film holds up a prospective mirror to contemporary U.S. society. The most significant ethical problems raised by a reproductive-genetic supermarket are seen on a macro, societal level: couple the supermarket with a lack of strict genetic privacy, and what is likely to result is an unlevel (and hence unjust) playing field of opportunity.

Harms to Individuals through RGTs?

Unlike many science-fictional worlds, Gattacan society feels close to home. Despite its being set in the "not-too-distant future," it feels as if we've been to *Gattaca*'s world before. There are no pointed ears or green-skinned aliens milling about. The look of the film is familiar, both from life and from art: the style of clothing and the design of furniture and automobiles are inspired by 1940s America. The buildings appear to have been designed by "neo-Bauhaus" architects. The film, in fact, has an important detective subplot, complete with Bordeaux-drinking, Gauloise-smoking characters who enjoy a night of dancing and piano jazz, evoking an America of film noir. The viewer is confronted with a world that is a strange combination of retro-style and cutting-edge science.

Also more familiar to us than many science-fictional worlds is the treatment of individual liberties. Unlike the early twentieth-century dystopia of Aldous Huxley's *Brave New World* (Huxley 1932/2004) in which the world elites practice eugenics by selecting the kind of offspring that will be produced (alphas, betas, gammas, etc.) in places like the "Central London Hatchery and Conditioning Centre," eugenics in *Gattaca* is done by individual couples who are offered genetic services that they can take or leave.

Here it is useful to make a few distinctions concerning the term *eugenics*, broadly understood as measures that "improve" the human race through genetic means. On the one hand, measures may be "eugenic in intent" (as they are in *Brave New World*) or "eugenic in outcome" (which is what happens in *Gattaca*). Buchanan et al. characterize this distinction in terms as one between the "public health model" or "personal services model" with respect to genetic technologies. Gattacan society is like that of a modern, liberal, industrialized society in that the use of genetic technologies to choose the traits of offspring takes the form of the "personal services" model (Buchanan et al. 2000): eugenic interventions are seen as services offered to individuals, to be taken advantage of, or not, rather than as a state-directed and mandated program.

But Gattacan society reveals that these distinctions are not as sharp as they first appear. While the eugenic outcome is not brought about through any explicit state program, nonetheless, the populace has generally internalized norms of genetic perfection that have become institutionalized (for example, the norms of "valid" and "in-valid" are involved in the criminal justice system as evidenced by how the police search for criminals, in employment practices, and in the insurance industries). The state does not need explicitly to direct the reproduction of its citizens in this world; the pressures put on would-be parents by societal structures act as a sort of eugenic "invisible hand."

The film is not explicit as to whether every person in society has access or equal access to these technologies, but it is suggested that the technology has become so cheap and routine it is within reach of couples with modest means, such as the parents of the film's protagonist, Vincent (played by Ethan Hawke), who decide to make full use of the services for their second child, Anton (played by Loren Dean), once they see the "imperfect" product that is Vincent.

There are two main (and related) warnings generally taken away from *Gattaca:*

1. The widespread use of RGTs to design children will likely result in a novel type of harm to the designed: the "burden of perfection" on the designed child.
2. A society that gains tremendous knowledge of the correlation between particular genes and predispositions to both desirable and undesirable physical and behavioral traits will (a) fall into a (false) belief in genetic determinism, (b) seek to control the genotype of its children as far as possible, and (c) attempt to gain access to and use genetic knowledge to competitive advantage in many other areas of life (including business, mating, the arts, etc.), all to the detriment of individuals and society in general.

Should those of us who live in technologically advanced societies take the above warnings seriously? Should we seek to regulate or even prevent a "genetic supermarket"? Some think not. Critics of the film argue first that the supposed harm to designed children (warning 1) is nothing new. Certainly, Jerome (played by Jude Law), "who was never meant to be one step down on the podium," cannot live up to the superlative expectations placed on him by his genome. Having failed in his suicide attempt ("I couldn't even get that right," he claims) he drinks himself into oblivion and is only consoled by the brotherly friendship of Vincent, who lends Jerome his authentically chosen dream. Although Jerome's plight is rather movingly and convincingly rendered in the film, Gavaghan, for instance, argues that this burden of perfection is nothing new (chapter 5); there are many parents who, without the use of RGTs, have high and often unreasonable expectations for their children (e.g., to be superlative athletes, pianists, business entrepreneurs, etc.) and who push their children in ways that cause psychological harm. Furthermore, he argues, it is entirely speculative whether RGTs would create any more harm than already results from pushy parenting. But, Gavaghan continues, even if RGTs do give rise to a more serious form of pushy parenting, because a liberal society does not *outlaw* this style of parenting, or place the children of such parents in foster care, the choice to use RGTs even with these possible harms should not be restricted. Fair enough.

Are there better reasons to regulate the use of such technologies? Another line of argument that one could take is that certain uses of reproductive technologies treat children in a manner similar to consumer products (to be chosen for certain traits much like a car or DVD player). In doing so, these technologies embody marketplace values of control and choice that threaten to undermine values at the core of family life, values such as acceptance of the unbidden and of largely unchosen obligations (Murray 1996).

Insofar as a technology threatens to undermine the norms of good parenting (e.g., that parents should try to bring out the best in their children while accepting and loving a child for who she is) then the use of RGTs for creating "perfect children" constitutes a legitimate public policy concern (Murray 1996). Perhaps this concern does not rise to the level of constituting grounds for a ban on the use of RGTs, but it gives good grounds for educating the public that this technology threatens to commodify children to the detriment of family life in general.

Lurking just around the corner for this view, however, is Parfit's "non-identity" argument. For Parfit (1984), unless these selected children would end up wishing that they were dead, one could not say that they were truly harmed at all by being so conceived, for the alternative to being conceived in this way is nonexistence for that child. In the case of Jerome, perhaps, one can justifiably say that he was harmed by virtue of being conceived through RGTs, for the burdens this placed on him leads him to prefer nonexistence to a life of disappointed expectations. Yet, in any case where a genetically selected child's life is seen by him to be worth living, which is bound to be the majority of cases, and constitutes the majority of cases in the film—to wit: Irene (played by Uma Thurman), Anton, and apparently all of the "valid" professionals at Gattaca—one cannot argue that a child has been harmed by being conceived through RGTs.

One problem with this Parfitian line of reasoning, however, is that it does not sit at all well with common sense. Take a plausible-enough case of seemingly wrongful conception: A woman has been warned by her doctor to refrain from conceiving a child for a couple of months while she is taking a particular sleeping medication. If she does conceive during that time, the child will almost certainly suffer some impairment (e.g., a withered arm or paralysis). The woman knowingly and voluntarily conceives a child while taking the medication, and she gives birth to a child who cannot walk. Common sense says that this woman has done something terribly wrong to her child. Now, it may be the case that we cannot logically say that she has wronged her child by bringing her into existence under these conditions. The child will, most likely, subjectively assess her life as worthwhile despite the disability. But we can say that the woman has done wrong in general (in a non-person-affecting way) by bringing about a situation that was much less good than the alternatives open to her, for she easily could have refrained from conceiving this child, knowing that this child would suffer and encounter many more obstacles in life (Brock 1995).

The relevant principle that captures the wrong committed by such a parent is stated nicely by Brock: "It is morally good to act in a way that results in less suffering and less limited opportunity in the world" (Brock 1995, p. 273). If the woman in the above example could have avoided bringing about more suffering and less opportunity in the world, without facing any significant hardship, she acted wrongly by not doing so.

It may be argued, however, that the case of conceiving the best children possible by way of RGTs is quite different: Notwithstanding the burden of perfection, these children were selected from a batch of in vitro fertilization embryos to bring about children with optimal potential to flourish in society. Insofar as genotype matters (and surely it does, even if "there is no gene for the human spirit" there are plenty of genes for other physical and behavioral traits) shouldn't all rational, responsible parents endeavor to choose the best genotype possible for their child? So the benefits of the use of RGTs might well outweigh the potential harms to children brought about by the burden of perfection and the change in the norms of parenting that might come with the commodifying move to choose "perfect" children. Perhaps the prospect of healthier, more intelligent, stronger, more musical, and more beautiful children is simply worth the psychological risks to children and families.

To see where the real harms to these children lie in Gattacan society, we need to take a step back from individual parents, children, and choices in this society and look at the collective irrationality that results from these individually rational choices. We need to look at the effects of many such choices on the societal level.

The Genetic Veil of Ignorance

John Rawls's notion of the "veil of ignorance" is one of the most famous thought-devices of political philosophy and plays a key role in the hypothetical social contract situation Rawls calls the "original position." Imagine sitting at a giant boardroom table, with a group of rational contractors who have come together to agree unanimously on the principles of justice for a society of people they're representing. The principles that all could reasonably agree to, will, by virtue of their agreement, be fair. Now, we are to imagine that each representative at the table wants to get the best deal for his or her constituents. Ordinarily, such a bargaining kind of situation will involve representatives trying to skew the principles to the advantage of his or her constituents. If the constituents are rural, the representative will try to ensure generous farm subsidies. If they are rich, tax breaks. If they are poor, a more progressive tax structure. In the ordinary bargaining situation, familiar to us in Congress, say, we have a political situation where power and the capacity to form alliances will determine the outcome, and it won't be unanimous.

Rawls places a fundamental constraint on the decision scenario, which he terms "the veil of ignorance": the contractors are charged with getting the best deal for their constituents in a choice of the principles of justice, but they won't know much of anything about their constituents. They will not know their sex, race, class, age, or any other characteristics about them. They won't know much more than that they desire a good life (however that may be construed), want the kinds of things that will enable them to lead good lives, and are capable of a sense of justice. Insofar as the contractors are ignorant of the kinds of people they are representing, they will seek to choose those principles that are not biased by any morally arbitrary factors (i.e., what social class you were born into, what your gender is, your race, your religion, age, etc.).

Ignorance, then, is key in this procedural device to determine fair principles of justice. Ignorance is the way in which the contractors are put "in the same boat" as it were. If we don't know where exactly our constituents might end up in society, as rich or poor, white or black, man or woman, clumsy or athletic, child or senior citizen, we'll all presumably want to ensure that wherever persons end up in the social lottery, it will be a guaranteed good place to be. Once we know who among us is actually poor, or rich, old or young, our interests tend to diverge. The self-interested solidarity promoted by ignorance is summed up nicely in Buchanan et al.: "People facing potential difficulties tend to have interests that are much more uniform in prospect and divergent after the fact. When each of us is ignorant of what may befall us but all consider ourselves vulnerable, we have a personal, self-interested stake in banding together for mutual support in the face of a common threat" (Buchanan et al. 2000, p. 326).

Ignorance about our genes puts us all in the same metaphorical boat. We don't know if we or our children are likely to get Huntington disease, or breast cancer, or Alzheimer disease; therefore, we all have an interest in joining forces to make a public investment in research for a treatment of these diseases. We are ignorant about our fellow citizens' risk for disease and disability; therefore, we join forces with each other rather indiscriminately in private and public insurance schemes, to share the risk, and ensure a guaranteeable level of welfare in case we're one of the unfortunate in this regard. Ignorance, however, is not always bliss: to make therapeutic use of genetic information, persons will need to know about their genetic endowments, and to make use of genetic selection technologies for one's offspring, knowledge is key as well.

In his original *Theory of Justice*, Rawls further suggests that because it is "in the interest of each to have greater natural assets" as this will allow people to "pursue a preferred plan of life" society has some kind of an obligation to take measures to improve the genetic endowment of descendants:

> In the original position . . . the parties want to insure for their descendants the best genetic endowment (assuming their own to be fixed). The pursuit of reasonable policies in this regard is something that earlier generations owe to later ones, this being a question that arises between generations. Thus over time a society is to take steps at least to preserve the general level of natural abilities and to prevent the diffusion of serious defects. These measures are to be guided by principles that the parties would be willing to consent to for the sake of their successors. (RAWLS 1971, P. 108)

Rawls seems to be saying that as a matter of intergenerational justice we owe our descendants "the best genetic endowment" we can leave them, which would seem to imply an obligation to use precisely the kinds of genetic services *de rigueur* in Gattacan society, such as preimplantation genetic diagnosis and embryo selection, to choose the best genetic inheritance for our children (in a society where the technology is available).[1] But does this obligation to choose "better children" conflict with the kind of ignorance needed for everyone in society to act in solidarity? Isn't it precisely the unchosen, lotterylike nature of genetic endowment that puts us all in "the same boat"? In the above passage, Rawls qualifies the societal obligation by calling for reasonable policies with regard to eugenics, "reasonable" meaning presumably those policies that would be chosen from behind a veil of ignorance that "the parties would be willing to consent to for the sake of their successors" (Rawls 1971, p. 108). To what extent is the use of RGTs consistent with reasonable eugenic policies?

Threats to Privacy

Most Western industrialized societies in the world have generous schemes of public health insurance and other social safety-net programs. In the United States, the state's role in providing health care is limited to those sixty-five or older, the very poor, veterans, and the disabled. Most Americans secure access to health care via private and employer-based insurance programs, and the premiums on these insurance programs have risen exponentially in the last few years. According to the Kaiser Family Foundation and the Health Research and Education Trust Study (2005), the year

2004 constituted the fourth straight that health insurance premiums rose in double digits. Employees are paying 48 percent more for their employer-sponsored health plans than they did in 2001.

Most Americans (minus approximately 45 million uninsured) gain access to health insurance through their employers, and businesses are increasingly feeling the squeeze to limit health insurance costs. How are they doing this? Many companies have tried the carrot approach to coax their employees into healthier lifestyles, in "wellness programs" offering financial incentives for employees who sign on to a comprehensive health assessment. One component of this kind of program is the health coach who will telephone periodically to see if you are keeping up with your exercise and eating right. In a recent article in the *Financial Times of London*, Mark Rothstein, director of the Institute for Bioethics, Health Policy and Law at the University of Louisville, commented on such a program at his university, saying, "Professors can afford to refuse to participate: but what about the janitors? They probably cannot pay the privacy tax for refusing to reveal their detailed health profile to a coach who may or may not tattle to their employer" (quoted in Waldmeir 1995).

Some major U.S. companies have been using the stick approach as well and have explicitly adopted a nonhiring policy for smokers (at least in the twenty-one states that do not have smoker's rights laws). For example, a Michigan company called Weyco, Inc.—a medical benefits administration company ironically—refuses to hire smokers outright and has implemented a no-smoking policy for employees that bans them from smoking even when they are away from the job, in the privacy of their own living rooms. The policy also requires that employees submit to regular urine testing for tobacco use. Now, according to the *National Law Journal*, "several attorneys say the policy . . . goes too far in that it aims to regulate legal activity—in this case smoking . . . they argue that it monitors what people do outside the workplace and discriminates against their lifestyles, a practice that is banned in 29 states that have smoker's rights statutes also known as 'lifestyle rights laws' which prohibit employers from discriminating against smokers" (Baldas 2005, p. 4).

Insofar as this practice is legal in those states that have not adopted such statutes, this means that, given two candidates, a smoker, Jones, and a nonsmoker, Smith. Even if smoking Jones is actually more promising, has better credentials, scored better on tests, and so on, Jones may be legitimately passed over for the nonsmoking Smith, because of statistical evidence that suggests that Smith as an employee will cost the company less than Jones in health care benefits.

We see the same logic, but with greater statistical precision, in *Gattaca,* as Vincent says, they have "discrimination down to a science": no matter how much he has studied the latest astronomy, no matter how actually physically fit he is (we see him doing incredibly strenuous sit-ups, running, outswimming his "valid" brother on one occasion), he will be passed over for any and all desirable jobs because his "real resume is in his cells."

Although illegal in *Gattaca,* all companies routinely practice "genoism" (genetic discrimination) to lower their training costs and to ensure that their workforce is as "fit" and productive as possible. Private schools as well refuse to accept a student whose genome predisposes him or her to health problems for fear of their insurance costs. The same kinds of pressures and cost-benefit analyses in *Gattaca* lead to a society where a routine and quick peek at one's DNA (through a urine sample for a substance test, for example) *is* the interview, and an "in-valid" is effectively barred from all but the most menial jobs, no matter how actually talented he or she is in the here and now. No employer is willing to share his risk with an "in-valid" employee (Figure 6.1).

Genoism

Not all discrimination of course is objectionable; some is justified on the basis of relevant characteristics. For example, a good case can be made that an airline does not discriminate against me for refusing to hire me as a flight attendant because I am petite in stature and cannot reach inside one of those overhead bins. My shortness does seem to be a relevant reason to disqualify me for the job. I do not possess the height necessary to do the job. Many others do possess those skills, and so it is perfectly legitimate for the airline to hire someone else. Discrimination, therefore, can be used in at least two senses, (1) in a descriptive sense as simply a discerning choice, or (2) in an evaluative sense, as an unjust choice, a choice that disadvantages someone for no good reason; in the hiring con-

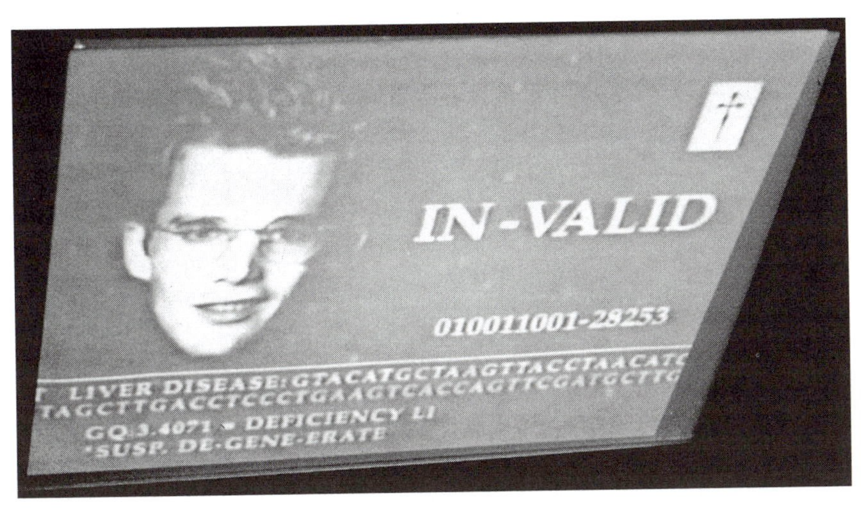

FIGURE 6.1 The "in-valid" profile of Vincent, played by Ethan Hawke, in *Gattaca*. *Source*: Columbia Pictures, The Kobal Collection, provided by The Picture Desk.

text, this evaluative sense of discrimination means that someone is passed over for no reason relevant to the performance of the job itself.

As is well known, the United States has a long history of objectionable discrimination, of companies refusing to hire African Americans or women for no reason relevant to the job itself, but, rather, due to prejudice or pandering to the prejudices of their customer base. It constitutes discrimination in the morally objectionable sense to choose based on a factor that is not relevant to doing the job, whether the factor concerns skin color, gender, hair color, and so on. But is Gattacan genoism morally objectionable in the same way as racism or sexism?

Just like skin color and gender, Vincent is certainly not responsible for the disadvantageous traits he has.[2] He had no hand in choosing them, so it seems blatantly unfair that he should be punished for the alleged "sins" of the parents (if sins they be). Thus, genoism in this regard seems to constitute a close parallel to racism or sexism, because his genes are at least out of the domain of his own control.

But, are Vincent's genes relevant to the performance of the job? Well, perhaps they are relevant. After all, it takes a lot of money and time investment to train a "navigator first class," the mission window is open only every seventy years, and there is a good probability that he will drop dead in space with the predictions of his 99 percent probability of heart failure and death at 30.2 years. However, the supposedly relevant factor here is still in the realm of probability, not actuality. It is possible that Vincent will live longer; it is possible that the only factors that Gattacan society looks at to determine someone's future diary are importantly incomplete. The film's final message is that there is no gene for the human spirit; as his name foretells, Vincent triumphs, he manages to beat the odds, against his brother in swimming contests and at the space center *Gattaca*. How much of a role character, training, and will play in Vincent's fitness is a live question in the film and is a large, unsettled question in science today. Gattacan society does not acknowledge the possibility that these factors, summed up by the word *spirit*, may be more determinative of Vincent's potential.

Is it unreasonable, however, to ask an employer to take the chance on Vincent, when there are plenty of other candidates out there who don't run the statistical risk? After all, Vincent's genetics, though unchosen by him, do suggest that he may not be able to perform the job as well in the future as a person with a healthier profile.

To see why genoism as practiced in Gattacan society is unfair, we need to see why it is reasonable for a society to ask all employers to share the risk of disease and disability by remaining ignorant of these risk factors. To do so, we need to look at a larger societal level of justice. The effect of many individual hiring and other choices in this society, where the veil has been lifted, is to create an unlevel playing field overall, and this is what the film portrays so well.

The playing field is so unlevel that Vincent cannot really partake in much of anything that will allow him to exercise his considerable talents and skills without cheating the system. His range of career and dating opportunities in the society is extraordinarily narrow, and far narrower than his actual talents in the here and now merit. No one behind a veil of ignorance, before one knows where one will end up, would agree to the social institutions that sanction this kind of genetic ghettoization. Society's institutions in *Gattaca* have effectively robbed many talented but genetically "inferior" people of any chance to develop their talents and to partake in the benefits of a cooperative framework. Thus, to allow the widespread use of RGTs without strict genetic privacy provisions would not constitute a "reasonable" eugenic practice, meaning, it would not be a policy chosen from behind a veil of ignorance that "the parties would be willing to consent to for the sake of their successors" (Rawls 1971, p. 108).

Many bioethicists focus, in the debate over genes and justice, on the unlevel playing field potentially created by unequal access to the eugenic technologies, which threatens to result in a kind of "genobility" for the well-to-do, and this is very important; but a subtler problem highlighted by *Gattaca* is the unlevel playing field potentially created by lack of ignorance, and the lack of solidaristic risk-sharing brought about by total genetic transparency.

When we look into the mirror held up to us by *Gattaca*, we see and feel the import of avoiding the illusion of genetic determinism, as environment, character, free will (a.k.a. the human spirit) all play a significant role in this film in making us who we are. In the possible world of *Gattaca,* we see and feel the effects of a transition that has taken place in the way children are viewed: formerly seen as gifts from nature, now children are akin to customized consumer items, to be controlled and selected for desirable qualities, rather than accepted and loved for who they are. By way of such a transition in procreation, we might succeed in pushing out the boundaries of human health, science, and art through the selection of incredibly robust, supersmart individuals and twelve-fingered pianists, but we also come to see in the film the risks of undermining the human bonds and relationships so vital to individual flourishing.

But *Gattaca*'s most pressing warning, I believe, is to be vigilant in protecting individual genetic privacy. Employers, insurers, and businesses of all stripes have a vested interest in gaining access to genetic information. The logic of the marketplace is such that businesses can gain access quite easily to the genetic information of would-be employees and ought to find out whatever is likely to be relevant to their bottom lines so long as doing so isn't illegal or the laws are not enforced. The forces intent on lifting the veil of genetic ignorance threaten to erode fair equality of opportunity. *Gattaca* admonishes us first and foremost to ensure that society puts the mechanisms in place to check this business imperative to discover whatever information (genetic or otherwise) might enhance competitive advantage.

Ironically, at the end of the film, it is the white-coated doctor, the genetic gatekeeper of the space agency, who provides the deus ex machina solution to the injustice of Vincent's situation. It is the doctor's personal solidarity with Vincent (why exactly, we never fully learn in the film) that allows our hero to exercise his talents and to fulfill his dream. The film offers sage advice: to use these genetic technologies, but only with better institutional safeguards than the lucky whims of individual gatekeepers.

QUESTIONS FOR CONSIDERATION

1. *Did* Gattaca *the space agency unfairly discriminate against Vincent in hiring practices? Why or why not?*

2. *The film* Gattaca *suggests that protecting genetic privacy is desirable but is a practical impossibility. Do you think this is true?*

3. *Why do you think the doctor at* Gattaca *helped Vincent to cheat the system?*

4. *If strict genetic privacy laws were in place, and were enforceable, would there be anything ethically problematic with widespread use of RGTs to choose the traits of children? In this case, would it be immoral for parents not to take advantage of these technologies if they had relatively easy access to them?*

ACKNOWLEDGMENTS

I thank Terrance McConnell, Colin Gavaghan, Steven Wagschal, and audiences at the Poynter Center for the Study of Ethics and American Institutions at Indiana University, at Hiram College, and at the Massachusetts College of Pharmacy and Health Sciences, for helpful discussion of themes in this chapter.

NOTES

1. I am indebted to Terrance McConnell for this point.

2. Although one might say *some* persons are to some extent responsible for the poor genetic profile he has: his parents. They are, of course, responsible for the fact that their child is a "faith birth," a "God child," an "in-valid" rather than a "vitro,"

a "made man," or a "valid." Crucially, however, there is no sense in which Vincent himself (the object of the discrimination) is responsible for his genes.

REFERENCES

Baldas, T. 2005. Heat Rises Over 'No Smokers Hired' Policy; Lawyers Debate If Ban, Nicotine Tests Are Legal. *National Law Journal* 26(20):4.

Brock, D. 1995. The Non-identity Problem and Genetic Harm: The Case of Wrongful Handicaps. *Bioethics* 9:269–75.

Buchanan, A., Brock, D.W., Daniels, N., and Wikler, D. 2000. *From Chance to Choice: Genetics and Justice*. Cambridge: Cambridge University Press.

Huxley, A. 2004. *Brave New World*. New York: HarperCollins Publishers. (Originally published in 1932)

Kaiser Family Foundation and the Health Research and Education Trust Study. 2005. At www.kff.org.

Murray, T. H. 1996. *The Worth of a Child*. Berkeley and Los Angeles: University of California Press.

Niccol, A. 1997. *Gattaca* [motion picture]. Culver City, CA: Columbia Pictures Corporation.

Parfit, D. 1984. *Reasons and Persons*. Oxford: Oxford University Press.

Rawls, J. 1971. *A Theory of Justice*. Cambridge, MA: Harvard University Press.

Waldmeir, P. 1995. Why Wellness Is Making Employees Feel Sick. *Financial Times of London*, February 17, 9.

SEVEN

Multiplicity

A Study of Cloning and Personal Identity

Troy Jollimore and Becky Cox White

Cloning provides an opportunity to create a new organism—one that is genetically identical to the original.[1] At present it is not possible to replicate fully formed human beings; only embryos can be cloned. In the popular imagination, however, clones are often depicted as precise duplicates of living individuals, fully capable of social interaction, and (frequently) capable of stealing the identity of the original individuals from which they were cloned. This mistaken concept is at play in the 1996 film *Multiplicity* (Ramis 1996), in which a working man who lacks time and energy to devote himself to both job and family clones himself—twice. We will use this film to illustrate and discuss many of the issues connected with the threat cloning is sometimes thought to present to personal identity.

The Film

The protagonist, Doug Kinney (played by Michael Keaton), is a construction worker who lacks the time and energy to meet the needs of both his job and his family. A serendipitous meeting with Dr. Leeds (played by Harris Yulin), a genetic engineer, suggests a miraculous solution: Dr. Leeds can create clones of Doug who will share his professional and domestic burdens. Doug opts for replication, and—at first, anyway—his life does indeed get better. (Note: From now on, we use "Doug-0" to refer to Doug before the cloning procedure, and "Doug-1" to refer to the "original" Doug—the one who has been cloned and is not himself a clone—follow-

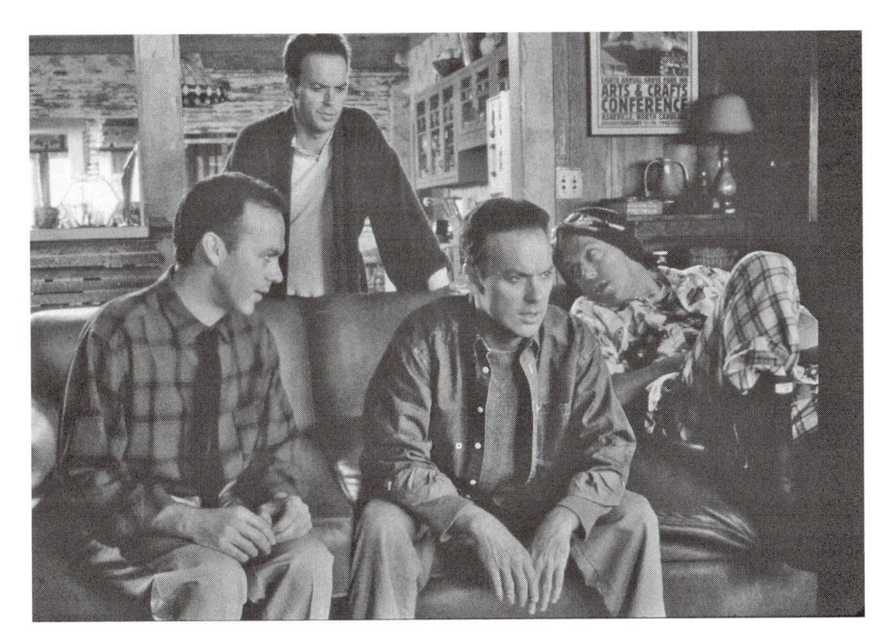

FIGURE 7.1 All of the Dougs, played by Michael Keaton, share a moment together, in *Multiplicity. Source*: Columbia Pictures, The Kobal Collection, provided by The Picture Desk.

ing the procedure. While many people might assume that Doug-0 and Doug-1 are the same person, we will not.)

Doug-1 turns over his job to his clone (Doug-2) and sets out to become an exceptional family man. But he soon finds himself longing for free time to pursue golf and other personal interests—in other words, time for *himself*. A second clone, Doug-3, is created to assume Doug-1's domestic duties. Doug-2 and Doug-3 live in an apartment over Doug-1's garage (see Figure 7.1). Initially the clones' main complaint regards the restrictions on their freedom necessary to keep their existence secret (particularly from Laura, Doug-1's wife, played by Andie MacDowell).

Circumstances begin to deteriorate. Doug-1, relieved of virtually all personal and professional responsibilities, finds himself with nothing to do. The life that defined him has been taken over by others, leaving him adrift. Meanwhile Doug-2, spending his time in the company of men at work or drinking beer in his room at night, becomes increasingly masculine and confrontational, while Doug-3, consigned to the family's domestic demands, becomes increasingly feminine. Ultimately, Doug-1 avoids his job sites completely and comes home only to sleep. But even these short "visits" lead to grief as Laura, attempting to finish conversations begun with Doug-3, becomes frustrated and angry with Doug-1's inexplicable behavior.

The inevitable drama arrives when Doug-1 sets off to redefine himself as a sailor. Doug-2 and Doug-3 break Doug-1's only prohibition: both sleep with Laura. The following day Doug-2, sick with the flu, sends Doug-3 to the job site. Doug-3, having never been involved in the project, is unable to answer the questions of a visiting inspector and, as a result, is fired. Doug-1 returns to find himself without a job and without a wife; Laura has thrown in the towel.

In the film's final act, the posse of Dougs remodels the house (fulfilling one of Laura's dreams), and the clones move to Florida and open a pizza place. Doug-1, with a reintegrated sense of self, persuades Laura to return. The credits roll, to the tune, "A Little Bit Me; A Little Bit You."

Cloning: Reality and Fantasy

At present, the prospect of creating exact replicas of fully formed, postbirth individuals remains a distant one.[2] But *genetic cloning*—creating genetic duplicates—of human embryos is currently possible. Human embryos are primarily cloned for research purposes (e.g., to produce stem cells that, scientists hope, can be stimulated to produce particular types of cells that might then be used to treat genetic diseases). Historically, the process of procuring embryonic cells destroyed the embryo, raising moral concerns about killing future human persons. Newer techniques may allow the extraction of a single cell from an embryo, procuring cells for research while preserving the embryo (Klimanskaya et al. 2006). Most countries have laws prohibiting cloning of and experimentation on embryos older than fourteen days, thereby minimizing moral concerns about experimenting on persons without their consent. The President's Council on Bioethics (2002) report on cloning addresses other moral concerns, as well as describing cloning procedures.

Even if it became possible to perform what we will call *full human cloning* (i.e., the creation of an exact genetic duplicate of a postbirth human being), reality would still fall short of the fantasy envisaged by this film and other such works in two significant respects. First, a clone would be younger than its original and would age at the normal human rate. (In Doug-1's case, his clones appear to be his age.)

Second, the procedure would replicate the original's *genetic* features, but not her *psychological* features. A person's memories, for instance, are determined by the experiences she has in her life (i.e., the things she remembers); they are not somehow programmed into her DNA. Because they are not part of the genetic code, they would not be installed in a clone. Because the clone would develop under different conditions, it would almost certainly never become a psychological near duplicate of the original. Thus, *Multiplicity*-type cloning, which produces a duplicate that is physically and psychologically indistinguishable from the original, will probably never become possible.

Personal Identity

According to a proclamation of the World Health Organization (WHO 1998, §1), "Cloning for the replication of human individuals is ethically unacceptable and contrary to human dignity and integrity." Such a statement raises several perplexing questions. What exactly are human dignity and integrity? What does respect for these purported attributes of persons require? And what reason is there to think that human dignity and integrity might be incompatible with the cloning of individual persons? The suggestions we will pursue here are that dignity and integrity are related to (and perhaps consist in) a person's *identity* and that one's identity is threatened by the prospect of cloning. But this only raises an additional, and very difficult, question: what does identity consist of?

Suggestion 1: Genetic Identity

Some have suggested that the genetic code built into your DNA makes you who you are. If this is so—if your and A's having the same genetic code means that you and A are the same person—then it is easy to understand why we would object to cloning: a clone, after all, would have as good a claim to being you as you do. The clone would be you.

But this position cannot be correct. After all, genetic duplicates happen naturally: we call them identical twins. Obviously, identical twins are two distinct people in what philosophers call the *numerical* sense: no matter how qualitatively similar they are (i.e., how hard it might be to tell which is which), two people, not just one, are obviously present. But in fact, so-called identical twins do not tend to be qualitatively identical, either. As Stephen Jay Gould writes:

> [H]ave we ever doubted the personhood of each member in a pair of identical twins? Of course not. We know that identical twins are distinct individuals, albeit with peculiar and extensive similarities. We give them different names. They encounter divergent experiences and fates. Their lives wander along disparate paths of the world's complex vagaries . . . Identical twins provide sturdy proof that inevitable differences of nurture guarantee the individuality and personhood of each human clone. (GOULD 1998, P. 48)

That identical twins occur in nature raises questions about WHO's claim that "Individuals have the right to retain control over their genetic identity" (WHO 1999, §8). What can this even mean, in cases in which one's genetic identity is shared with another? If my twin lends his DNA out for research, is he lending my genetic identity as well—and if so, can I hire a lawyer to stop him? At any rate, identical twins do not typically believe that they are lacking an identity in any meaningful sense: they regard themselves as distinct individuals. Nor do they tend to see their genetically identical siblings as interlopers. These psychological facts about human beings strongly suggest that, whatever sense we might be able to make of the idea of our "genetic identity" and our rights over it, "genetic identity" is just not the same thing as "personal identity."

Suggestion 2: Physical Resemblance and Physical Continuity

Physical appearance is an important component of many people's self-conception. Yet we clearly cannot ground personal identity in physical appearance in any substantial way. Identical twins often look alike, some so much so that others cannot tell them apart: Witness the accounts of identical twins who go out on each other's dates or attend classes for each other.[3] The mere fact that Doug-1's clones share his physical appearance does not seem to inspire in him any deep soul-searching regarding his own identity (We do not see him late at night, head buried in his hands, moaning to himself, "Who am I? Who am I?"). And why should it? As we will suggest later, there may be other aspects of this case that ought to be at least somewhat disturbing to Doug-1; but the mere fact that his clones *look* like him hardly seems deeply worrisome.

Physical resemblance is neither sufficient nor necessary for identity. Suppose you undergo a radical physical change—for instance, you are burned beyond all recognition. Although your life would be different in many ways, there seems little reason in such a case for saying that you are no longer you. Of course, a person who made his living by his appearance—a model or actor, for example—might say such a thing. But while we would understand what he was trying to express, the claim still would not be literally true. After all, someone underwent the accident and someone is struggling to deal with its consequences; and who could that someone be if not the person who was burned and who, before being burned, had a different physical appearance? Although appearance may be a common and typically successful method for identifying persons—or at least for distinguishing them from each other—it does not seem to be what constitutes personal identity.

A more promising suggestion might arise from the burn-accident case. Why think that the person after being burned is the same person as before? What does it even mean to say this? A straightforward answer focuses on the body: although the body is not qualitatively the same as before the fire (it has been badly burned), it is still the same body in the sense of being physically continuous with the body before. There is, crucially, a sufficient degree of physical continuity.

The physical continuity account is promising, at least as an account of identity over time. (However, it doesn't function at all as an answer to the "Who am I?" question one might ask in a therapist's office.) But even with respect to identity over time, is physical continuity really what we *mean* by identity, as opposed to merely being (like physical appearance) good *evidence* of identity? Scientists tell us that over a period of seven years, every molecule in the human body is replaced. Does this mean that seven years from now, we will no longer exist, but will have been replaced by new people?

We might also doubt that physical continuity is *sufficient* for identity.

Many would say that a person who as a result of a serious trauma loses all her memories and takes on new behavior patterns is quite literally no longer the same person as before. This is so even though her body is physically continuous with the body before the trauma. So perhaps physical continuity, like physical appearance, is really just an indicator of personal identity over time.

Suggestion 3: Memory-Based Accounts

Imagine that tomorrow morning when you look into your bathroom mirror, you discover that overnight you have been transformed into the spitting image of Henry VIII. This would be surprising. After all (we are imagining), you do not remember going to bed looking like Henry VIII. Part of what it is to imagine yourself waking up looking like Henry VIII is to imagine ("from the inside") a person who has your memories waking up looking like Henry VIII. Thus, we might identify you in terms of your memories: you are you because you possess your unique collection of memories.

Again, though, problems arise with this account. As time passes, memories tend to fade or disappear altogether, even as new ones are added. It will matter a great deal, then, how the memory account is defined: which particular memories must one continue to possess to remain oneself? We must also determine whether one's memories must be accurate. As the controversy over planted false memories demonstrated in the 1990s, it is actually quite common for people to think that they remember some event that it turns out they could not possibly remember. Can memories of this sort ground a person's identity?

Let us call the suggestion that a person's set of memories, and nothing more, makes him the person he is, the simple memory account, or SMA. (We already know that SMA won't work, because your memories change over time even while you remain the same person; but it might be worth seeing what else is wrong with it.) When Doug-0 is duplicated, Doug-2 (the clone) has all of Doug-0's memories, and insists, on that account, that he must be the original Doug. "I remember coming in here," he states. "I remember putting this thing on. I remember getting the shot." To which Dr. Leeds replies: "Of course. You have all of Doug's feelings and his quirks, all of his memories right up to the moment of cloning. But from now on, to whatever extent you have different experiences, you'll begin to diverge."

According to SMA, Doug-2 and Doug-1 are the same person! Well, for a moment they are—as soon as they begin to have divergent experiences, they will start to diverge in memory. But for a long time, it seems, they will be mostly the same person—if the idea of being "mostly" the same person makes any sense. Moreover, suppose that both of them were unconscious for several hours following the operation, during which time they did not form any new memories. The SMA theorist would be committed to saying that there was only one Doug during these hours. (He could say that there were two *copies* of the one Doug, but not that there were two distinct *persons.*) Suppose, moreover, that some problem with the cloning procedure rendered both Doug-1 and Doug-2 unable to form new memories. In this case, SMA would imply that they would both be the same person for the rest of their lives. All these claims seem counterintuitive.

It might seem easy enough to repair the account. We need only require that a memory be formed in the right way: whether a given mental state in A's mind, which appears to be a memory, actually counts as a memory (and not as a mere *quasi-memory,* as some philosophers have termed it) depends on whether it was formed in A's brain as a direct result of her having the experience the memory seems to be a memory of. Call this the *modified simple memory account*, or MSMA. By this criterion, Doug-1's are the real memories: he remembers his wedding, for instance, because he was there and experienced it and formed memories as a result of it. But Doug-2's memories are only quasi-memories: he does not remember the wedding, because he was not there. He only seems to remember it. Because Doug-2's apparent memories are not real memories, MSMA will say that he and Doug-1 are different people. (And because Doug-1 is the one with the real memories, MSMA will likely count him as the real Doug.)

But this account raises a new problem: to say that Doug-1's are the *real* memories, we have to already know who is who. Thus, MSMA seems to hold the following:

1 Doug-1 and Doug-2 are different people because, although they seem to share the same memories, Doug-1's memories are real and Doug-2's memories are not.

2 The explanation of why Doug-2's memories are not real memories is that he is not the person who originally formed them; rather, Doug-1 originally formed them.

But number 2 assumes that we already have some account for saying that Doug-1 is a different person from Doug-2, and that Doug-1, not Doug-2, is the person who originally formed the memories in question. (What type of account? Presumably a physical account—despite the problems we have observed with these, the most obvious explanation for our intuitions in this case seems to be that Doug-1 is, or occupies, the *body* that was physically present at the wedding that both Doug-1 and Doug-2 both seem to remember.) On its own, then, MSMA seems circular: it attempts to show that it provides the proper account of personal identity, but it must presuppose some other account of personal identity in that explanation. Nor is it obvious how to create a memory-based account that will not presuppose some sort of independent criterion.

The "Real" Doug?

A common intuition, with respect to the case, is that Doug-1 really is Doug—some might even say that he is the real Doug—and that this cannot be said of the clones. Thus, Doug-1 is literally identical to Doug-0, while the other clones are not. It is not entirely clear, however, just how this intuition is to be supported. Indeed, many of the candidate criteria for personal identity will not seem to support it. Consider the moments shortly after the creation of the first clone, Doug-2. In these first few moments, Doug-1 and Doug-2 are almost perfectly identical, both psychologically and physically: they have the same genetic identity, physical appearance, personalities, and even, for the first few moments, memories (and their memories will be mostly similar for a considerable time to come). Again, as Dr. Leeds says to Doug-2, "You have all of Doug's feelings and his quirks, all of his memories right up to the moment of cloning."

Of course, the perfect qualitative identity between Doug-1 and Doug-2 will not last very long. Because the two occupy different positions in space and thus experience the world from different perspectives, the memories they form following the cloning procedure will not be identical; in time, they will diverge significantly. But while different constellations of memories can distinguish the Dougs from each other, they do nothing to establish which one is the real Doug. After all, if anything distinguishes the "real" Doug from the others, it must be facts that precede the cloning procedure and, as Dr. Leeds makes clear, Doug-1's memories of life up to that point will be exactly identical to Doug-2's! Similarly, while differences in behavior might be observed (Doug-2's machismo versus Doug-3's domestic passivity, for instance), why should any pattern of behavior be privileged as the pattern belonging to the "real" Doug? After all, Doug-0's behavior might have changed over time even if he had not been cloned.

In the film, Dr. Leeds resolves the identity issue by pointing to a red "2" tattooed behind the ear of Doug-2, indicating that Doug-2 is the newly created individual (i.e., the clone). One might wonder, though, whether this is really good enough. Consider the identical twin case: no one wants to say that the twin who is born first is the "real" child, and that the other twin is therefore unreal or illegitimate in some sense. Indeed, rather than risk the implication that one of the Dougs is a "fake" Doug (or, worse, a fake human being) some might suggest that we should avoid settling the question of which Doug is "real." Consider an analogy. Suppose that a cell, *C*, undergoes fission and splits into two cells, *C1* and *C2*. Is there any reason to say that we must be able to determine which cell, *C1* or *C2*, is the "real" *C*? And might we not see what happens to Doug as very similar to this? Presumably some of the biological material that makes up Doug-0's body ends up in Doug-2. Why not, then, just consider cloning a case of fission?

Suppose we accept this position. What, then, should we say happened to Doug-0? If Doug-1's claim to be identical with Doug-0 is no better than that of Doug-2, then either both are identical with Doug-0, or neither is. The former option is unattractive. (Suppose both Doug-1 and Doug-2 are identical with Doug-0; and suppose that Doug-2 is killed the following day in an accident, while Doug-1 lives another twenty years. When does Doug-0's life end?) So it appears that we should say that neither Doug-1 nor Doug-2 is identical with Doug-0. But this implies that Doug-0 went into the hospital and never came out! Can this be so—can the process of making a copy of a person amount, in essence, to that person's death?

These implausible implications render the fission view somewhat unattractive, even in the light of our reservations about how to choose which Doug is "real," and what this might imply for the other Doug.

Does Full Human Cloning Have Moral Implications?

To ask about the moral implications of a belief, action, or policy is in large part to ask what its effects will be for human well-being. Modern moral outlooks tend to hold that all persons are equally worthy of consideration and should be treated accordingly and therefore to rule out actions or policies that will hinder the flourishing of human individuals.

The eighteenth-century German philosopher Immanuel Kant argued that because they could engage in rational and moral reasoning, human beings were worthy of respect and should be considered as "ends-in-themselves" (Kant 1785/1990, p. 46 [428]). Roughly (very roughly!) this means it is always wrong to treat a person merely as a means to some end, or as a mere tool for your own purposes. Perhaps creating a clone with a particular purpose in mind is incompatible with treating the clone as an end in itself.

Using someone as a *mere* means requires discounting the dignity, decisional authority, or welfare of the person so used—treating that person, to an objectionable degree, as a tool to be put to use. But the mere fact that Doug-1 has reasons for creating Doug-2 does not imply that Doug-2 is being used as a mere means. After all, parents often express instrumental reasons for having children: to carry on the family name or genetic lineage, for instance. If Doug-1 had been prepared to force the clones into playing assigned roles, whether they wanted to or not, or if he insisted on scripting every detail of their lives, leaving them no choices about how to carry out these assigned roles, then he could be accused of using of them as mere means: clearly under such conditions he would not be respecting the clones' autonomy. But if Doug-1 grants Doug-2 the authority to make this choice (even as he hopes that Doug-2 will happily choose to play the role assigned to him), he cannot reasonably be accused of treating Doug-2 as a mere means.

More generally, it is simply not true that human cloning (whether genetic or full) would make possible violations of autonomy that are not possible now. A person might indeed create a clone for a specific purpose and fail to respect the clone's free decisions. But this is already perfectly possible: a parent, for instance, can decide to have a child for a specific purpose that fails to respect the child's wishes and judgments. The fact that the former case involves a clone rather than an "ordinary" child makes no important moral difference at all.

What of the claim that cloning involves stealing the identity of the "original"? This claim is hard to make. No one stole Doug's identity or DNA, as he undertook to replicate himself of his own volition. Of course, if someone were cloned without her consent, this would more plausibly constitute a wrongdoing. Still, exactly why this is wrong is unclear: the "stealing" metaphor seems threatened by the fact that even after the "theft," the victim still has his genetic code. (If someone removes money from my wallet and keeps it, I have been robbed; but can I say the same thing if someone takes the money, photocopies it, and puts it back?)

Perhaps the worry is that while the act of cloning is not itself an act of identity stealing, it does enable a particularly frightening and egregious form of theft: a perfect duplicate of a person would be able to steal that person's very life. Moreover, this might happen even if the clones are not completely indistinguishable. Once Laura learns to distinguish between the clones, for instance, she might well decide that she prefers the more masculine Doug-2 or the sensitive Doug-3—as might Doug-1's friends, employer, or children. The "theft" metaphor may perhaps do nothing more than capture a certain sort of anxiety—the worry that one may end up competing with one's near duplicates.

But does this anxiety ground a moral objection to cloning itself? The fact that duplicating oneself would be risky and thus unwise does not mean that would necessarily involve a moral wrong. As divorce rates demonstrate, people change spouses with some frequency, so even if Doug-1's being left by his wife amounted to a serious wrong (an indication of her fickleness, perhaps), it would have little intrinsic connection with the ethical status of cloning. The real danger here may be that of making too much of the metaphor of theft.

Still, certain forms of "identity theft" really *do* constitute a form of theft, and a physical duplicate might be particularly well suited to engage in such crimes. If Dr. Leeds decided to use Doug-2 to drain Doug-1's bank account, he would surely be guilty of a serious wrong.[4] But again, identity theft of this sort is already possible, albeit by different technical means—rather than duplicating the customer, the thief duplicates the customer's commercial identity. So while full human cloning would surely facilitate certain forms of identity theft, it is much harder to conclude that it would involve some sort of new type of identity theft in any fundamental sense.

Perhaps, though, things are not quite so simple here. A physical duplicate could get away with things that (almost) no one else could. Doug-2 can pass for Doug-1 not only at the bank but also at home; indeed, both Doug-2 and Doug-3 repeatedly fool Laura into taking them for Doug-1. (In particular, each has sex with her while pretending to be her husband, which raises the thorny question of whether those acts would constitute rape.) It is uncertain whether this constitutes a moral wrong against Doug-1, but it surely represents a moral wrong against Laura, who has been deceived and taken advantage of.

Again, though, these types of wrongful action do not really originate with cloning. As we noted above, some identical twins have admitted to switching with one another without their friends' or romantic partners' knowledge. The advent of full human cloning would increase the possibilities for deception between persons; but deception is a moral phenomenon as old as human society itself and would not be fundamentally changed by the new technology.

We have discussed several types of morally bad situations that might arise in connection with human cloning. In each case the wrongful action identified was a type that already existed: the particular actions that turn out to be morally worrisome turn out to be nothing more than variations on morally worrisome actions that already exist in our world and that we must already face. We have not yet found reason to think that cloning would *necessarily* involve or even lead to any bad moral consequences at all; at worst, cloning would make these abuses more likely or frequent. Like any technology, cloning is capable of being used for bad purposes. But this hardly shows that cloning in itself is wrong or bad, any more than the fact that it is possible to deliberately run someone over shows that automotive technology is inherently wrong or bad.

Perhaps, however, we will judge differently when we turn our attention away from the interests of the "original" (Doug-0, in *Multiplicity*) and parties closely related to the original (Laura, the children, etc.) and instead concentrate on the clones themselves. As we have seen, defending a compelling version of the claim that cloning robs the original of his identity is more difficult than one would at first expect—even when full human cloning is under consideration. But what about the clone's identity?

The film glosses over this. When Doug-2 discovers that all of his memories are only quasi-memories, and that he is actually only a couple hours old, he doesn't seem to find this exceptionally disorienting. But imagine discovering such a thing in your own case. Imagine, that is, being convinced that despite all your apparent memories of having had years of life, you had in fact only been created a few hours before. Imagine discovering that you have actually never even met the people whom you love most in all the world, that you only seem to remember them because your brain was built to seem to remember them. Imagine being Doug-2, lying on a bed with a head full of happy memories of marriage to Laura, staring at Doug-1 and being told that all these happy memories were memories of Doug-1's wife. Don't Doug-2 and Doug-3 ever miss Laura? Wouldn't it be at least somewhat painful, being confined to the small apartment above the garage just a few hundred feet away from the bedroom of the woman you clearly and distinctly remember loving and being happily married to?

Of course, the film is meant as a lighthearted, entertaining comedic fantasy and understandably avoids such questions.[5] In truth, though, even a little imagination will show that the situation depicted would give rise to the mother of all existential crises.[6] As discussed above, while there are serious problems with basing personal identity *entirely* on memory, it is nevertheless true that the typical person's memories are very tightly and extensively bound up with her conception of who she is. The news that nearly all of one's memories of a pleasant and fulfilling life that one valued and wished to continue were in fact false is not something one could accept and incorporate into one's set of beliefs while remaining sane.

What Doug-2 and Doug-3 lack, in terms of personal identity, is a history—and history does seem to be essential to personal identity. There is, then, a strong case against full human cloning, based not on the interests of the person cloned or of any third party, but on the interests of the clone. Finding oneself in such a situation would be psychologically devastating. It is questionable whether a person would ever recover from it and develop a genuine sense of self. One could, of course, lie to the clone about his history. But that this sort of deception could ever be justified is doubtful; or at least, it is doubtful that one could ever be justified in bringing into existence an individual whom one would have to deceive in this way. The most serious moral worries that arise about full human cloning, then, seem to arise in connection with the interests and identities of the clones themselves.

Identity and the Ethics of Genetic Cloning

The best moral case we have found against full human cloning, as imagined in films like *Multiplicity,* argues that the procedure would result in the creation of individuals who occupy an untenable psychological situation, and whose pervasively false memories would imply the lack of a stable identity. That is, it is concerns about the clone's situation that do the work, not concerns for the cloned person. In the latter case, it is not clear (largely because the very concept of personal identity is itself not clear) that worries about identity are relevant or substantial enough to support moral objections to cloning (let alone to justify a ban on the procedure).

But these sorts of worries about full human cloning cannot possibly justify prohibiting genetic human cloning. A genetic human clone does not have false memories, any more than an identical twin has false memories; rather she, like most of us, will have memories based on her actual experiences. (Some will be more accurate, of course, and some less so; but the set will be accurate enough, on the whole, to allow her as much of a stable sense of identity as any of us have.) So the worry about the clone's existential predicament arises from the science-fictional aspects of full human cloning; and while the moral case against that sort of cloning may be quite strong, it gives us no reason whatsoever to object to genetic cloning.

Similarly, whatever worries we might have about Doug-2's being able to deceive Laura by passing for Doug-1 will not apply to typical cases of genetic cloning: a clone of an adult human being will both be and appear to be years younger than the original and so will be unable to pass for him. Of course, if we genetically cloned an infant, the two clones might be able to pass for one another; but this, again, would be nothing more than an artificially induced case of identical (near) twins, and it is not clear what ought to be deeply morally worrying about this.

As with full human cloning, the most serious worries here may have to do with treatment of the clones themselves. It is a mistake to regard clones as less than fully human; this is no more plausible, after all, than claiming a naturally occurring identical twin is less than fully human. This mistake, however, may be one that many people are prone to make; and this might increase the likelihood that cloned human beings would be treated in ways that we would regard as deeply inappropriate with respect to nonclones. The idea of "farming" clones to serve as potential organ donors for nonclones, for instance, is horrifying not because such clones would lack identities in any deep sense—they would be fully distinct, independent human beings—but because it is surely impossible to imagine an arrangement that could meet this purpose while at the same time respecting the clones' equal claim to dignity and respect.[7]

Similarly—though somewhat less seriously—some have worried that genetic human cloning might lead parents who had, for instance, lost a child to illness or accident to bring their child "back to life" by creating her clone. It should be clear by now that creating a clone of a dead person does not amount to bringing that person back to life but is the creation of a new and distinct individual who happens to be genetically identical with the original.[8] Again, the moral worry about such cases is not that the clone would lack her own identity in any literal sense but that the misguided parents, through misunderstanding the concept of personal identity or the nature of human genetic cloning, would believe that their clone was somehow identical to the child that had died, which could lead to various forms of unjustifiable treatment (and, perhaps, to deep disappointment should the parents eventually grasp the truth of the situation).

These sorts of moral concern are genuine and compelling. However, they have nothing essentially to do with the concept of personal identity. That concept is, if we are correct, largely irrelevant in the social context within which actual cloning techniques must be addressed and evaluated. Putting aside the science-fictional fantasies of the movies, it seems safe to assert that the moral issues surrounding human cloning, while serious and difficult, seem to have little if anything to do with the still inadequately understood notion of personal identity.

QUESTIONS FOR CONSIDERATION

1. *How could the World Health Organization's position that persons have a "right to retain control over their genetic identity" stand up to the objection that there cannot be such a human right insofar as identical twins share a genetic code, which seems completely unproblematic from a moral standpoint?*

2. *The physical continuity account of personal identity seems promising except for the fact that scientists tell us that over seven years every molecule in our bodies will be replaced. If this is true, does this finding constitute an objection to the physical continuity account of personal identity? Why or why not?*

3. *The authors of this chapter claim "But if Doug-1 grants Doug-2 the authority to make this choice [whether to play the role assigned to him in Doug 1's life] . . . he cannot reasonably be accused of treating Doug-2 as a mere means." Even if Doug-2 is "free" to leave the arrangement, hasn't Doug-1 treated Doug-2 as a mere means? Explain why or why not.*

ACKNOWLEDGMENTS

We thank Cynthia Watson and Kendra Wright for suggesting that *Multiplicity* was worth analysis.

NOTES

1. Actually this simplifies matters. The nuclear DNA of a clone will be identical to the original, but the mitochondrial DNA will come from the embryo into which the nucleus is implanted. See Harris (2004), pp. 8–9.

2. An embryo is the postfertilization stage lasting from uterine implantation of the zygote (one egg and one sperm) to eight weeks' gestation.

3. An intriguing film that trades upon the physical identity of twins is *Dead Ringers* (Cronenberg 1988), in which Jeremy Irons plays twin gynecologists, both of whom date—and terrify—Genevieve Bujold.

4. This is *not* to say that Doug-2 should have no right to take money from Doug-1's account. The film also avoids many related problems that would have to be

dealt with if full human cloning became a possibility. For instance: what are Doug-2's rights over Doug-1's property? The film seems to assume that Doug-2 has no property rights at all; he is allowed to live in the room above Doug-1's garage but seems to have no claim on even this minimal accommodation. One might argue this is appropriate: after all, when people have children, the children do not immediately gain rights to some specified portion of the parents' property (though the parents are, of course, expected to maintain the children at a decent level of comfort and security—a responsibility which, it could be argued, Doug-1 meets with respect to Doug-2). But the situation of a newborn infant, who doesn't know what property is and doesn't desire or, for the most part, need any, is a far cry from that of a newly created adult, who both has a conception of property, and seems to remember owning a fair share of it. Isn't Doug-2 crushed to discover that, despite his apparent memories of being fairly well off, he has no house, car, or bank account?

5. See note 4.

6. Several recent films have explored, at least to a degree, the psychological hazards of manipulated or otherwise unreliable memories. See, for instance, *Total Recall* (Verhoeven 1990), *Memento* (Nolan 2000), and *Eternal Sunshine of the Spotless Mind* (Gondry 2004).

7. For a fascinating exploration of this topic, see Ishiguro (2005).

8. For similar reasons, those who hope to achieve immortality by cloning themselves would seem to be in for a tremendous disappointment.

REFERENCES

Cronenberg, D. 1988. *Dead Ringers* [motion picture]. Los Angeles: Morgan Creek Productions.

Gondry, M. 2004. *Eternal Sunshine of the Spotless Mind* [motion picture]. Los Angeles: Anonymous Content.

Gould, S. J. 1998. Dolly's Fashion and Louis's Passion. In *Clones and Clones: Facts and Fantasies about Human Cloning*, ed. M. C. Nussbaum and C. R. Sunstein, 41–53. New York: Norton.

Harris, J. 2004. *On Cloning*. London: Routledge.

Ishiguro, K. 2005. *Never Let Me Go*. New York: Knopf.

Kant, I. 1990. *Foundations of the Metaphysics of Morals*, 2nd ed., trans. L. W. Beck. Indianapolis, IN: Bobbs-Merrill. (Originally published 1785)

Klimanskaya, I., Young, C., Becker, S., Lu, S. J., and Lanza, R. 2006. Human Embryonic Stem Cell Lines Derived from Single Blastomeres. *Nature*. At www.nature.com/nature/journal/vaop/ncurrent/abs/nature05142.html.

Nolan, C. 2000. *Memento* [motion picture]. Beverly Hills, CA: Newmarket Capital Group.

President's Council on Bioethics. 2002. *Human Cloning and Human Dignity: An Ethical Inquiry.* At www.bioethics.gov/topics/cloning_index.html.

Ramis, H. 1996. *Multiplicity* [motion picture]. Culver City, CA: Columbia Pictures Corporation.

Verhoeven, P. 1990. *Total Recall* [motion picture]. Beverly Hills, CA: Carolco Pictures.

World Health Organization. 1998. Ethical, Scientific and Social Implications of Cloning in Human Health. At www.who.int/entity/ethics/en/WHA51_10.pdf.

———. 1999. Cloning and Human Health. At www.who.int/entity/ethics/en/A52_12.pdf.

EIGHT

Is Ignorance Bliss?

Star Trek: Nemesis, Cloning, and the Right to an Open Future

Amy Kind

One consideration that comes up frequently in discussions about cloning—in both philosophical and public discourse—concerns the clone's potential for a happy and fulfilling life. Opponents of cloning worry that the clone's individuality, and even her very identity, will be threatened by the fact that she is a copy of an already-existing individual. The fear is, at least in part, that the clone and her achievements won't be considered in their own right, for her entire existence will be measured against that of the person from whom she was cloned. In some sense, neither her successes nor her failures will be her own. And in every choice the clone makes, she'll be burdened by the pressure to meet expectations that have been generated by our knowledge of the life that has already been lived. How could the clone of Marie Curie, for example, choose to pursue a career in Hollywood instead of capitalizing on her native scientific gifts? Surely whoever was raising this clone would steer her toward the laboratory at the earliest opportunity.

This point is often put by noting that, in important respects, the clone's choices have already been settled—that she has lost her right to an open future. As such, the clone also loses what Hans Jonas called the *right to ignorance*: The fact that the clone already knows so much about herself (as do others) is "pernicious to the task of selfhood" (Jonas 1974, p. 162). Ignorance, according to Jonas, is "the precondition of freedom" (Jonas 1974, p. 159). As Leon R. Kass put it, the clone is "saddled with a genotype that has already lived" (Kass 2005, p. 226).

Opponents of cloning thus offer what we might call the ignorance argument. Their claim, in essence, is that too much knowledge is a dangerous thing. But what should we make of this argument? And what should we make of the assumption of genetic determinism—the claim that genotype fixes identity—that seems to underlie it? These questions were explored in a particularly interesting way by the movie *Star Trek: Nemesis* (Baird 2002). Set in the late twenty-fourth century, the film depicts a showdown between the Federation and one of its longtime enemies, the Romulans. As the film opens, all the members of the Romulan Senate are killed in a violent coup that brings Shinzon of Remus to power, installing him as praetor. Shortly thereafter, when the Federation's flagship, the U.S.S. *Enterprise*, is summoned to the planet Romulus, the crew makes an astonishing discovery: the new Romulan leader is a much-younger clone of their own captain, Jean-Luc Picard. Picard and Shinzon are genetically identical—they share mannerisms, a tendency toward early balding, and a rare genetic disease known as Shalaft syndrome. But they have led very different lives. Thus, despite all they have in common, they have turned out to be very different men.

In what follows, I examine the plausibility of the ignorance argument through the lens of *Star Trek: Nemesis*, using the case of Picard-Shinzon to explore the importance of the role that ignorance plays in the life of a clone—and in the lives of us all. In particular, I attempt to unravel the role that ignorance plays in our identity formation. Though ignorance may be bliss, the kind of knowledge that clones would have about their future would not prevent them from finding happiness and fulfillment. Ultimately, then, we shall see that the ignorance argument does not present a decisive objection to the morality of cloning.

The Alleged Importance of Ignorance: A First Look

In 2001, President George W. Bush created the President's Council on Bioethics (PCB) to serve an advisory role with respect to ethical and policy issues emerging from recent advances in science, medicine, and technology. The council chose cloning as the subject of its first investigation. Ultimately, having concluded that cloning for reproductive purposes "is not only unsafe but also morally unacceptable, and ought not to be attempted," the PCB unanimously recommended a permanent ban on reproductive cloning (President's Council on Bioethics 2002).[1]

The PCB based these conclusions on five different categories of moral concern about reproductive cloning. First, troubled family relations might result if parents elect to clone themselves to produce children—for example, a woman who clones herself would be both mother and identical twin to the newborn clone, thereby complicating the parent-child relationship. Second, reproductive cloning is perceived to pose a threat to human dignity and the value of human life. Cloned children are "manufactured," rather than "begotten." Thus, such children might come to be viewed more as products or things than as people. Third, reproductive cloning might lead us down a slippery slope to a more pervasive eugenics program. Fourth, reproductive cloning could have widespread effects on society, for example, in the way that children are viewed or, more generally, in the way that relationships are formed between one generation and the next. Finally, the council worried that clones might face problems with their identity and individuality.

Of these five concerns, the last is central to the ignorance argument. According to the PCB, cloning poses a "unique and possibly disabling challenge to the formation of individual identity" (President's Council on Bioethics 2002). The basic thought goes as follows. Most of us, as we live our lives, enjoy a blissful ignorance of our futures. For us, the future is truly unknown, with all possibilities wide open. For the clone, however, this fails to be the case. The life that the original has already lived gives the clone a glimpse of her own likely future. The original's successes and failures constrain the clone's ability to make her own free choices, to find her own way in the world. As Jonas put it, "The simple and unprecedented fact is that the clone knows (or believes to know) altogether too much about himself and is known (or is believed to be known) altogether too well to others. Both facts are paralyzing for the spontaneity of becoming himself, the second also for the genuineness of others' consorting with him" (Jonas 1974, p. 161).

One question naturally arises in response to this argument. What if the cloning process were done entirely covertly? Suppose, for example, that neither the clone nor anyone around her knew that she was a clone or knew anything about the life of the original. In such a case, it is hard to see how she would suffer from any special problems of identity and individuality. The mere fact that an individual is a clone cannot be what threatens identity formation and the right to an open future. Rather, the threat can arise only as a result of *knowledge* of the life already lived.

These considerations suggest that even if the ignorance argument were wholly successful, it would not show us that cloning is wrong in principle but only in certain circumstances. If it were possible for us to produce a clone so that she and everyone around her were entirely in the dark about her status as a clone, then how could we have jeopardized the open nature of her future?

Proponents of the ignorance argument attempt to respond to these considerations by suggesting that it is implausible to suppose that the clone's true nature can be kept a secret from both the clone and those around her. In the case of reproductive cloning, for example, when an individual deliberately clones herself to produce a "child," even if it were possible to keep the clone in the dark about her true nature, it would obviously be impossible to keep this knowledge from the "parent." Or suppose we were to clone someone of particular distinction to attempt to reproduce that person's accomplishments. Here too it is hard to see how the clone's true nature could be kept entirely a secret. As Jonas notes, "The day must come when the (presumably not stupid) copy makes the connection between himself and the publicly enshrined original" (Jonas 1974, p. 162). He goes on to argue: "The choice between being told early or discovering later is one between two unacceptable alternatives. The only remedy against the certainty of the second would be random cloning from the anonymous and insignificant: but then, why cloning at all?" (Jonas 1974, p. 162).

Jonas's response is not entirely successful. Even if, at present, there seems to be no reason for anonymous cloning, we can imagine all sorts of doomsday scenarios that could motivate it. After some worldwide disaster, for example, the earth's population might have dwindled to such low numbers that the few remaining humans scavenge random samples of DNA from databanks and produce a nursery of clones to repopulate the planet. The circumstances of their creation might not be shared with the clones—but even if they discovered their true nature, the original DNA's being random and (let's suppose) untraceable would prevent clones from having to live in the shadow of their originals. This sort of imagined scenario reinforces our point above: the ignorance argument poses an objection to cloning only if we assume that the life of the original is known, either by the clone or by those around her. The ignorance argument alone cannot show us that cloning is intrinsically wrong.

This does not mean, however, that the argument is not worth considering. Even if cloning is not morally wrong in principle, there could be many circumstances in which cloning would be morally unacceptable. The ignorance argument, if sound, could be helpful in sorting out exactly which circumstances those are.

Mirror, Mirror

At this point, it will be useful to turn more directly to *Star Trek: Nemesis*, and to see what light the case of Shinzon can shed on the soundness of the ignorance argument. Early in the film, when the two men meet for the first time and it becomes clear that Shinzon is Picard's clone, Shinzon asks Picard to dinner so that they can have a private conversation. "Come to dinner tomorrow on Romulus," he says. "Just the two of us. Or should I say: just the one of us." In issuing the invitation this way, Shinzon is presumably speaking at least partially in jest, taunting the older man who is attempting to come to grips with the newfound knowledge that he has been cloned—and attempting to come to grips with his relationship to Shinzon. But behind the jest lurks a more sinister worry about a clone's sense of self—one of the very worries highlighted by the PCB.

It is important, however, to note that the reasons behind Shinzon's creation were quite different from the ones that the PCB had in mind when they considered (and condemned) reproductive cloning. As imagined, the typical case occurs when a person wants a biological child but is unable to produce one via the normal procreative route. In this case, however, the "parent" had no knowledge of the existence of the "child."[2] As Shinzon tells Picard when they first sit down, one-on-one, he was created as part of a Romulan plot to infiltrate the Federation. Having somehow acquired some of Picard's genetic material, the Romulans hoped to create a clone and then covertly substitute him for Picard, thereby giving them a spy in perfect position at the helm of their enemy's flagship. The plot, however, was shelved during a change in Romulan regime, and Shinzon ended up spending most of his life in hard labor, working the dilithium mines on the neighboring planet Remus.

The story of his creation gives Shinzon some baggage that the typical clone would presumably lack. But many of the burdens that Shinzon faces are exactly those that the PCB imagines the typical clone would face. As the PCB notes, "Cloned children may experience serious problems of identity . . . because the expectations for their lives may be shadowed by constant comparisons to the life of the 'original' " (President's Council on Bioethics 2002). Shinzon's remarks in a later conversation with Picard strongly support this worry. At this point in the film, Shinzon has captured Picard, and the captain is trying to reason his way out of the situation. "What is this all about?" Picard asks. "It's about destiny," says Shinzon. As the conversation continues, Shinzon's resentment towards Picard bubbles over. "My life is meaningless as long as you're still alive," he seethes. "What am I while you exist? A shadow. An echo."

In this speech, Shinzon gives voice to some of the prime concerns that motivate proponents of the ignorance argument. Shinzon was created to substitute for Picard, to be his replacement. In *Nemesis*, the reasons behind the clone's creation are nefarious, but the sense that the clone serves as a substitute for the original remains even in cases where there is no malicious intent. In all cases of reproduction, parents are in at least some sense looking to recreate themselves—it is called *reproduction*, after all—but this seems even more evident in the case of cloning, where we have exact genetic replication.[3]

As *Nemesis* illustrates, however, this genetic replication does not entail that the clone will be exactly like the original in all respects. When Shinzon catches Picard staring at him during their one-on-one dinner, Picard admits that Shinzon's face is not quite the one he remembers. "A lifetime of violence will do that," Shinzon remarks. And the scars Shinzon bears, scars that distinguish him from Picard, are not only on the outside.

The Ignorance Argument and Genetic Determinism

Despite the fact that Picard and Shinzon share their genetic makeup, they are very different men, with very different motivations, plans, and sensibilities. Their differences call into question the notion of genetic determinism, the claim that genotype fixes identity. This in turn calls into question the ignorance argument, which seems to rely on the assumption of genetic determinism. To sort out these issues, we need to get clearer on exactly what is involved in the claim of genetic determinism and exactly what role this claim plays in the ignorance argument.

If one's identity were not in some way fixed by one's genotype, then it is hard to see how being a clone would pose a special threat to one's sense of identity and individuality. Presumably, any identity problems that would arise for a clone would stem from her sense of herself as a distinct individual. She might believe that she derives her selfhood from the person from whom she was cloned—or even that she shares her selfhood with that person. This makes sense only against the background assumption that one's genotype wholly fixes one's identity. Otherwise, two individuals who share the same genotype could have distinct identities.

But this raises an interesting question. What exactly does it mean to have the same identity as someone else? Some of the exchanges from *Nemesis* are relevant in this regard. Early in the film, when Picard and Shinzon are attempting to forge a relationship, both between themselves as individuals and between their peoples, Shinzon questions Picard's faith in him:

> SHINZON: You don't trust me.
>
> PICARD: I have no reason to.
>
> SHINZON: You have every reason. If you had lived my life, and experienced the suffering of my people, you'd be standing where I am.

The "you" here is not meant to be generic. Shinzon is not saying that *anyone* who had lived his life would be standing where he is. Rather, he is commenting on the similarities between himself and Picard. Had Picard grown up in the Reman mines rather than in a vineyard in France, wouldn't he be the man that Shinzon is? This point resurfaces much later in the film, in a climactic confrontation between the two men:

> SHINZON: You are me. The same noble Picard blood runs through our veins. Had you lived my life, you'd be doing exactly as I am. So look in the mirror. See yourself. Consider that, Captain. I can think of no greater torment for you.
>
> PICARD: Shinzon, I'm a mirror for you as well.

These exchanges between Shinzon and Picard seem to suggest that, at least from the younger man's perspective, the two men do share an identity. When Shinzon tells Picard "You are me," or refers to himself as a mirror for the older man, he seems to be equating their identities. Understandably, this troubles Picard. After all, Shinzon is hell-bent on executing a plan that, if successful, will result in the total annihilation of the population of Earth.

But consider also a later conversation between Picard and one of his colleagues, Lieutenant Commander Data.[4] Data tries to set Picard's mind at ease, arguing that the two men should not be viewed as having the same identity:

PICARD: He said he's a mirror.

DATA: Of you, sir?

PICARD: Yes.

DATA: I do not agree. Although you share the same genetic structure, the events of your life have created a unique individual.

In this way, I think the film is helpful in showing us that there are two different senses of identity that we might care about. In one sense, an identity is *dispositional*, such that two people have the same identity if they are disposed to react in the same way to certain situations. In another sense, however, an identity is *categorical*. A person's identity in this sense is built out of the actual experiences she has, the actual life she leads. We might contrast the two this way: the first sense of identity construes identity as a kind of potentiality; the second sense of identity construes identity as the actualization of that potentiality. Let's call these two senses $identity_P$ (for potentiality) and $identity_A$ (for actualization).

Shinzon seems to understand the notion of identity as $identity_P$. It is this sense of identity that most plausibly ties in with genetic determinism—one's genetic makeup lays down the framework of one's potentiality. And in this sense, Picard and Shinzon can be said to share an identity. Data, in contrast, seems to understand identity as $identity_A$. In this sense, Picard and Shinzon have very different identities indeed. Though they share the same potential, the circumstances of their lives have led them to actualize that potential in very different ways.

The conflation of these two senses of identity seems to me to play a significant role in a lot of the discussion of the ignorance argument. But once we disambiguate these two senses, we can see that the argument requires us to understand identity in terms of $identity_P$.[5] Because the circumstances of one's environment and one's upbringing play a significant role in identity_A formation, there is no reason to think that the clone's identity_A is seriously threatened by the fact that he is clone.

Granted, one's identity_P will lay down certain constraints on one's identity_A. This means that we can expect the clone to have much in common with the original person from whom she was cloned, no matter what the circumstances of her life. Despite having been raised in very different environments, for example, Shinzon and Picard share not only a strong physical resemblance but also certain mannerisms, character traits, and a fondness for hot tea. But it is hard to see how these kinds of commonalities alone would pose any serious threat to the clone's sense of self. After all, these are exactly the kinds of commonalities shared by identical twins, who share an identity_P without sharing an identity_A. Twins live their lives contemporaneously, so they do not have to grow up shadowed by an original who has already lived, but a twin still learns something about her own identity_P from her knowledge of the other's successes and failures. Given that identical twins do not have disabling problems with identity formation, why should there be any reason to think that clones, who share an identity_P without sharing an identity_A, should have such problems? Insofar as they would, the problems must simply be the result of confusion or misinformation.[6] Were clones really to understand the role that one's genetic makeup plays in shaping one's life, there would be no reason for them to have identity issues of the sort imagined by the proponents of the ignorance argument.

The Alleged Importance of Ignorance: A Second Look

The considerations of the previous section suggest that we should reject the ignorance argument. But proponents of the argument would undoubtedly respond that we have not adequately understood its subtleties. The real cause of the threat to one's identity, they would argue, comes not from the fact that one shares an identity with the original, but from *expectations* generated by the life that the original has lived. As the PCB argued:

> However much or little one's genotype actually shapes one's natural capacities, it could mean a great deal to an individual's experience of

> life and the expectations that those who cloned him or her might have. The cloned child may be constantly compared to "the original," and may consciously or unconsciously hold himself or herself up to the genetic twin that came before . . . Living up to parental hopes and expectations is frequently a burden for children; it could be a far greater burden for a cloned individual. The shadow of the cloned child's "original" might be hard for the child to escape, as would parental attitudes that sought in the child's very existence to replicate, imitate, or replace the "original."
>
> (PRESIDENT'S COUNCIL ON BIOETHICS 2002, P. 103)

And as Jonas wrote:

> Note that it does not matter one jot whether the genotype is really, by its own force, a person's fate: it is *made* his fate by the very assumptions in cloning him, which by their imposition on all concerned become a force themselves. It does not matter whether replication of genotype really entails repetition of life performance: the donor has been chosen with some such idea, and that idea is tyrannical in effect.
>
> (JONAS 1974, P. 161)

If this is what's really behind the ignorance argument, however, then it seems that the problem facing the clone is no longer one stemming from a lack of ignorance. If genetic determinism is false and the clone is not saddled with a genetic destiny, then there is no reason to believe that the clone will have special knowledge of her own future. Insofar as cloning deprives her of the right to an open future, then, it is not by depriving the clone of her ignorance. Rather, the clone's future is purportedly closed by the unfair expectations put on her by others (and perhaps also by herself).

This, however, is a much weaker argument. As the PCB itself notes in the passage quoted above, almost all children are forced to grapple with parental expectations. And while it may be true that a clone child might face greater expectations than other children, there is no special reason that this need be the case. Consider the young clone of Andre Agassi versus the young son of Andre Agassi and Steffi Graf. Would the expectations we have for the former really be that different from the expectations that we have for the latter? One might even be tempted to think that in this case we would have greater and more burdensome expectations for the procreated child than for the clone child. Consider also the expectations that have been placed on Prince William since his birth. Could the expectations be any greater or more burdensome for the clone of Prince Charles? In fact, because the clone of Prince Charles would not be in direct line for the throne of England, it seems reasonable to suppose that the expectations on Prince William are weightier.[7]

Granted, some people who choose to create a clone may well have sinister attitudes. Their decision to clone may well be guided by intentions that are ethically questionable. But some parents who choose to procreate also do so with intentions that are below the moral bar. This fact does not lead us to condemn procreation as morally wrong; nor should it lead us to condemn cloning as morally wrong. For the above interpretation of the ignorance argument to get off the ground, we must assume that those who would choose to clone must in principle be driven by improper motives, that the decision to clone is in principle a "tyrannical" one. But there seems no reason to buy into this assumption.

All of us get glimpses of our future from time to time. Some of these glimpses are relatively minor, as when someone sees her mother's graying hair and wrinkled brow. Knowing that she too will one day get gray and wrinkly does not seem to threaten her sense of self. Some of these glimpses are more significant, as when someone sees her mother suffering from a congenital heart defect for which she too has the gene. The knowledge that she will one day experience similar symptoms will undoubtedly affect her life. But such effects, however significant, would not likely be viewed as paralyzing to her sense of self.

The clone, depending on how much knowledge she has of the life of the original, gets more of these glimpses than the average person. But why should they be any more threatening, just because she is a clone? Some of the glimpses, in fact, may be helpful. The clone of Michael Jordan may not have to go through the endless soul-searching that the typical college basketball player goes through in deciding whether and when to turn pro—he knows that he has the potential to be good enough to make it (see Tooley 2005, p. 237). The clone of Sandra Day O'Connor need not worry about whether she is cut out for a career in law. For many twenty-somethings, it's the indecision about what to do with their life that's paralyzing. A little knowledge may well be the antidote to that paralysis, rather than the cause.

As we can see, then, the knowledge that a clone has about her future is not really so different from the knowledge that we all have about our futures. Just like all of us, the clone must choose what to do with that knowledge—it can be stifling, or it can be liberating. But as Data puts it in *Nemesis*, what really matters is that we aspire to be better than we are, and for this, ignorance is no prerequisite. Thus, as *Nemesis* helps to show us, we should reject the ignorance argument. In the end, even the clone has what she needs to boldly go where no one has gone before.

QUESTIONS FOR CONSIDERATION

1. *Proponents of the ignorance argument seem to presuppose that individuality is something to be valued. How might they argue for this claim? How might their opponents argue against it?*

2. *The ignorance argument raises an objection to cloning based on the fact that the clone would have too much knowledge about her identity. Supposedly, such knowledge places her at an unfair disadvantage. In response, opponents of the ignorance argument might make the case that the clone's knowledge should be prized, rather than feared. How could they support this claim?*

3. *Proponents of the ignorance argument focus on the ways that the existence of the "original" poses a threat to the clone's sense of self. Might they also argue that the existence of the clone poses a threat to the original's sense of self? For example, how might Picard's sense of self be threatened by the existence of Shinzon?*

NOTES

1. The council did not reach similar unanimous agreement about the ethical ramifications of cloning for the purposes of biomedical research.

2. The fact that Picard did not consent to being cloned raises a different kind of objection to cloning, one that is beyond the scope of this chapter.

3. In fact, there are already real-life cases of cloning, though not of the human variety, that bear directly on this issue of substitution. Consider the people currently

using the services of the company Genetic Savings and Clone to clone their beloved cats (or to bank their dog's DNA for some future time when dog cloning becomes technologically feasible). As of 2006, a cat cloning cost $32,000. Though the company's promotional materials stress that cloning will not "raise an animal Lazarus-like from the dead," the customers are clearly looking for at least partial replacements for their "one-in-a-million" pet. See www.savingsandclone.com. The company does stress that they cannot guarantee a perfect replacement: "The best dog or cat you've ever known had a genetic code that provided the foundation for its success. Training, experience, and loving care did the rest. Those factors can't be replaced, but the foundation can be replaced by cloning."

4. A secondary plotline of *Nemesis* concerns some identity issues faced by Data, an android. Early in the film, the crew of the *Enterprise* discovers an android named B-4, who at least outwardly appears identical to Data. I do not have the space here to consider the relationship between Data and B-4, but it is an interesting question to consider what light this parallel plotline sheds on the issue of the identity of clones.

5. Even the PCB and other proponents of the ignorance argument seem to recognize the importance of identity_A. The PCB notes, "Of course, our genetic makeup does not by itself determine our identities" (President's Council on Bioethics 2002). Kass makes a similar point, "True, [the clone's] nurture and his circumstance in life will be different; genotype is not exactly destiny" (Kass 2005, p. 226). These remarks make sense only if we understand identity as identity_A.

6. See Tooley (2005) and Brock (1998).

7. I'm not sure exactly how clones would enter into the royal line of succession, but I am assuming they do not get to jump the queue.

REFERENCES

Baird, S. 2002. *Star Trek: Nemesis* [motion picture]. Hollywood, CA: Paramount Pictures.

Brock, D. 1998. Cloning Human Beings: An Assessment of the Ethical Issues Pro and Con. In *Clones and Clones,* ed. M. Nussbaum and C. Sunstein, 141–64. New York: Norton.

Jonas, H. 1974. *Philosophical Essays: From Ancient Creed to Technological Man.* Englewood Cliffs, NJ: Prentice-Hall.

Kass, L. R. 2005. The Wisdom of Repugnance. In *Applying Ethics,* ed. J. Olsen, J. C. Van Camp, and V. Barry, 221–33. Belmont, CA: Wadsworth. (Originally published in L. R. Kass and J. Q. Wilson, eds., *The Ethics of Human Cloning.* Washington, DC: AEI Press, 1998)

President's Council on Bioethics. 2002. *Human Cloning and Human Dignity: An Ethical Inquiry.* At www.bioethics.gov/reports/cloningreport/index.html.

Tooley, M. 2005. The Moral Status of Cloning Humans. In *Applying Ethics,* ed. J. Olsen, J. C. Van Camp, and V. Barry, 233–44. Belmont, CA: Wadsworth. (Originally published in J. M. Humber and R. F. Almeder, eds., *Human Cloning.* Totowa, NJ: Humanities Press, 1998).

PART THREE

The Good Life

NINE

"Blessed Are the Forgetful"

The Ethics of Memory Deletion in *Eternal Sunshine of the Spotless Mind*

Andy Miah

How happy is the blameless vestal's lot!
The world forgetting, by the world forgot.
Eternal sunshine of the spotless mind!
Each pray'r accepted, and each wish resign'd.

ALEXANDER POPE, "ELOISA TO ABELARD,"
QUOTED BY MARY IN *Eternal Sunshine of the Spotless Mind*

Eternal Sunshine of the Spotless Mind (Gondry 2004) pursues a perennial problem within the philosophy of medicine: whether society should limit the pursuit of biological modifications that have no clear therapeutic purpose. In the context of memory modification, the origin of this question has its roots in two crucial bodies of literature. The first concerns the mind-body problem, which involves attempting to ascertain their relationship. In large part, the entire practice of medicine is concerned with this question, which eludes any definitive answer. Nevertheless, various perspectives have emerged over the centuries from René Descartes' deduction that mind and body are separate or, more specifically, that we can consider human consciousness as separate from the physical world. His Cartesian dualism has been challenged by more recent philosophical thought, though one might ask whether recent discussions in relation to mind modifications, including the alteration of memories, constitutes some level of revival of these ideas (Hacking 2006). Within bioethics, these questions have become pertinent to legislation surrounding end-of-life issues, what rights should one, where it is necessary to decide, afford a person who is in a persistent vegetative state? Locating the individual in such notions as *personhood* or *psychological connectedness* (Parfit 1971, 1984) remains an important question within philosophical psychology (Reid 2005). Moreover, these debates have informed attempts to establish the moral status of embryos and inquiries into what defines humanness.

The second body of literature that informs our debate involves the ethics of neurological enhancements (neuroethics), crucial at a time when medicine seems to be stretching far beyond what some would see as its traditional role, as safer forms of biological modification become possible and commercially available (Whitehouse et al. 1997; Wolpe 2002).

Rather than presenting us with a biological modification that offers superhuman capabilities, *Eternal Sunshine* questions what should be considered as an enhancement. It invites the viewer to consider how the brain constructs identity and what components of this identity are essential to being the same person over time. Crucially, it invokes this conundrum in normative terms, which again offers rich material for ethicists to consider. Thus, the viewer is encouraged to identify "psychological connectedness" as a valuable or constitutive criterion of the "good life." In this sense, we also see how the film engages with a number of other bioethical debates, such as the use of psychotropic drugs that Elliott (1998) considers troubling because they have the potential to break the continuity of our identity in a way that limits our capacity to claim autonomy of action. The film pursues these issues by exploring the possibility of neurological modification, specifically, the deletion of memories. In this capacity, *Eternal Sunshine* usefully problematizes the value of enhancement technologies.

The modification that is pursued in *Eternal Sunshine,* however, is not clearly denoted as a form of enhancement. Indeed, the film's narrative urges us to avoid seeking happiness via technological solutions and dwelling too much on how we might engineer a good life. It is an intriguing and complex story, precisely because the desire to seek technological fixes to unhappiness resonates with present-day methods by which medicine aims to relieve such suffering. Today, pharmaceutical products, psychological counseling, and even the self-help movement are used to offer such resources through which people might overcome trauma. However, the additional challenge from the film is that the form of trauma it describes does not easily fit within a biomedical definition of trauma but is a regular occurrence in most people's lives—the break-up of a romantic relationship. As such, it also raises a question about how much we demand from technology in solving social and intrapersonal problems. From watching the movie, it would be easy to imagine that memory deletion is the next stage of medical therapeutic interventions. In such an era, the question arises as to whether humanity should seek such neurological transformations or rely mostly on our learned ability to cope with whatever life may bring us.

The futuristic science implied by *Eternal Sunshine* is articulated within a recognizable, present-day period, where the environment of isolated American diners, chilly train stations, and dowdy waiting rooms challenge the assumption that high technology is located exclusively within the genre of science fiction or, indeed, within a distant or even near future. Indeed, *Eternal Sunshine* celebrates the natural and the every day, which reinforces its antitechnological and dystopian narrative. Many of the scenes are located within nature, with frequent depictions of the frozen Charles River in Boston and snow-covered beaches in Montauk, Long Island. Even director Michel Gondry's style of shooting resonates purist ideals, eliminating special effects and, as such, any connections that might be made between the future and high technology. These elements are inextricable from the ethical dilemmas that are presented throughout the film where the depiction of nature and technology inhabits a moral space.

Yet, despite these warnings about too much technology, the moral narrative of *Eternal Sunshine* is ambiguous in many respects, because it confronts our uncertainty about how best to overcome difficulties in life. The optimist's view that technology could improve human happiness is reflected through the character of Mary (played by Kirsten Dunst), who at first finds value in memory deletions. As she remarks when witnessing the procedure: "It's amazing . . . what Howard [Dr. Mierzwiak] gives to the world . . . to let people begin again . . . it's beautiful . . . Howard just makes it all go away." Mary embodies the optimism of those who argue on behalf of enhancement technologies. Yet, she ultimately comes to symbolize the naivety or impracticality of these views because, on discovering that she has been an unwitting participant in a memory-deletion procedure herself, she finds it an abhorrent affront to her dignity. More will be said about this later.

After watching *Eternal Sunshine*, one is left feeling that the best solution to dealing with human suffering already resides within our learned capacities. There is also a sense that leaving this merely for time to heal is inadequate and that we are quite right to seek more effective, efficient, and gentle means. The difficulty, though, is that *Eternal Sunshine* portrays memory deletion as anything but gentle.

This chapter will pursue these ambiguities in detail, exploring the range of ethical issues presented through the movie. In particular, it outlines how *Eternal Sunshine* successfully links philosophical with ethical questions about enhancement. It invites reflection on what we might define as a human enhancement and, subsequently, what we might then ask medical science to do to enable it. As such, it engages with one of the fundamental and timely questions within bioethics, which concerns its proper role in a time of expanding autonomy. Underpinning each of these parameters is a question about the good life and utopia: is a good life one in which we are free to call on medicine to alleviate any form of suffering we might encounter?

I begin by offering a brief synopsis of the movie to clarify how the philosophical relates to the ethical within the story. Subsequently, I discuss the neuroscience of *Eternal Sunshine* and the recent bioethical context for the debates it raises. Finally, I offer an ethical analysis of memory modification in the movie from the perspective of the medical profession and, more briefly, of the individual consumer.

Remembering the Film

As was suggested earlier, *Eternal Sunshine* is an accomplished bioethical text due to its careful composition of the aesthetic alongside the ethical.[1] It reminds the viewer that visions of the good life are often difficult to separate from ideas about beauty. Yet, like all great works of art, it does not pursue any moral or social agenda aggressively; instead it stumbles over a set of complex issues arising from quite simple premises. Its main characters are visually and metaphorically vivid, signified by Clementine's brightly colored hair and Joel's contrasting, depressive presence. Throughout the film, these strong motifs reappear, which continually reinforces the idea that the subject matter is of moral concern, invoking matters of hope, desperation, anxiety, and excitement.

The film begins with Joel (played by Jim Carrey) waking in his bed on Valentine's Day morning, seemingly surprised at his circumstances. Within moments, he flees from his apartment and takes the Long Island Railroad to Montauk without knowing why he is going there. He walks the snow-covered beaches noticing the figure of the, then, unknown Clementine (played by Kate Winslet), whom he sees again moments later in a diner by the beach. Their first encounter within the film takes place at the Montauk train station, while they both await the return train. She is drawn to him, and it is apparent that their meeting is inevitable. However, this inevitability is not merely a structural necessity for the movie—it is not just that we need for them to meet in order for there to be a story—but a literal claim that writer Charlie Kaufman and director Gondry are seeking to reveal. For Joel and Clementine *have* met before; they are just not aware of it yet.

As the film progresses, we are drawn into a series of disjointed, but connected, scenes in which two timelines overlap. The first tells of Joel and Clem's initial relationship, which ends with Clem erasing all memories of Joel, and Joel's subsequent revenge deletion of his own memories. A considerable part of the film depicts the process of Joel's procedure, taking us into his mind as he recalls, in reverse order, every memory of Clementine, each of which is deleted one by one. During this process, Joel also changes his mind and attempts to break free from the procedure by hiding Clem in other memories. Throughout this timeline, we see first how they broke up and finally how they first met. The second timeline explains their subsequent and inevitable reunion, which began as I have already described. This timeline begins on the morning after Joel's memory deletion. We learn later that his compulsion to head off to Montauk has something to do with a residual memory of Clem that was not completely erased.[2]

The film functions on several levels. While our interest here is to consider the ethics of biomedical modifications, Martin-Jones offers an interpretation that assists in revealing the values that, I suspect, are at stake in the analysis of legitimate action. Thus, he articulates the film as an explicit post–9/11 trauma narrative, which adopts a moral stance on how to respond to feelings of trauma. As he notes, "Rather than being defined by a traumatic loss from their recent past its protagonists decide to rework this loss. Instead of seeking a triumphal revenge over the recent past, they consciously choose to recreate the situation that led up to their trauma, and to reexamine their own role in creating it. They determine that if they can avert the trauma this time they can break out of the vicious cycle of triumphalism, a cycle rendered in the film as the actions of brainwashed automatons" (Martin-Jones 2006, p. 157).

Martin-Jones's analysis locates the moral cause of *Eternal Sunshine* in the characters' initial failure to choose the right course of action in dealing with loss and their subsequent recognition of the inadequacy of this decision, which culminates in the film's final, distraught scene; a moment of profound enlightenment. It also acknowledges the motif within the film that can be reduced to the commonly held belief that failure to remember the past necessitates our being doomed to repeat it. Yet, it also extends this belief by allowing its protagonists the opportunity to change "the conditions that led to the past trauma" (p. 181), thus advancing the idea that memories (as truth claims about the past) do not constitute the entirety of history. Rather, they are, at best, critical moments within a longer historical narrative that is often perpetually open to rewriting.[3]

Each of the protagonists is unsatisfied, incomplete, and naively innocent—a "blameless vestal," as character Mary describes—and the story is as much about self-discovery, as it is about the impossibility (and unimportance) of engineering utopia via technology. Their incompleteness of character and the voids in their memories connect the overarching narrative about the importance of experiencing loss in life and the value of conflict in human relationships. For instance, in one part of the film we watch Joel remembering a time when he and Clem are having lunch. The viewer is taken into the scene via Joel's memory, where he reinhabits himself as if acting out a role in a play. Each character plays out the scene as it originally occurred, though the viewer is conscious of Joel's awareness that he is within a memory. Joel's experience of this is portrayed in a way that is akin to the playfulness one feels on realizing that one is dreaming. At some point midway through their lunch, Clem sarcastically asks Joel if he wouldn't mind "cleaning the goddamn hair off the soap after using the shower," which reveals that this is another tense exchange. Yet, Joel's encounter with this memory is one of happiness; he relishes knowing what she is about to say and displays affection, rather than irritation, for her unapologetic, direct, and perhaps aggressive character. This scene offers a moment for questioning the value we attribute to memories, as either positive or negative. In this instance, the unpleasant encounter is recalled with a rich and deep happiness, which conveys something of the value in accepting the, often, crippling unpleasantness experienced in personal relationships.

"There's No Such Thing as This"

The procedure of memory deletion in *Eternal Sunshine* is portrayed as reasonably straightforward and of limited risk. Patients are asked to bring any artifacts that remind them of the person they want to forget, which would be destroyed by the clinic after the procedure. By monitoring the client's brain responses to these "mediated memories" (Van Dijck 2004), the scientists create a mental map using brain scanning technology. Once this is complete, the scientists visit their clients at night and assault them into a comalike state to perform the memory-deletion procedure. The client wakes up the next morning with no recollection of the procedure's having ever taken place or of the deleted memories.[4]

The technology demonstrates some appreciation for research on brain structure and links between emotions and memory. As Damasio notes, "The essence of feeling an emotion is the experience of such changes in juxtaposition to the mental images that initiated the cycle" (Damasio 1994, p. 145), which corresponds with how memory is imagined within the film. Indeed, the process of eliminating the links between these images is critical to the process of forgetting. Moreover, the idea that specific memories occupy material space within the brain is also consistent with both Damasio's and Sacks's (Sacks 1985) observations of memory. Nevertheless, Baxendale (2004) notes that the frequent portrayal of memory loss within films doesn't often take into account the distinction between "amnesic syndromes with a psychiatric basis and those with an underlying neurological cause." *Eternal Sunshine* manages to disguise its science to a great extent, which limits any (rather dull) criticism of its failure to portray adequately whether memory deletion could ever be a possibility.

Nonetheless, perhaps the most pressing scientific question is to ask how long it will be before such science is available. In part, the science presented extends from present-day approaches to conceptualizing and treating traumatic memories. For instance, Kolber (2006) discusses how propranolol is an FDA-approved drug that has been shown to dampen memories associated with an event when taken within six hours of its occurrence. Beyond this, there are high expectations about the future of neuroscience to deliver memory modifications. Indeed, Farah et al. note that some are predicting that the "twenty-first century will be the century of neuroscience" (Farah et al. 2004, p. 421), and the ethical implications of this are neatly characterized in *Eternal Sunshine*. Yet, crucial metaphysical questions are still unresolved in neuroscience, which have the potential to undermine the way that *Eternal Sunshine* imagines memory-altering procedures. For instance, it remains unclear whether memory can be isolated from other forms of knowledge, though we are reasonably clear that "the brain stores emotional memories very differently from unemotional ones" (Johnson 2004). Thus, one of the problems not resolved by the film is whether it is possible to delete something that cannot easily be defined. To draw a parallel between neuroscience and genetics: it is difficult to point to a gene and say, "Let's enhance that," precisely because most genes perform many functions. Similarly, the functions of memory are multifaceted; suggesting that it is possible to isolate them within a brain space is problematic.

One might also question the suitability of a cinematic lens to portray memories. The viewer is inevitably looking into the memory as a spectator, and this requires its construction as a familiar visual form. The conceptualization of the brain itself also corresponds with established ways of representing brains, often as computerlike in their construction (Van Dijck 2005). This is reflected both in the way in which the technicians in the film are presented as computer geeks and in the way that memories are displayed as small dots within regions on the brain scan, rather like individual bits within a computer's hard drive. This way of imagining what memories look like is useful but nevertheless contrived.

One might also say something about the problem with Joel's witnessing the deletion of his memory, and how that process would generate a new memory to confound the initial deletion. These ideas are approached by Reason (2003), who draws attention to the distinction between lived experiences and recordings as markers of reality. While the direction and script attempt to attend to the "detritus" of memory—by presenting details that are witnessed only through the subconscious—this is certainly difficult to convey through cinema. Indeed, the two protagonists' resignation to living in the "present" somehow confirms the important distinction between recorded and lived experiences, where the latter is presumed to offer some guarantee of greater correspondence to a truthful existence.

A further difficulty involves the claim that memories of particular objects or people can be isolated from all other memories. Again, *Eternal Sunshine* sidesteps this problem by neglecting to engage with it. We do not sense, for example, whether Joel has lost two years of all other memories or just those that involve Clem. However, there are moments where this problem is suggested. For instance, when trying to hide in another memory to avoid its deletion, Joel says to Clem, "I can't remember anything without you." This gets to the very heart of the scientific problem: our memories of others are not located merely in our physical interactions with them; we often spend time thinking of others when they are not there, or even dreaming about them. It is unclear from the film whether these indirect memories must also be deleted for the procedure to be complete.[5]

Finally, the problem of inevitability is never fully addressed by *Eternal Sunshine*. When Joel and Clem are informed that they once knew each other, this constitutes a new act, rather than simply the replaying of the same past. This intervention implies a challenge to the fatalistic stance of the movie and could be seen as monumental in determining where they go next. They now have knowledge of their future and this alone might be enough for them to alter it. Indeed, we are reminded that, but for their "complicity" (Martin-Jones 2006, p. 177), at every point in their relationship, there was an opportunity to change and be more flexible with each other. This possibility of minute changes offers a challenge to the overall thesis of the film, that we are destined to repeat our actions if we do not remember the past. This is confirmed at the end of the movie when both Joel and Clem agree to start again. Despite their inevitable repeated separation, there is still a sense of hope that this need not happen and that they will overcome any differences that should arise.[6]

Layered Ethical Narratives

It is possible to analyze the ethics of *Eternal Sunshine* from at least two perspectives. The first involves an assessment of the medical professionals within the film, as they undertake a practice that is ambiguously defined as health care. The second, concerns the choices sought by the protagonists in their attempt to improve their happiness through employing quick-fix technology to change their memories. I focus on the ethics of the profession within this analysis, though offer some brief comments on individual ethics.

The Ethics of Lacuna

The organization offering memory deletion services within *Eternal Sunshine* is called Lacuna and is led by Dr. Howard Mierzwiak (played by Tom Wilkinson). It appears to employ three other staff members, two of whom—Patrick and Stan—have a mixed professional role, which might be characterized as medical assistants or biostatisticians. The other, Mary, is the clinic's receptionist. In each of the cases, the characters' performative function extends well beyond their professional titles. Indeed, one of the major sources of ethical concern resides within the clumsy character of their organization. Lacuna is a low-tech outfit, operating from dull and simple premises. There is no visible high-technology within the clinic. Rather, the technology of memory deletion is obscured by the invisibility of its digital form. This makeshift character is given gravitas by Dr. Mierzwiak, who, we are reminded by Mary, should one day "be in Bartlett's" (book of famous quotations) for his work in developing this technology.[7]

A series of ethical questions precedes the general practice of their work, the first of which concerns whether this technology resides (or should reside) within the profession of medicine at all. This question is more broadly contextualized in debates about the proper role of medicine. For example, it is similar to discussions over the status of cosmetic surgery as a medical speciality. Clearly, Lacuna's work encompasses a therapeutic role for many of its clients—which includes an elderly lady seeking to overcome the death of her dog. However, it also seems nontherapeutic, enhancing or merely nonmedical, in that it is used by individuals for means that are medically questionable—such as the customer who asks Mary whether it is possible to receive the procedure three times in one night. Although she indicates that this is not their policy, the dialogue alludes to the challenge arising from commercial models of medical provision, where consumer demands may conflict with medical advice. The confused status of the medicine is further compounded by the behavior of Lacuna's employees. Throughout the film, we learn that Dr. Mierzwiak has previously had an affair with the receptionist Mary but that all memories of this were deleted—at her request—to overcome the trauma it created after his wife discovered them. It would not be particularly difficult to characterize this as a conflict of interest! The two assistants are equally unprofessional in their practice. For instance, during Joel's procedure, they are drinking, taking drugs, and dancing on his bed. One of them even passes Joel's memory objects off as his own to get Clem to fall for him.

Yet, to dwell too much on these details would be to miss the more interesting and complicated ethical issues the film presents. Indeed, the movie allows us to dismiss the possibility that memory deletion might simply be an unethical use of science. For, as I have argued, if we accept that the technology is therapeutic, then it is reasonable to consider Lacuna's work as just another form of alleviating trauma, comparable to perhaps psychiatry, the use of psychopharmacology and so on. However, if we do *not* regard it as therapeutic, then we are also informed that there are no grave concerns about the practice anyway. Indeed, when asked by Joel whether the procedure involves "any risk of brain damage," Dr. Mierzwiak informs him that, "technically, it is brain damage" but that it is "on a par with a night of heavy drinking." In this statement, we learn that Lacuna's work is justified on behalf of an argument from precedent—the brain damage involved from memory deletion is equivalent to the damage arising from acceptable current practices. This argument is familiar to many debates surrounding the ethics of enhancement technologies, though its legitimacy is contested.

As Parens argues, two sets of problems arise from arguing from precedent. The first is that one cannot assume moral equivalence to different means through which we might pursue a particular end or moral equivalence to different ends. The second problem is that different means can "embody and/or express different values," so again it does not follow that they are simply the same as the previous case (Parens 1998, p. 13).

At least, we might conclude that memory deletion is not obviously unethical from a medical perspective, but we might also accept that it is not medicine at all. The implications of this are significant, for it matters how one characterizes specific applications of technology, particularly with regard to the regulatory structure underpinning it and the funding mechanisms through which it is provided. Indeed, one initial conclusion from *Eternal Sunshine*, which can inform more general debates about the ethics of enhancement, is that a radical new ethical framework is required to address how medicine can be administered to healthy subjects. The fundamental assumption that such procedures would contradict the ethical principle of nonmaleficience is brought into question when the technology is made sufficiently safe.

A final set of ethical issues surrounding Lacuna's work concerns privacy and confidentiality. When Lacuna deletes memories, it recognizes that it is not sufficient merely to delete the client's own memories. For the procedure to be effective, it is crucial that all of the client's significant others refrain from mentioning the deleted person, as this could trigger the memory or create further trauma. Thus, the film takes into account the cultural life of memories. Lacuna's answer to this is to send letters to all of Clem's close friends and relatives, which read, "Clementine Kruczynski has had Joel Barish erased from her memory. Please never mention their relationship to her again."

In this way, one might argue that confidentiality functions as a truly relational concept (Meyers 1989; Donchin 1995; Sherwin 1998; Mackenzie and Stoljar 2000). Indeed, turning traditional ethical issues surrounding privacy on their head, privacy is ensured *only* by telling other people. Thus, privacy is afforded by all parties respecting the patient's wishes to keep the truth from them, rather than by others not knowing. Patients/clients must waive their entitlement to confidentiality but are also predisposed to disvalue what could be described as a traditional notion of privacy. Again, this issue is critical to contemporary bioethics, where debates over the confidentiality of something like genetic information continue to raise new questions. The only difficulty is that the film also shows us that such openness is not protected from abuse. For example, I have already mentioned that Mary had an affair with Dr. Mierzwiak, which was subsequently deleted from her memory. However, I did not mention that she learns of this after a second indiscretion with him that takes place on the night of Joel's procedure. If we are to believe that Lacuna protects the integrity of the procedure by ensuring that all friends are aware of what not to mention, then it is unclear how Mary could find herself in this situation for a second time. For while Dr. Mierzwiak might feel obliged to say nothing and allow her to continue working, it is harder to believe that his wife will have been comfortable with the situation. Indeed, it is more likely that Mary would have been dismissed from the organization. These circumstances characterize the difficult position within which the friends of the client are placed and the broader conflict of interests that will ensue.

This is articulated in the scene where Joel's friend gives up trying to lie about the circumstances and shows him the letter sent by Lacuna. The entire process creates a range of ambiguous situations in which friends and family will struggle to know how best to protect the client, ultimately undermining this dispersed model of confidentiality. Indeed, this entire problematic situation is ethically intriguing insofar as the usual rules of morality, such as truth telling, are overturned as concerns the deleted memories and persons. A friend will have to decide whether to respect the truth or respect the friend, where the two, formerly, should have coincided.[8]

Doctor, Will You Fix My Broken Heart?

Blessed are the forgetful, for they get the better even of their blunders.

FRIEDRICH NIETZSCHE, *Beyond Good and Evil*,
QUOTED BY MARY IN *Eternal Sunshine of the Spotless Mind*

The other perspective one can take on the bioethics of *Eternal Sunshine* concerns the actions of its protagonists, Joel and Clem. One of the difficulties within the film is its bias—we have little choice but to conclude that memory deletion is a bad idea. For instance, the fact that Joel appears to seek memory deletion almost as revenge for Clem's having done it does not sit particularly well for anybody seeking to argue that such choices are empowering acts of autonomy and self-authorship. Clementine's decision is presented in equally negative terms. When Joel first finds out what she has done, a mutual friend tells him that Clem probably did it "as a lark," so both characters are described as having done this without much careful consideration.[9] Again, the fact that this is of no concern to Lacuna, who "provide the possibility" of moving on and "starting again," further diminishes the organization's professionalism. Indeed, Lacuna's mode of practice constitutes perhaps the one major futuristic narrative, insofar as it presents an era where medical treatments occupy a commercial social space, where all boundaries of medical professionalism and care have been transcended. Thus, Lacuna functions in a time where health care is consumer led and based on a very loose definition of health as a vague form of well-being. The protagonists claim an unquestioning entitlement to the procedure to help them overcome a difficult time in their life, and perhaps the only characteristics in their favor are the protagonists' familiar circumstances. Neither of them exhibits the usual hubris of the scientist seeking to control nature and push the frontiers of human capabilities. Rather, their choice to use the technology is relatively understated; one might even say normal.

In this sense, *Eternal Sunshine* does not encounter the typical characteristics of movies in which high technology is associated with limitless wealth and liberty—a kind of frivolous autonomy. It is not obvious that Joel and Clem are acting immorally toward each other when deleting their memories. Rather, the problem is determining whether our moral commitment to others extends to our *memories* of them, rather than simply our *actions* toward them. While the film suggests a positive response to this question, it stops short of conveying it as an obligation. My suspicion is that there should be no obligation to remember others, but that there could be good reasons to preserve even those memories we would prefer to be without. In the case of the latter, the desire not to hold the memory should more properly be described as the desire for the event not to have occurred. Nevertheless, one must admit an incomplete knowledge in understanding what the relevant memories are in order to enable the greatest flourishing in life.

Eternal Sunshine avoids being forced into making any such claim by characterizing the consequences of memory deletion as traumatic. In this sense, it offers a passionate, intuitive appeal to the idea that such a practice would be wrong in itself by demonstrating the "pain and heartbreak" (Grau 2006, p. 119) that will inevitably result. Moreover, it appeals to notions of authenticity and selfhood by showing the altered mind to be devoid of meaning. As Herzog notes, "Memory is what distinguishes a particular human being from being in general" and is the "inner narration of the search for freedom" (Herzog 2005). So conceived, it is also difficult to neglect the moral content of this pursuit and the need to retain the integrity of one's memories. In contrast, Mary's quote from Nietzsche suggests that there is value in seeking to forget. In this sense, the ethics of memory deletion are "beyond good and evil," as the quote might attempt to convey.

Conclusion

The bioethical issues raised through *Eternal Sunshine* permeate a number of crucial questions arising from emerging medical technologies. On one level, it discusses the ethics of medical science, portraying several challenges posed by a commercial model of medicine and the difficulty with modifying the biology of healthy subjects. It also encompasses a critique on the ethics of enhancement and the value of pursuing neurological modifications. More broadly, the movie situates bioethical debates within philosophical questions about the irrelevance of fatalism and the importance of remembering. Toward the end of the movie, these issues are foreshadowed when the protagonists realize that they are doomed to be separated, but that they are *also* doomed to fall in love. Their response is to resign themselves to both states of affairs and to accept the inevitable highs and lows of life, which seems to be all they can do.

In the world of *Eternal Sunshine*, where it is possible to delete unwanted memories, it also becomes clear that people are generally capable of overcoming the trauma of those memories through their own volition. This provides a persuasive argument against the use of medical technology to alleviate some forms of suffering, no matter whether we sympathize with the sufferer. Indeed, *Eternal Sunshine* attempts to derive clear limits to the use of medicine, to encourage the viewer to seek alternative ways of dealing with suffering, and to accept that happiness is in part constituted by the absence of guaranteeing a life free from suffering. Even where medication might make our lives better, we would suffer at the hands of technology from being deprived of characteristics that make us human. It suggests that, without grief and suffering, we are unable to achieve the kind of intimacy that binds people together.

However, *Eternal Sunshine* also obscures a balanced evaluation of memory modification, by relying on the assumption that it is impossible to characterize neurological enhancements as improvements. As such, it never satisfactorily attends to the fact that people are unavoidably positioned within a locus of decision-making that compels them to alleviate human suffering by whatever means are available to them. In such circumstances, it is hard to imagine that people would be satisfied with relying on their own capacities, should alternative means be available. Moreover, it is not obvious that anybody is harmed by the use of such technology, even though the practical ethics of employing such means are incredibly difficult to resolve.

Both a beautiful production and a subtle (and stormy) romance, *Eternal Sunshine* engages bioethicists through a confrontation with questions about the good life and utopia. Its narrative is a warning about runaway individualism and the problem of having too much choice and control over ourselves. However, there are various nuances that allow *Eternal Sunshine* to occupy the space of a genuine ethical issue, which leaves the viewer uncertain about how to reconcile the intuition to alleviate human suffering by whatever means are available and the concern that human suffering might also be fundamental to our appreciation of happiness.

QUESTIONS FOR CONSIDERATION

1. *If memory deletion were possible, how would you decide which memories to keep and which to erase?*

2. *In what way can memory deletion be characterized as human enhancement?*

3. *Do we have a moral responsibility to remember?*

4. *How does the professional contact (or lack thereof) of Lacuna employees correspond with general medical ethics?*

NOTES

1. This is reflected at one point in the film when Mary compares Dr. Mierzwiak to a surgeon or a concert pianist, invoking metaphors of healer, creator, magician, or deity. From this, one can derive claims about "playing God," which are so prevalent within many discussions about the limits of medical ethics.

2. This is one of many moments when the complexity of the human mind is

shown to be superior to the complexity of a technological intervention that seeks to disrupt it.

3. This reinforces Martin-Jones's (2006) claim that the film "smuggles in a political critique" (p. 157) by offering a chance to consider 9/11 as a pivotal moment for addressing global relations in U.S. foreign policy, rather than concluding that it represented the impossibility of reconciling ideological difference.

4. The quote at the beginning of this section is from Joel, on learning about the science. I will use the terms *patient* and *client* interchangeably throughout this chapter, without saying too much about the film's capacity to raise questions about the collapse of these concepts within medicine.

5. The film alludes to these unresolved problems by indicating that remnants of memories remain within the minds of our protagonists, thus suggesting that the procedure was not completely flawless.

6. In this way, the tapes they receive of their consultations at Lacuna then constitute a performative, reconciliatory function, which is much closer to contemporary psychiatric practices.

7. One might offer various interpretations of why Howard's colleagues consider that he is worthy of entry into Bartlett's book of quotations. Perhaps there is some attempt here to connect the doctor with Mary's citation of Nietzsche's *Beyond Good and Evil* or even Alexander Pope's poem from which the "eternal sunshine" title derives. Alternatively, perhaps they believe he will be remembered for all time, just like Pope and Nietzsche.

8. An additional ethical ambiguity on behalf of Dr. Mierzwiak arises here again when, on playing her consultation tape to herself, we hear the doctor say, "We agreed it was for the best" (for Mary to delete her memories), which raises questions about his integrity, but also whether one can truly enter into such technology with a strong sense of empowerment, because it seems always and only to be moments of deep suffering that bring people to this technology.

9. This signifier is also used later in the film, when Joel is reminded that this is also a characteristic that he loves about Clementine, further advancing the claim that affection and anxiety are so closely related that it would be foolhardy to seek the deletion of one.

REFERENCES

Baxendale, S. 2004. Memories Aren't Made of This: Amnesia at the Movies. *British Medical Journal* 329:1480–83.

Damasio, A. R. 1994. *Descartes' Error: Emotion, Reason and the Human Brain.* London: Papermac.

Donchin A. 1995. Reworking Autonomy: Toward a Feminist Perspective. *Cambridge Quarterly of Healthcare Ethics* 4 (9): 44–55.

Elliott, C. 1998. The Tyranny of Happiness: Ethics and Cosmetic Pharmacology. In *Enhancing Human Traits: Ethical and Social Implications,* ed. E. Parens, 177–88. Washington, DC: Georgetown University Press.

Farah, M. J., Illes, J., Cook-Deegan, R., Gardner, H., Kandel, E., King, P., Parens, E., Sahakian, B., and Woolpe, P. R. 2004. Neurocognitive Enhancement: What Can We Do and What Should We Do? *Nature Reviews (Neuroscience)* 5, May: 421–26.

Gondry, M. 2004. *Eternal Sunshine of the Spotless Mind* [motion picture]. Los Angeles: Anonymous Content.

Grau, C. 2006. *Eternal Sunshine of the Spotless Mind* and the Morality of Memory. *Journal of Aesthetics and Art Criticism* 64: 119–33.

Hacking, I. 2006. The Cartesian Body. *BioSocieties* 1:13–15.

Herzog, A. 2005. Levinas, Memory, and the Art of Writing. *Philosophical Forum* 36 (3): 333–43.

Johnson, S. 2004. The Science of *Eternal Sunshine* [hypertext document]. At www.slate.com/id/2097502/.

Kolber, A. J. 2006. Therapeutic Forgetting: The Legal and Ethical Implications of Memory Dampening. *Vanderbilt Law Review.* San Diego Legal Studies Paper No. 07–37.

Mackenzie, C., and Stoljar, N., eds. 2000. *Relational Autonomy: Feminist Perspectives on Autonomy, Agency and the Social Self.* Oxford and New York: Oxford University Press.

Martin-Jones, D. 2006. *Deleuze, Cinema and National Identity.* Edinburgh: Edinburgh University Press.

Meyers D. 1989. *Self, Society, and Personal Choice.* New York: Routledge.

Parens, E. 1998. Is Better Always Good? The Enhancement Project. In *Enhancing Human Traits: Ethical and Social Implications,* ed. E. Parens, 1–28. Washington, DC: Georgetown University Press.

Parfit, D. 1971 Personal Identity. *Philosophical Review* 80: 3–27.

———. 1984. *Reasons and Persons.* Oxford: Clarendon Press.

Reason, M. 2003. Archive or Memory? The Detritus of Live Performance. *New Theatre Quarterly* 19 (1): 82–89.

Reid, M. D. 2005. Memory as Initial Experiencing of the Past. *Philosophical Psychology* 18(6):671.

Sacks, O. 1985. *The Man Who Mistook His Wife for a Hat.* London: Picador.

Sherwin, S. 1998. A Relational Approach to Autonomy in Health Care. In *The Politics of Women's Health: Exploring Agency and Autonomy,* ed. S. Sherwin, x–xx. Philadelphia: Temple University Press.

Van Dijck, J. 2004. Mediated Memories: Personal Cultural Memory as Object of Cultural Analysis. *Continuum: Journal of Media and Cultural Studies* 18(2): 261–77.

———. 2005. From Shoebox to Performative Agent: The Computer as Personal Memory Machine. *New Media and Society* 7(3):311–32.

Whitehouse, P. J., Juengst, E. T., Mehlman, M., and Murray, T. H. 1997. Enhancing Cognition in the Intellectually Intact. *Hastings Center Report* 27(3):14–22.

Wolpe, P. R. 2002. Treatment, Enhancement, and the Ethics of Neurotherapeutics. *Brain and Cognition* 50:387–95.

TEN

Hacking the Mind

Existential Enhancement in *Ghost in the Shell*

Paul J. Ford

Controversies surrounding medical enhancement continue to gain significant attention in bioethics, both in the popular press and in academic journals. Advances in the uses of genetics, pharmacology, prosthetics, surgery, and computer chips toward enhancing human function prompt vigorous debates concerning fair play in sports, justice in resource allocation, unreasonable health risks, and abuse of individuals through commodification (Murray 2002; Conrad and Potter 2004; Kamm 2005; Lauritzen 2005; Mehlman 2005; Ford 2006). In general, an underlying assumption persists that improving an individual's functional abilities, which in turn makes her more independent and functionally better than others, is at least a good thing for the individual being enhanced. This seemingly straightforward assumption is challenged in director Mamoru Oshii's 1995 anime film *Kôkaku kidôtai*, distributed in English-speaking countries as *Ghost in the Shell*. Through a science fiction cyberpunk story set in the not-too-distant future, *Ghost* challenges our valuation and categorization of enhancement technologies. The film reflects on the values associated with certain individual, governmental, and societal goals of enhancement technologies. Simply put, *Ghost* posits that a focus on individual functional enhancement and the uniformity it brings wrongly ignores the value of integration and heterogeneity, both for the community's good and for an individual's own progressive evolution. The way to enhance one's existence is to become more integrated and closer to others rather than more separate and distant.

Although the philosophical issues raised by *Ghost in the Shell* may at first seem similar to those raised in the *Matrix* trilogy of films, the film goes beyond questions of mind-body, authenticity, or purpose of life (Holt 2002; McMahon 2002; Wrathall 2005). It pushes the audience to reexamine the views and goals of biological enhancement with respect to the existential and moral challenges of increased individualized function. *Ghost* suggests the possibility of self-preservation and the relief of existential suffering through a paradoxical loss of individual self leading to a higher evolution of being. The film likewise suggests that true enhancement occurs through a continuation of self as assimilated into a larger and novel connectedness with another self.

This chapter explores the ways in which *Ghost in the Shell* challenges the contemporary bioethics of enhancement through philosophical discussions of self, meaning, and value. The idea of an enhanced self requires a nuanced understanding of the nature of the self. To further explore the themes of *Ghost* with respect to enhancement, I turn to three figures from American pragmatism and phenomenology who paid careful attention to the nature of the self. From these twentieth-century thinkers, three ideas concerning the self are of particular import: the notions of the social self, of spheres of meaning, and of connectedness with the past. I also discuss briefly the autobiography of Jean-Dominique Bauby, whose narrative of disability following a stroke sheds additional light on the nature of the self.

Ghost in the Shell: The Story

Ghost in the Shell is an adaptation of a manga written by Masamune Shirow, which tells the story of Major Motoko Kusanagi (the Major). The Major is a statuesque female whose body has been largely replaced by cybernetic parts. Although the Major began life as a wholly organic human, only a portion of her brain remains from her original body. This cyborg body allows her to be stronger and faster than noncybernetic humans. As a cyborg, she is also able to "jack into" electronic networks to parse data through a direct neural interface. She can almost fully immerse herself in the digital sphere of meaning, although this interface appears more observational than truly immersive. She can look through and find data but does not have a presence in the digital world. We find that the Major feels disconnected from the physical and social worlds in which she finds herself immersed. Other characters in the story play foil for her character, given their varying degrees of synthetic bodies. These range from the almost completely organically human to the completely artificial. In the Major's society, the "ghost" is the unique pattern or element that distinguishes a human person from a machine no matter how mechanized the person becomes or how seemingly real the machine acts. In this way, as long as the Major and others continue to have a unique, nondecaying "ghost" they are persons of moral worth and respect. Because of neural interfaces implanted in most people, it is possible to break into and modify human "ghosts" in the same way that hackers can break into computer systems. In *Ghost* this is referred to as a "ghost hack" and can be thought of as the ultimate type of brainwashing.

At the beginning of the film, we find the Major leading an elite squad of covert government police. The primary action of the story centers on finding a ghost hacker whose code name is the Puppetmaster. This code name is given because he hacks into people's ghosts and controls their memory and volition, as if they were puppets.[1] During the search for the Puppetmaster, the audience encounters many isolated and sad individuals who believe their lives have purpose and integration only because of having been ghost-hacked. The ghost hacker's use of these lonely people highlights the Major's own loneliness and feelings of being owned by the government. For instance, the ghost-hacked garbage collector is made to believe he has a family to motivate him to act in certain ways. In reality, he has no significant human relationships, and his existence is portrayed as lacking meaning because of this. In a pivotal scene, the Major waxes philosophical about her existence while diving underwater for pleasure. Engulfed in the sea that could kill her given her lack of buoyancy, she claims to feels connected with life and living in a way she cannot attain during her daily existence.[2] In spite of being motor and memory enhanced, the Major experiences a decreased connectedness to the world in which she interacts. This is exacerbated as she recognizes that the government agencies that employ her continue to deceive her, use her as a pawn in political games, and deprive her of a true social network. The enhancement technology has been developed and implemented with the aim of political usefulness and does not reflect attention to the needs of the self who was to be enhanced.

The Puppetmaster, developed by the government, is an artificial intelligence (AI) who unexpectedly gained self-awareness and acquired a ghost of his own. With this acquisition of a ghost, he developed a desire to create and procreate as a way of achieving meaning through permanence, evolution, and connectedness. After escaping from government computers, the Puppetmaster attempts to accomplish this procreation, which he understands as distinct and different from replicating digital copies of his ghost. When the Puppetmaster finally makes an appearance in the film, he inhabits a freshly manufactured, statuesque female cyborg body. He uses this body to communicate his circumstances and propose a merger with the Major.

During the climax of the movie's action, the bodies of both the Major and the Puppetmaster are physically destroyed. At that moment of destruction, their ghosts merge and make a virtual escape. During the denouement, this merged consciousness is "downloaded" into a little girl's body, from which the ghost(s) is (are) left to explore a new existence. The new life is portrayed as a dynamic melding of the previous characters that provides a refreshed experience of existence. Although the movie ends on a somber note, it is filled with hope and expectation about the unknown but novel life. The movie intimates that the merged selves will struggle but will gain existential satisfaction. Their existence is enhanced.

Enhancement, Bioethics, and Selves

The bioethics debate over enhancement has usually focused on individuals' functional improvements through genetics, surgery, or pharmaceuticals, including debates over surgery and steroids in sports, drugs like Ritalin in academics, and genetic manipulation in eugenic pursuits. The discussions have been framed in terms of costs to nonenhanced or disabled individuals, costs to society, or conflicts of individual liberty versus community control (Murray 2002; Conrad and Potter 2004; Kamm 2005; Lauritzen 2005; Mehlman 2005; Ford 2006). A good example is the debate over preimplantation genetic testing, in which embryos are tested before in vitro implantation for certain genes that parents want to select for or against (Sandel 2004). Even broad-stroke arguments of the transhumanists, those who believe that technology will provide the next step in a Darwinian evolution of humankind, have rarely suggested that the improvement of a particular function might in fact be a denigration for the individual rather than an enhancement.

One notable exception to this in the general dialogue about enhancement technologies is the concept that individual functional enhancement might break "solidarity" between people. For example, Robert (2005) emphasizes solidarity in terms of social inequities, yet his argument is in the same realm of the discussion in *Ghost in the Shell* regarding technologies as potentially distancing the functionally enhanced individual from others in society. This distancing then leads to a denigration of existence both for the enhanced and all others around him. Although the critique of the negative influence of technology on social interactions is not new (Forster 1970; Lachs 1981; Zuboff 1988; Ford 2000), the concept that an improvement in core body function can be socially distancing is a much rarer discussion.

George Herbert Mead

George Herbert Mead (1863–1931) was an American pragmatist whose works resonate strongly with the phenomenological tradition. Mead's writing deals extensively with the experience of individuals within a social context. He posits that the self, properly understood, has two important components, "me" and "I," both of which are understood only in relationship to other people. The "I" is evoked through the responses of others, while the "me" is the organized attitudes of others that are incorporated within the self (Mead 1934/1967, p. 175). The "I" includes the innovative portions of a self that are private. This would be the portion we see during the Major's underwater diving. The voice-over provides reflection of the inner self. However, the "I" still makes reference to and arises in the context of other people and environments in which she interacts. This is the individual's response or experience mediated by interactions with all factors. The "me" is defined and can be known by others because it consists in the understanding and expectations created by the melding of the judgments and interactions of others. The Major's "me" is composed of all the other characters' actions and attitudes toward her. This distinction between "I" and "me" does not map on neatly to a first person versus third person perspective on an individual, however. The "me" is part of the self's understanding as much as the "I." Both aspects of the self are defined in light of or through other community members. "When a self does appear it always involves an experience of another; there could not be an experience of self simply by itself" (Mead 1934/1967, p. 195).

It is clear in this understanding of a self that the primary organizing factors of an individual are found in the community of others. "The organized community or social group which gives to the individual his unity of self may be called 'the generalized other.' The attitude of the generalized other is the attitude of the whole community" (Mead 1934/1967, p. 156). In this way, for Mead, the richest or most enhanced community is one that facilitates diversity and expression of impulses. It is when communities create moments of self-expression for an individual that she finds her true value. "The situation in which one can let himself go, in which the very structure of the 'me' opens the door for the 'I,' is favorable to self expression" (Mead 1934/1967, p. 213). Simply put, an integrated social setting that yet allows for unique expression provides an important satisfaction for a self. Through these situations and expressions, the self becomes fulfilled as an individual and fulfills valued social functions. "Now if this situation is such that it opens the door to impulsive expression one gets a peculiar satisfaction, high or low, the source of which is the value expression of the 'I' in the social process" (Mead 1934/1967, p. 213).

Throughout *Ghost in the Shell,* the Major emphasizes the importance of diversity on her team. A mix of old and new, as well as organic and machine, creates the possibility for plasticity and creativity. This openness to diversity allows for evolutionary processes to protect populations from devastating events like viruses. This diversity also provides meaning and uniqueness to the individual. The ability to be more than mere "robots" provides benefit both to the individual and to the society even if at first it appears to be a weakness or inferiority. The unique propagation created by the merge of Major and Puppetmaster creates the possibility for a novel expression of self. Susan Napier, an Asian studies scholar at Tufts University, commenting on the film, identifies one aspect of this merge as a way of freeing from stereotypes imposed by the government (Napier 2001, p. 114). One could read this as the Major and the Puppetmaster both being allowed to express their "impulsive expression" through the merge that otherwise would have been suppressed by their community.

Alfred Schutz

Alfred Schutz (1899–1959) was a phenomenologist who explored varieties of styles of meaning and interactions found in the experiences of everyday life. He discusses these in terms of provinces or spheres of meaning. Each person, according to Schutz, has multiple provinces of meaning depending on social circumstances, tasks at hand, and roles to be played. "The transition from one province of meaning to another can only be accomplished by means of a 'leap' (in Kierkegaard's sense). This 'leap' is nothing other than the exchange of one style of lived experience for another" (Schutz and Luckmann 1973, p. 24).

Schutz here refers to the type of leap that Sören Kierkegaard (1813–1855), a nineteenth-century Danish philosopher, postulates as being necessary to have a belief in God in spite of a lack of physical evidence. These types of shifts are clearly dramatized in a number of instances in *Ghost,* including when the Major jacks into the information network during the swimming scene and even when characters get ghost-hacked. In many ways, the integration of the Puppetmaster and the Major is not an abandonment of a single reality, but rather it is an alternation in spheres of meaning. For Schutz, the digital is not virtual but is real because of its associated meanings. In this way, unreal are those spheres of meaning that do not engage fully the attention of the self.

Spheres of meanings are not without some hierarchy or moral substance, however, and Schutz's philosophy does not collapse into a complete relativism, with every sphere of meaning being equally real or good. Schutz has very specific ideas about the reasons for which a person cannot (or at least should not) persist in a world of pure fantasy: "As long as I live in fantasy worlds, I cannot 'produce,' in the sense of an act which gears into the external world and alters it. As long as I tarry in the world of fantasy I cannot accomplish anything, save just to engage in fantasy" (Schutz and Luckmann 1973, p. 29). This idea of production has wrapped up in it an idea of obligations to others and the value of creating something that is tangible. Schutz at least begins to create a vocabulary to open a discussion of the meanings imposed by the physical and digital worlds.

Although the Major-Puppetmaster union may be criticized as encouraging an irresponsible enhancement because the meld appears to advocate abandoning what Schutz might call "the sphere of meaning of everydayness," the new combined self still resides within a physical reality—the little girl. The child's body is much more vulnerable and physically inferior to those the Major and the Puppetmaster possessed before the meld. The action of their reintegration into society through such novel means can be reflected in real-world scenarios. In our contemporary society we see a re-embodying of alienated persons into virtual communities via the Internet that involve gaining responsibilities and meanings (Ford 2003). The richness of such people's experience depends less on their actual physical activity than it does on the richness of meanings they acquire throughout their experiences—digitally mediated and physically mediated.

William Ernest Hocking

William Ernest Hocking (1873–1966) was an American idealist and pragmatist who strongly emphasized the context and role of the individual. Given the strong themes of histories and evolution in *Ghost,* it is interesting to note Hocking's explanation of the role of heredity and the body with relation to the self. "We must regard the body not as an appendage of the mind nor as a detachable instrument, but as an inseparable organ. The self is a system of meanings, but not of meanings without facts" (Hocking 1928, p. 95). The self incorporates and, in part, *is* the physical element of the body; so this is not a strictly dualist picture of two separate things, mind and body. For Hocking, the facts that give shape to the self are deeply influenced by history and heritage. The self is connected to an archive of the past. "The body, then, is a portal, not a possession. And through this portal the self peers out into a dark and cavernous background in which the perspectives of its living past merge insensibly with the vast shapes of physical nature" (Hocking 1928, p. 110).

So, the self is a set of meanings that draw from the past history and lineage, expressed through a physicality. That physicality is always in the context of the past, the present, and the future, with death and birth being the linkage. Michael Pinsky, an English professor and film critic, makes a great deal out of ghosts, death, and existence in comparing the themes of *Ghost* with several other anime films. In many ways death through merging, as with the two main characters in *Ghost,* brings meaning that allows progression of family lines through chance. The film has several important references to history and heritage. In the battle directly proceeding the merging of the Major and the Puppetmaster, the screen is filled with a stone carving of a family tree, which is obliterated by gunfire during the scene. This scene emphasizes the importance of a structured line of progression and a connectedness with the past, while also demonstrating traditional ways being overcome through the destruction. The linkage of heredity is both acknowledged and done away with at the same time.

Just as a child is a new body that merges the heredity of two selves, so does the new merging of two characters into one create a new corporality of existence with a different type of heredity. The new self is enhanced not by being free of a body but by still having a physical portal to the outside with a new and more robust heredity to draw on.[3] The memory of this new heredity is preserved and does not rely on only the traces lingering in the growing body of a child. Yet the body's growth plays an important role in giving a portal through which the self may be expressed.

Jean-Dominique Bauby

In his best-selling book, Jean-Dominique Bauby (1952–1997) describes his life after a stroke left him in a physically "locked-in" state (Bauby 1997). After a career as a magazine editor, Bauby found himself in a condition wherein eye blinking became his only significant means of communication. He lost the physical ability to move the majority of his body voluntarily. During his stay in a rehabilitation hospital, he dictated a short autobiography by blinking his eye as his secretary moved a pointer across a board containing letters of the alphabet. Letter by letter he described his thoughts and understandings of himself in his new state of being: His mind was like a butterfly and his body a diving suit.[4] In his writings, Bauby demonstrates a significant movement of self away from a definition based on bodily function toward that of intellectual understanding. There is a tension between having to redefine himself as a completely different self and a desire to retain the spheres of meanings he previously experienced. Even with very little bodily movement, he remained a self with a richness of mental experience. The physical interactions between Bauby and others changed, and the meanings of these interactions changed.

Bauby's story is a striking way to explore the value placed on enhancement of his life through human interactions. Denise Dudzniski (2001), a bioethicist, makes much of his adaption to his new set of meanings in "re-membering" himself. This play on "member" as a part of the physical body and of memory as a cognitive activity brings attention to the richness of possibilities in redefining and recognizing the importance of our connectedness with others. Although Bauby's life was not enhanced by the stroke, it was significantly altered in such ways as to produce a valuable text that is now used as a teaching tool about the diversity of lives and selves. Through this experience, he was alienated and reintegrated at the same time, which speaks to the kinds of plasticities possible for an individual self. In *Ghost in the Shell,* the destruction of the body and the re-embodying brings about a shift in thinking. The "butterfly" for Bauby and the "ghost" for the Major both survive and flourish in spite of the costs to physical function exacted by Bauby's stroke and by the Major's merge with the Puppetmaster.

Misogynist or Feminist Subtext

In writing an essay on *Ghost in the Shell,* I would be irresponsible not to directly address the idealized and eroticized female bodies as well as the dismemberment of these bodies. On the surface, the film appears to be an adolescent male fantasy of violence and sex. Although no characters actually engage in explicit sexual interaction, the film is peppered with projections of Barbie Doll–like female bodies that are slowly panned by the camera, often in some state of undress. In the first scene, the Major is scantily clad, disrobes, and then turns invisible. In the opening credits we see a naked robot body being created. When the Puppetmaster and the Major "merge," their arms and legs have been in some way destroyed, leaving their idealized half-naked torsos. There is even a shot during the movie of naked female mannequins, which end up dismembered or destroyed in some way or another. These scenes easily reinforce the unrealistic Western stereotypes of idealized female bodies and demonstrate considerable violence toward female characters. This film may in itself reinforce the denigration of women, which has a significant history in film.

In defiance of this stereotype, *Ghost in the Shell* has a strong subtext that challenges the very idealized and sexualized female bodies that it portrays. It figuratively and literally attempts to destroy these idealized bodies both in form and in the valuing of these types of beauty enhancements. Although the large-breasted, thin-waisted bodies are portrayed as ideal and enhanced, these bodies are also the very selves who appear most distanced from happiness. They appear to have the least enhanced state of being. In the end, the Major abandons her idealized body that both set her physically apart from others and made her the generically idealized female form in her community. In these ways, the apparent enhancement of the body turns out to be precisely the opposite of this and a denigration of experience and meaning. Read in this light, the film strongly argues against ideal and uniform bodies. The violence in the film then could be read as violence toward the idea of the artificial and denigrated enhanced female form rather than against women in general. However, the reading of this is open as to whether the subtext justifies the possibility of a misreading that reinforces the opposite meaning.

Conclusion

At the beginning of the film, the cyborg character of the Major demonstrates a type of technological evolution that enhances her physical and cognitive ability. In spite of, or because of, this, she experiences significant existential moral suffering or angst about her body modifications. The story explores ideas of an ultimate evolution as a complete loss of any particular physical enhancement and a gain of enhancement through distributive relationships that still have a physical presence. Simply, true enhancement of existence happened only when a character gave up the pursuit of physical enhancement to maximize the social connections that give rise to richer spheres of meaning. These ideas concerning the interrelationship of physical, moral, and existential modifications can be found in many of the film's characters. In fact, the themes are carried into, and enhanced in, the sequel entitled *Kôkaku kidôtai 2: Inosensu* (2004), distributed in English as *Ghost in the Shell: Innocence*, in which the main protagonist's relationship with a basset hound highlights his loneliness. The self that is most enhanced is not one that has its potential maximized organically nor mechanically. Rather, it is one that has enriched the important interconnectedness with others in a sphere of meaning that allows a great amount of individual unique expression.

Ghost calls into question the limits and challenges in contemporary biomedicine through the interplay between characters and through the repetition of the motif or refrain of "hacking" found throughout the film. Philosophically this refrain continually challenges the selection of appropriate enhancement goals for individuals and communities during technological shifts. The implications of "enhancing" a self in one aspect must take into account the expected effects in the social contexts in which the self has interplay. One can frame this discussion in terms of the multiplication of spheres of meanings within which each person interacts. These spheres exist within a history and future composed of varieties of individual selves and shape values. Independent of the framework in which one reads this *Ghost in the Shell,* it richly challenges our concepts regarding which enhancement goals are worthy of pursuit.

QUESTIONS FOR CONSIDERATION

1. *Could this unrealistic science-fictional occurrence depicted in* Ghost *be an allegory for another type of melding of persons? What current technologies could parallel the idea of two selves merging (beyond traditional procreation)?*

2. *What criteria would you use to judge when enhancing one trait or aspect of a person causes greater harm to the integrated whole of the person or community?*

3. *What is the difference between enhancement and eugenics when looking at reproductive or merging technologies?*

4. *Given the potential for the film to reinforce violence toward women as well as the display of idealized women's bodies as commodities, does the existence of this film in itself enhance or denigrate our social interactions?*

NOTES

1. In referring to the Puppetmaster, gendered pronouns become difficult. The Puppetmaster takes over a female cyborg body yet often speaks with a masculine voice.

Using *it* to refer to the Puppetmaster would be contrary to the postulate of the film that the Puppetmaster is a self, not a simple object or possession. The English dub of *Ghost* uses the masculine pronoun *he*. This convention is adopted for the current chapter for ease and consistency. The point should not be lost, however, that during the climactic "merging" scene, it is two female bodies that are connected. The imagery strongly suggests a critique on the value of a procreative joining of two females and hence could be seen as challenging contemporary heterosexual biases regarding relationships. This could be read as referring to lesbian relationships or the irrelevance of gender in important types of novel creations of self.

2. Clearly these ideas of integration with nature have strong Eastern themes. The juxtaposition of Eastern philosophy with Western technology and political structures creates a tension that runs throughout the film but is outside the scope of this chapter.

3. I take an opposite position on this point to Susan Napier, who understands the film as one of transcending corporeality (Napier 2001, pp. 37 and 104). However, Napier does rightly observe the strong theme of human connectedness, and loss of it, in her exploration of *Ghost* (Napier 2001, p. 106). We appear to disagree about the resolution of this lack of connectedness with relation to the physical body.

4. The popular English translation of *le scaphandre* is "diving bell." However, the direct translation of "diving suit" seems to be a much closer metaphor for his intention.

REFERENCES

Bauby, J. D. 1997. *The Diving Bell and the Butterfly*, trans. J. Legatt. New York: Alfred A. Knopf.

Conrad, P., and Potter, D. 2004. Human Growth Hormone and the Temptations of Biomedical Enhancement. *Sociology of Health and Illness* 26(2):184–215.

Dudzinski, D. 2001. The Diving Bell Meets the Butterfly: Identity Lost and Re-Membered. *Theoretical Medicine* 22:33–46.

Ford, P. J. 2000. Virtual Shifts in Disabling Realities: Disability, Computer Mediated Environments, and Selves. PhD diss., Vanderbilt University.

———. 2003. Virtually Impacted: Designers, Spheres of Meanings, and Virtual Communities. In *Virtual Morality*, ed. M. Wolf, 79–93. New York: Peter Lang Publishers.

———. 2006. From Treatment to Enhancement in Deep Brain Stimulation: A Question of Research Ethics. *The Pluralist* 1(2):35–44.

Forster, E. M. 1970. The Machine Stops. In *The Eternal Moment and Other Stories*. New York: Harcourt Brace.

Hocking, W. E. 1928. *The Self: Its Body and Freedom*. New Haven: Yale University Press.

Holt, J. 2002. The Machine-Made Ghost: Or, the Philosophy of Mind, Matrix Style. In The Matrix *and Philosophy,* ed. W. Irwin, 66–74. Chicago: Open Court.

Kamm, F. M. 2005. Is There a Problem with Enhancement? *American Journal of Bioethics* 5(3):5–14.

Lachs, J. 1981. *Intermediate Man*. Indianapolis, IN: Hackett.

Lauritzen, P. 2005. Stem Cells, Biotechnology, and Human Rights: Implications for a Posthuman Future. *Hastings Center Report* 35(2):25–33.

McMahon, J. L. 2002. Popping a Bitter Pill: Existential Authenticity in *The Matrix* and *Nausea*. In The Matrix *and Philosophy,* ed. W. Irwin. Chicago: Open Court.

Mead, G. H. 1967. *Mind, Self, and Society*. Vol. 1. Chicago: University of Chicago Press. (Originally published 1934)

Mehlman, M. J. 2005. Genetic Enhancement: Plan Now to Act Later. *Kennedy Institute of Ethics Journal* 15(1):77–82.

Murray, T. H. 2002. Reflections on the Ethics of Genetic Enhancement. *Genetics in Medicine* 4(6 Suppl): 27–32S.

Napier, S. J. 2001. *Anime from Akira to Princess Mononoke: Experiencing Contemporary Japanese Animation*. New York: Palgrave.

Oshii, M. 1995. *Kôkaku kidôtai* [English title: *Ghost in the Shell;* motion picture]. Tokyo: Bandai Visual Company.

———. 2004. *Kôkaku kidôtai 2: Inosensu* [English title: *Ghost in the Shell: Innocence*; motion picture]. Tokyo: Bandai Visual Company.

Pinsky, M. 2003. *Future Present: Ethics and/as Science Fiction*. Madison, NJ: Fairleigh Dickinson University Press.

Robert, J. S. 2005. Human Dispossession and Human Enhancement. *American Journal of Bioethics* 5(3):27–29.

Sandel, M. J. 2004. The Case against Perfection: What's Wrong with Designer Children, Bionic Athletes, and Genetic Engineering. *Atlantic Monthly,* April, 51–62.

Schutz, A., and Luckmann, T. 1973. *Structures of the Life-World,* trans. by R. Zaner and H. T. Englehardt. Evanston, IL: Northwestern University Press.

Wrathall, M. A. 2005. The Purpose of Life Is to End: Schopenhauerian Pessimism, Nihilism, and Nietzschean Will to Power. In *More* Matrix *and Philosophy Revolutions and Reloaded Decoded,* ed. W. Irwin, 50–66. Chicago: Open Court.

Zuboff, S. 1988. *In the Age of the Smart Machine: The Future of Work and Power*. New York: Basic Books.

ELEVEN

Commodification, Exploitation, and the Market for Transplant Organs

A Discussion of *Dirty Pretty Things*

Clark Wolf

> The hotel business is about strangers. And strangers will always surprise you, you know? They come to hotels in the night to do dirty things, and in the morning it's our job to make things all pretty again.
>
> SNEAKY, *Dirty Pretty Things*

In the film *Dirty Pretty Things* (Frears 2002), one of the main characters, Okwe (played by Chiwetel Ejiofor), discovers that his employer, "Sneaky" (played by Sergi Lopez), is running a peculiar business. During the day Sneaky seems an ordinary hotelier. But on the side he runs a service to provide counterfeit passports for illegal immigrants who wish to remain in Britain. He arranges for poor immigrants to "donate" one of their kidneys, which he sells to people in need of a transplant. In return, he provides the "donors" with forged passports or immigration documents. Unfortunately he employs an incompetent physician to perform the surgery. We never discover how many of those who participate in Sneaky's scheme die after their kidneys are removed. But what we discover about the procedure gives us reason to believe that few could survive.

In the course of the film, we discover that Okwe is in fact a surgeon from Nigeria. Over time, Okwe finds himself drawn further and further into Sneaky's world: Sneaky uses Okwe's own goodness as a weapon to manipulate him by showing him pictures of a little girl he (Sneaky) says will be saved by the pending kidney transplant (Mills 1995). Okwe is also drawn in because of his friendship with a Turkish immigrant, Senay (played by Audrey Tautou), and his concern to protect her from Sneaky's incompetent surgeon. It is Okwe's own virtue that tempts him to participate in Sneaky's scheme. As Okwe's friend Guo Yi (played by Benedict Wong) says, "There's nothing more dangerous than a virtuous man."

The film raises many different issues, only some of which will be discussed here. One important issue that occupies center stage is the specific problem of whether it is morally permissible for people to sell and buy transplant organs. While the arrangement described in the film is horrific, some people urge that the main problem with the existing transplant organ system is the *absence* of a legitimate market, rather than the existence of a black market. Another issue addressed in the film is that of commodification or marketization: Are there some things that simply should not be bought and sold on an open market, even when the participants are consenting adults? Can we legitimately prohibit people from selling things they own or control, like their kidneys? Like sex? Finally, there is the problem of exploitation: Sneaky exploits people who are willing to take an enormous risk only because they are desperate. Is their choice to sell their kidneys *voluntary*, or do the circumstances in which the choice is made undermine its freedom? If one judges that the risk of selling her kidney is worth taking, do we nonetheless have a right to interfere?

A Market for Transplant Organs? (Is Sneaky Selling Happiness?)

> If you were just some African, the deal would be simple. You give me your kidney; I give you a new identity. I sell the kidney for 10 grand, so I am happy. The person who needs the kidney gets cured, so he is happy. The person who sold his kidney gets to stay in this beautiful country, so he is happy. My whole business is based on happiness.
>
> SNEAKY, *Dirty Pretty Things*

As I write this sentence, more than 90,000 people in the United States are waiting for transplant organs (Institute of Medicine 2006). About 66,000 of them are waiting for kidneys (Postrel 2006a, 2006b). By the time you read it, the number will almost certainly be much larger, because people are added to the list much faster than they leave it. Some people leave the list when they receive a transplant. But many more will leave the list because they will die waiting for one. Every year between four and six thousand people in the United States die waiting in vain to receive the transplant they would have needed to survive. Today alone more than a dozen people will die in the United States because they were unable to acquire an appropriate organ for transplant. We have a shortage of transplant organs, and because of this shortage people are dying every day.

Where might the missing transplant organs come from? Some transplant organs, like hearts, can come available only at the death of the donor. Others, like kidneys, can be donated by living individuals. As long as one's remaining kidney is functioning normally, a person can live as well with one as with two. Donation does increase the donor's risk, however: in the event that a donor herself later develops kidney disease, she may have given away what would have saved her life. But every year, more than ten thousand people die whose organs would be appropriate for transplant, but of these only about half actually donate their organs. The problem might be solved and lives saved if we could provide a motive or an incentive for those who have *not* made arrangements to donate their organs.

What are your options if you are one of those people whose survival depends on getting a transplant organ? If you need a kidney transplant, you can get on the waiting list and hope that a kidney becomes available before your situation becomes critical. If you are fortunate, you may have a friend or family member willing to donate an organ to save your health or your life. But what if you can't wait that long? What if you know that you are among the four thousand who will die this year if you don't receive a transplant, and what if the likelihood that you will receive what you need is slim?

If you are wealthy, then you may not need to wait and hope. There is an alternative available for you: you could purchase your kidney in a thriving international black market. In 2004, the *New York Times* published a detailed account of an international market that connects poor organ donors with wealthy Americans in need of organ transplants:

> When Alberty José da Silva heard he could make money, lots of money, by selling his kidney, it seemed to him the opportunity of a lifetime. For a desperately ill 48-year-old woman in Brooklyn whose doctors had told her to get a kidney any way she could, it was. At 38,

> Mr. da Silva, one of 23 children of a prostitute, lives in a slum near the airport here, in a flimsy two-room shack he shares with a sister and nine other people. "As a child, I can remember seven of us sharing a single egg, or living for day after day on just a bit of manioc meal with salt," Mr. da Silva said in an interview. He recalled his mother as a woman who "sold her flesh" to survive. Last year he decided that he would, too. Now, a long scar across his side marks the place where a kidney and a rib were removed in exchange for $6,000, paid by middlemen in an international organ trafficking ring.
>
> (ROTHER 2004)

The movie *Dirty Pretty Things* is a work of fiction. But the problems it addresses are real problems that real people face every day. Is it morally defensible to allow poor people to sell their organs to rich people? We might object that such arrangements are exploitative in the sense that they take advantage of the unfortunate predicament of the donors. But some might respond that these donors would be better off if they were able to sell their kidneys than they would be if they were unable to do so. Those who accept payment must value the cash more than they value what they're giving up, or else they wouldn't be willing to make the exchange. Are there some things that just shouldn't be bought and sold on the market? And what right do we have to interfere in a voluntary exchange between consenting adults? Should people have a right to decide for themselves which risks they should take and which they should avoid, or do we have a right to intervene and make the decision for them?

Perhaps the reason we prohibit people from selling their kidneys for transplant is that this procedure involves risks for the donor. Still, under most circumstances people are responsible for their own risks, and other people have no right to intervene to prevent them from taking risks they themselves have considered and accepted. If I wish to run risks by biking to work (which involves much greater personal risk than driving a car would), or to spend my leisure time climbing cliffs, the decision is my own. In these cases, you could pay me to take the risk in question without violating the law. But in the United States, if you pay me to have my kidney removed, you (and I) have violated the law. What is the difference between these cases? If the risks are comparable, why do we allow the law to intervene in one case and not in the others?

Consider the arrangement from the perspective of the donor: Alberty da Silva received six thousand dollars for his kidney. As long as he was appropriately informed about the risks he undertook, what right have we to tell him that the risk is too great? The woman who received Mr. da Silva's kidney was apparently out of options. She told Larry Rother, of the *New York Times,* "My doctors told me to 'get a kidney any way I could' or expect to die" (Rother 2004). Several economically strapped countries now advertise themselves as good places for surgical operations; large numbers of wealthy Americans and Europeans now go abroad to South Africa or to India for surgery that would be prohibitively expensive in their home countries (Alsever 2006). This facilitates the flow of money and resources from the developed world toward cash-strapped nations in the global South. Economists urge that such trade arrangements are more effective than international aid packages that seek to promote economic security in poor countries. If these arrangements are advantageous for everyone involved, if they save the lives of people who would otherwise die, then what justification can we give for the laws that prevent them? No justification for such prohibitions seems immediately apparent; however, if these trade arrangements involve organ donation from the desperate to the well-heeled, the practice in this case seems exploitative.

According to John Stuart Mill's famous "harm principle," state intervention in individual behavior is justified only to prevent harm to others. When other people make choices we disapprove of, we may let them know; but if their questionable choices are harmless, or harm no one but themselves, we have no right to interfere. However, one need not accept Mill's harm principle to think that legislation that limits people's liberty must be justified by very good reasons, especially when we are preventing people from doing things that will save lives. The prohibition on kidney sales interferes with people's voluntary choices and prevents them from engaging in a life-preserving exchange. Unless there are very strong reasons to justify interference with such exchanges, we should not interfere.

Persuaded by this argument, many economists and bioethicists urge that we should change the existing practice by opening up a legal, regulated market for transplant organs (Boudreaux and Pritchard 1999; Morley 2003; Roth et al. 2004). In the case of organs like kidneys, which can be given by living donors, this could involve a direct market linking donors who would sell their organs to the recipients who would buy them. But arrangements could also be made for the post-mortem sale of transplant organs: donors could arrange for payment to be made to their families and heirs at the time of death. In this way, organ donation could become an additional life-insurance policy benefiting bereaved families who may need resources to help compensate from lost income due to a wage-earner's death. For some families, such a benefit could be very important indeed, so this might provide a powerful incentive to donate for people whose organs would otherwise be buried with them.

Sneaky claims, in the quotation at the head of this section, that his "whole business is based on happiness." Of course, he is lying: his business is based on blood and death, not on happiness. Because he doesn't care about the welfare of the penniless and powerless donors, he is able to exploit them for their organs without concerning himself with their welfare. Some—perhaps most of them—pay for their forged passports and identification papers with their lives. But defenders of a legal and regulated market for transplant organs would not regard this as an objection to their position: if we leave such arrangements to the black market, or force them underground with legislative prohibition, we should expect that the market will be managed by unscrupulous criminals like Sneaky. To avoid this, we would need to regulate the practice of organ transfer and to insure appropriate care for donors and recipients. But regulation will only become possible when the practice itself becomes legal.

If these arguments are correct, then the following would be true: (1) An appropriately regulated market for transplant organs could improve the situation of everyone involved in it. (2) Only if such markets are legal can they be appropriately regulated. (3) Unregulated markets will exist even if the sale of transplant organs is declared illegal, because some desperate people will do whatever they can to preserve their lives, and because there are plenty of people who would be willing to provide transplant organs on the black market.

These considerations constitute a powerful argument in favor of a policy that would open up a legal and legitimate market for transplant organs. To evaluate the argument more fully, we would need to articulate the details of the policy with precision. Then we would need to compare it with the status quo and with other plausible alternatives. We would also need to address specific objections that would apply to any such policy—objections that are brilliantly explored in the film under consideration.

Here we will consider two such objections: the first urges that some things simply should not be bought and sold—should not, by their very nature, be turned into commodities. The second common objection appeals to considerations of justice: it urges that a market for transplant organs would facilitate the exploitation of the weak and poor by the strong and the wealthy. The next two sections of this chapter will address each of these concerns.

Questionable Commodification of Sex and Kidneys (Selling What Should Not Be Sold?)

TRANSPLANT ORGAN COURIER: How come I've never seen you people before?

OKWE: It is because we are the people you do not see. We are the ones who drive your cabs, who clean your rooms, and suck your cocks.

It is often argued that there are some things that just shouldn't be bought and sold—shouldn't be turned into "commodities" (Radin 1996). Consider sex first: Juliette (played by Sophie Okonedo) is a "sex-worker," a prostitute who provides sexual services to anyone who can afford to pay. Like a kidney, sex is often regarded as something that should not be exchanged for money, and indeed many nations and states have laws prohibiting prostitution for just this reason.

Different reasons can be given in defense of laws prohibiting prostitution: Sometimes it is argued that such laws promote gender equality, because women who are prostitutes do not interact on equal terms with those who pay them for sex. Or it may be argued that prostitution often involves serious risks to health, and other risks as well, because prostitutes are often the victims of criminal violence. It may also be argued that prostitution alienates people from their own sexuality, changing the meaning of sex from an expression of tenderness and affection into a mere market exchange (Nussbaum 1999).

The character of Juliette invites us to question all of these assumptions: she is presented as a strong and sensitive person with a powerful sense of self-respect. Her strength, humor, and compassion make it possible for her to comfort Senay after Senay has been abused and (arguably) raped by Sneaky. In many respects, Juliette appears to be the strongest and most well-adjusted person in the film.

Of course, Juliette is a fictional character and represents a common stereotype: a well-adjusted "hooker with a heart of gold" appears in many films. The stereotypic image may be appealing in part because it provides false comfort for people who would rather not think about the squalid, dangerous, and unfortunate lives many prostitutes endure. In the real world, prostitution exposes women to very serious risks, both physical and psychological. And it seems plausible that these dangers do stem from the problematic commodification of the body that prostitution involves. It would be better from the moral point of view if people expressed tenderness and affection in their sex lives instead of turning them into mere exchanges. But even if we grant all of these points it would not follow that laws prohibiting prostitution are justifiable: In most circumstances, people have a right to engage in mutually consensual though morally questionable relationships with each other, and third parties do not have a valid claim to interfere. Beyond this, it is quite clear that laws prohibiting prostitution "punish the victims," because the penalties fall hardest on those who engage in it, not on their customers (Nussbaum 1999). Laws criminalizing prostitution cannot possibly be justified on grounds that they protect or benefit the women who are or who would otherwise become prostitutes.

In a similar vein, it can be argued that people should not commodify their bodies and their internal organs. This reasoning is often used to justify the prohibition on organ sales. Arguably, there is something morally problematic about viewing our bodies or body parts as commodities to be bought and sold. But to urge that commodification is morally problematic is not enough to show that other people are justified to interfere with those who are forced by circumstances to make tragic choices. Just as it seems to be worse for poor women when prostitution is made illegal, it may be worse for poor people when they are unable to make their own decisions whether or not to turn their spare kidneys into cash.

Perhaps there really is something morally problematic about the commodification of bodily organs. Maybe people shouldn't consider their body parts as marketable items ready to be sold to the highest bidder. But if so, then the badness of such commodification must be set against the competing reasons that militate in favor of legal and regulated markets for transplant organs: in particular, the possibility that such markets might improve the situation of everyone involved and might save the lives of thousands of people who need transplants. It is not obvious that this point about commodification provides any conclusive reason against either laws prohibiting prostitution or laws prohibiting a market for transplant organs. It is legally and socially permissible to sell some body products, including human eggs, blood, and sperm. If we are not bothered by markets for these items, then isn't the concern about the commodification of transplant organs overblown?

Some things should not be available on a market at any price: the prohibition on slavery means that we can't buy people. The prohibition on some other things, like child sex, is uncontroversial. It seems clear that people and children should not be commodified in these ways, and we have good reasons that underlie our concerns in these cases. But where we object that it is inappropriate to commodify some item, we should be able to articulate the moral reasons that lie behind our objection. It is not enough to use the commodification objection as a conversation stopper, especially where people's lives and well-being are at stake. In this case, since people are literally dying every day because of the lack of transplant organs, the commodification argument must be supported with the strongest underlying reasons and argument. Unless we have such an argument, the claim that we should not commodify our bodies is not by itself a strong enough reason to forbid a market for transplant organs.

Injustice and Exploitative Offers (Leveraging Personal Advantage from the Poor and Desperate?)

> For you and me, there is only survival.
>
> OKWE

> Financial incentives [for transplant organs] might disproportionately affect the poor or other marginalized groups, and might also cause a drop in donations for altruistic reasons if people see donated organs as goods with a certain market value. And nonfinancial incentives, such as reciprocity agreements, might disadvantage those who are less informed about organ donation and therefore increase existing social inequality.
>
> INSTITUTE OF MEDICINE REPORT

Why does Senay consent to trade her kidney for a passport? It is because she is absolutely desperate. Why did Alberty da Silva sell his kidney for six thousand dollars? Because he was very poor and needed the money. It is worth asking whether such exchanges are impermissibly exploitative in the sense that they take advantage of people who are very poor and who would not be willing to put their lives and health at risk if they were not desperate. When Okwe tells Senay "For you and me, there is only survival" he drives home the point that they have few options. Senay's life in London is intolerably bad. She concludes that her only option, the only thing she can do to pursue her hope for a decent life, is to sell her kidney to Sneaky. If people are willing to sell their kidneys only because they have no other options, is their decision even voluntary? In such a situation, is a purchase offer exploitative?

To understand the sense in which these arrangements may be impermissibly exploitative, we need to distinguish between at least two different senses of the term *exploitation*, which will be explored below.

> *E1-Exploitation*: A exploits B when A intentionally causes B to fall into an unfortunate predicament, and then uses B's misfortune as a lever to manipulate B into doing what A wants B to do.

E1-exploitation is the classic sense of the term found in the writings of Karl Marx (1818–1883). Marx regarded capitalists as not only the cause of the misery of workers but also as persons who take advantage of the misery they have created to increase their own wealth and power. An example may help to make the moral objection to E1-exploitative arrangements clear:

> *Example:* Alph meets Beth at a bar, and she tells him she's planning to drive out into the desert. While she's in the bathroom, Alph sidles out to Beth's car, slashes the spare, and puts a slow leak in one of the tires. Then as Beth heads out for the desert, Alph quietly finishes his beer, planning to go out to find Beth after the tire goes flat and after enough time has passed that her life is in danger from the heat. On finding desperate Beth, Alph offers to sell her his spare provided that she signs over the deed to her house and pays him all the money in her savings account.

The existing black market for kidneys is not E1-exploitative unless those who arrange for the sale of transplant organs intentionally put the prospective donors into the desperate predicament that renders them willing to sell. In the case of Alberty da Silva and others involved in the South African transplant ring discussed above, da Silva's poverty was not caused by those who offered to buy his kidney. And in *Dirty Pretty Things,* the desperation of the poor immigrants who sell their kidneys is not caused by Sneaky; he just takes advantage of their plight. We need another sense of exploitation to identify the problem:

> *E2-Exploitation:* B is in an unfortunate predicament, for which A is not responsible. But A takes advantage of the unfortunate predicament of B, using B's misfortune as a lever to manipulate B into doing what A wants B to do.

Once again, an example may make this clear:

> *Example:* Alph is driving through the desert and by chance finds Beth stuck on the road in a desperate and life-threatening situation with a flat tire and no spare. Alph offers to sell Beth his spare tire provided that she signs over the deed to her house and pays Alph all the money in her savings account.

In this case, Alph does not intentionally *cause* Beth's misfortune; he just takes advantage of it. While his offer may save her life, clearly he doesn't deserve any praise for making it. While there is clearly something seriously wrong with arrangements like this one, it does not follow that anyone else has a right to interfere with E2-exploitative arrangements unless they are also willing to do something to improve the predicament of the person who is exploited (Sample 2003). Legislative prohibition of E2-exploitative arrangements would certainly be misplaced if the object of such legislation were to improve the situation of the exploited.

One might be inclined to regard Sneaky's exploitation of poor immigrants as E2-exploitation. Sneaky doesn't directly or intentionally cause the poverty and desperation of those he exploits. If their predicament is unjust (as it certainly is), he is no more responsible than others—no more responsible than we are, for example—for the initial injustice that leaves them willing to take an enormous risk. E2-exploitation leaves its victims better off than they would otherwise be. But because his surgeon is incompetent, because Sneaky doesn't care whether the donors live or die, those who sell their kidneys to him are much worse off as a result. So even if we accept the view that third parties usually have no business interfering with E2-exploitative arrangements, it would certainly not follow that we should leave Sneaky to continue to exploit (and murder) his victims.

What is peculiar about E2-exploitation is that the exploitative offer actually improves the situation of the person who is exploited. This is not the case for E1-exploitation. If we were to prohibit Alph from selling the tire to Beth in this outrageous offer, as a result she will be even worse off than she already is. Some people take this fact as a conclusive argument that E2-exploitation is not unfair to those who are exploited. Thus, Sally Satel writes, in the *New York Times*:

> Some critics worry that compensation for kidney donation by the living would be most attractive to the poor and hence exploit them. But if it were government-regulated we could ensure that donors would receive education about their choices, undergo careful medical and psychological screening and receive quality follow-up care. We could even make a donation option that favors the well-off by rewarding donors with a tax credit. Besides, how is it unfair to poor people if compensation enhances their quality of life? (SATEL 2006)

Satel's argument radically understates the moral problems involved. We should be troubled by the case of Alberty da Silva, whose poverty drove him to give up his kidney. It is certainly unfair in an ordinary sense that some people are born to poverty and cruelly limited opportunities. A world that includes unfairness of this kind is *unjust* in a significant sense. If we could eliminate the injustice that left Mr. da Silva in this predicament, then perhaps he would be less willing to sell his kidney. We should at least expect that he would demand a higher market price.

The relatively well-off citizens of wealthy nations do not intentionally cause the poverty of people like Alberty da Silva. It follows from this that their interactions with him are not E1-exploitative. But it would be a mistake to assume that the wealth and security enjoyed by people in economically strong nations is unconnected with the predicament of people in poor countries. As Thomas Pogge (2002) pointed out, our wealth is supported in part by institutions that impose serious disadvantages on poor people in authoritarian nations.

One such institution is the "international borrowing privilege," which allows dictators in poor countries to obtain money and credit on the international market and to assign the debt to their *nation*. Thus, a dictator might borrow money in the name of the nation and use these funds to secure power and to forcefully eliminate political opposition. Obviously the people of the nation gain no benefits from this borrowing: the benefits are entirely private and enjoyed by the dictator. But if he is later deposed, the subsequent regime inherits the obligation to pay off the debts of the previous regime. Thus, the system of international lending and debt can sometimes operate to fund the oppression of the poor people in a poor country, who then inherit the obligation to pay for the cost of their own earlier oppression.

While we may not participate directly in this institution of international lending and what is known as odious debt, these lending practices have a decisive impact on the strength of First World economies and the rate of interest available within the United States. If you have a credit card or pay a mortgage, then in a direct way you enjoy benefits that are created, in part, by an institution that facilitates the poverty and oppression of poor people who live under repressive political regimes. While we do not directly or intentionally cause these people's poverty and desperation, neither are we unconnected or uninvolved third parties. Our situation relative to people who live in poor countries would seem to be intermediate between the two concepts of exploitation identified above. This fact is significant from the moral point of view: to the extent that we are implicated in the poverty of those with whom we interact—that is, to the extent that our wealth depends on institutions that cause them harm—we have positive obligations to rectify the injustices involved. But if we take advantage of the poverty of people who are badly off because of institutions that benefit us, our relationship with them comes much closer to being E1-exploitation and is even more problematic from the moral point of view.

Ideally, we might wish to provide Mr. da Silva with opportunities that his life does not now present. Arguably, justice requires that we do this. But if we are unable to address the underlying injustice that caused his poverty and the poverty of millions of others like him, then we are not justified in stepping in to prevent him from exercising the problematic opportunity that presented itself to him—the opportunity to sell his kidney in a problematic and (probably) exploitative arrangement. If he is appropriately informed about the risks involved (Rother 2004 provides evidence that da Silva was not appropriately informed), if he nonetheless judges that the risk associated with donating a kidney is worth six thousand dollars to him, who are we to tell him that he is making the wrong choice? Unless we are willing to step in and eliminate the initial injustice that leaves him in a situation where he is willing to accept this problematic offer, we have no right to prevent him from improving his situation by accepting such an offer.

If we were to put in place a legal and regulated market for transplant organs, we would need to insure that those participating in this market had a clear understanding of the risks involved. We would need to insure that people whose kidneys (or other organs) are removed must receive proper follow-up care and that the arrangement in which they participate does not take advantage of their ignorance or poverty. Those who would argue for the elimination of the present system should be prepared to offer a specific proposal to insure appropriate regulations to protect the interests of everyone involved in such transactions.

Conclusion

Where do these considerations leave us? If you are one of the 66,000 people who are waiting for a transplant organ, the current situation is bad indeed. Unless the system is dramatically changed, most of the people who are presently waiting on that list will die waiting. Their deaths, inevitable under the current U.S. system, could be avoided if we could increase the number of transplant organs available. Providing financial incentives for donors would almost certainly accomplish this.

Above we have considered several important reasons that are typically used to justify the current system. Some of these reasons are significant from the moral point of view: perhaps it *is* unfortunate and undesirable for people to commodify their bodies. And certainly we should do what we can to promote justice and to avoid exploitative arrangements.

However, we need to decide whether these reasons are sufficiently weighty to justify the deaths of those who die every day waiting for a transplant organ.

> Paying for organs, from the living or deceased, may seem distasteful. But a system with safeguards, begun as a pilot to resolve ethical and practical aspects, is surely preferable to the status quo that allows thousands to die each year. As the International Forum for Transplant Ethics put it: "The well-known shortage of kidneys for transplantation causes much suffering and death. If we are to deny treatment to the suffering and dying, we need better reasons than our own feelings of disgust."
> (SATEL 2006)

Those who argue against the development of a market for transplant organs must face the fact that the system for which they argue is responsible for a massive number of unnecessary deaths. But those who regard the present system as unjustifiable also have a burden to bear: It must be shown that a market for transplant organs can effectively and appropriately protect the interests of everyone involved in it. Then we need to persuade our politicians to put it in place.

QUESTIONS FOR CONSIDERATION

1. *If you were in Senay's shoes, would you sell your kidney given the nature of the bargain in the film? To what extent is Senay's choice free or coerced? In what way would you say that she is being exploited by the arrangement?*

2. *If permitting a legal, regulated market in kidney sales would, for reasons given by Pogge, constitute a legal sanctioning of the exploitation of poor persons in the developing world, wouldn't this be reason enough to prohibit such a market? Explain why or why not.*

3. *Are there some things that just shouldn't be commodified, like kidneys or sex? Come up with the best moral argument you can make for why some things should not be allowed to be bought and sold. Should the law also prohibit such commodification, on the moral grounds you describe? Why or why not?*

REFERENCES

Alsever, J. 2006. Basking on the Beach, or Maybe on the Operating Table. *New York Times,* October 15.

Boudreaux, D. J., and Pritchard, A. C. 1999. Organ Donation: Saving Lives through Incentives. *Viewpoint on Public Issues.* Midland, MI: Mackinac Center for Public Policy. 99(34).

Frears, S. 2002. *Dirty Pretty Things* [motion picture]. London: British Broadcasting Corporation.

Institute of Medicine of the National Academies. 2006. *Organ Donation: Opportunities for Action.* Washington, DC: National Academies Press.

Mills, C. 1995. Goodness as a Weapon. *Journal of Philosophy* 92(9):485–99.

Morley, M. T. 2003. Increasing the Supply of Organs for Transplantation through Paired Organ Exchange. *Yale Law and Policy Review* (Winter 2003):221.

Nussbaum, M. 1999. Whether from Reason or Prejudice: Taking Money for Bodily Services. In *Sex and Social Justice,* ed. M. Nussbaum, 276–98. Oxford and New York: Oxford University Press.

Pogge, T. 2002. *World Poverty and Human Rights.* Cambridge: Polity Press.

Postrel, V. 2006a. Cash for Kidneys. *Los Angeles Times,* June 10.

———. 2006b. "Unfair" Kidney Donations. *Forbes Magazine,* June 6.

Radin, M. J. 1996. *Contested Commodities.* Cambridge, MA: Harvard University Press.

Roth, A., Sonmez, T., and Unver, M. U. 2004. Kidney Exchange. *Quarterly Journal of Economics,* May: 457–88.

Rother, L. 2004. Tracking the Sale of a Kidney on a Path of Poverty and Hope. *New York Times,* May 23.

Sample, R. 2003. *Exploitation: What It Is and Why It's Wrong.* Lanham, MD: Rowman & Littlefield.

Satel, S. 2006. Death's Waiting List. *New York Times,* May 15.

TWELVE

"She's DNR!" "She's Research!"

Conflicting Role-Related Obligations in *Wit*

Terrance McConnell

The HBO movie *Wit* (Nichols 2001)—based on Margaret Edson's (1995) Pulitzer Prize–winning play of the same title—features the plight of Vivian Bearing (played by Emma Thompson), a university literature professor who has stage IV ovarian cancer. There are many themes in *Wit*: Vivian's experiences of suffering and dying; Vivian's examination of her own life and how she treated others; her relationship with her mentor, E. M. Ashford; and her relationship with her primary nurse, Susie. This chapter, however, will focus on Vivian's relationship with two physicians: Harvey Kelekian, her oncologist (played by Christopher Lloyd), and Jason Posner (played by Jonathan M. Woodward), a resident and fellow studying with Dr. Kelekian. *Wit* is set in a major university hospital that clearly has multiple missions: it administers medical treatment to patients, it conducts cutting-edge medical research, and it trains residents and interns. Similarly, Dr. Kelekian has multiple roles: as an oncologist, he provides care to seriously ill patients; as a researcher, he conducts clinical trials; and as a teacher, he trains residents and medical students.

At the outset of *Wit,* Professor Bearing is informed of her diagnosis, though nothing about her prognosis is mentioned. Dr. Kelekian recommends "an experimental combination of drugs," describing it as "the most effective treatment modality" available. Later Dr. Kelekian says, "This treatment is the strongest thing we have to offer you. And, as research, it will make a significant contribution to our knowledge." From the outset, then, Vivian Bearing is both a patient and a research subject.

General versus Role-Related Obligations

Does Dr. Kelekian do anything wrong in his interactions with Vivian Bearing? Let us begin by distinguishing between two types of moral obligation.[1] *General obligations* are moral requirements that individuals have simply because they are moral agents. That moral agents are required not to kill, not to steal, and not to assault others are examples of general obligations; each moral agent is bound by these requirements. By contrast, *role-related obligations* are moral requirements that agents have in virtue of their role, occupation, or position in society (McConnell 1997, p. 19); for example, that lifeguards are required to save swimmers in distress, that health care providers are required to maintain confidentiality, and that teachers are required to educate their students are examples of role-related obligations. It is likely, of course, that anyone who is in a position to do so ought to save a drowning person. Certainly if I could save someone's life merely by tossing him a life preserver, I ought to do so. But lifeguards have obligations to help swimmers in distress even when most others do not because of their abilities and contractual commitments.

General obligations and role-related obligations can, and sometimes do, conflict. When a health care provider has a patient who is dangerous to others, her general obligation to prevent harm to innocent persons may conflict with her role-related obligation of confidentiality. If one of these two types of obligation always took precedence over the other, perhaps these conflicts would not be worrisome. But that does not appear to be plausible; for intuitively it seems that in some cases of conflict general obligations are stronger, while in other cases role-related duties prevail. Moreover, different role-related obligations can conflict. For example, a health care provider's role-related obligations to her patients may on occasion, because of unexpected contingencies, conflict with her role-related obligations as a parent.

Conflicts

As was noted earlier, Dr. Kelekian has three different roles in *Wit*. He is an oncologist. In that role, he has a therapeutic obligation to recommend to patients what he believes is medically best for them (Miller and Brody 2003, p. 20). Even when we reject the excessive paternalism of the past and accept instead a more collaborative model of the health care provider–patient relationship, we still expect physicians to recommend to their patients what they think is medically best.

Dr. Kelekian is also a researcher. While we don't know if he is the principal investigator in the protocol that he recommends to Vivian, he clearly is a key player. The main role-related obligation of researchers is what Maria Merritt calls "scientific duty" (Merritt 2005, pp. 310–11). This is an obligation to produce generalizable knowledge. This requires researchers to conduct clinical trials in a way that produces valid results in a timely manner.

Dr. Kelekian's third role is that of an educator. He teaches medical students, residents, and interns. This role gives him obligations both to the students and to the institution that employs him. In this context, his primary obligation is to prepare his students to be competent practitioners of medicine. Kelekian's role as an educator is further complicated by the fact that he is a mentor to fellows like Jason Posner, and in that role he is responsible for training good researchers.

The university hospital in which *Wit* is set also has different obligations in virtue of its multiple missions. As a provider of patient care, the hospital has an obligation to adopt and enforce policies that promote the well-being of patients and the ethical practice of medicine. As an institution that conducts medical research, the hospital is required to support and encourage the generation and dissemination of generalizable knowledge while protecting human subjects. And as a teaching facility, the hospital has a duty to its students and to the public to ensure that those whom it trains will be competent practitioners of medicine.

These various role-related obligations to which Dr. Kelekian and the university hospital are subject can on occasion conflict. When they do, it may be disadvantageous for people who are patients or subjects or, as in the case of Professor Bearing, both. This is one of the lessons that viewers of *Wit* learn vividly.

Teaching Hospitals

It is no surprise that patients in a teaching hospital may be at a disadvantage. While their attending physician will be a full-fledged doctor, they will also be examined and treated by residents, interns, and medical students. Even if this arrangement does not compromise care, it is apt to be annoying. The argument in support of such a setup is broadly utilitarian. Residents and interns must receive adequate training before they set out on their own. In a university hospital, they are carefully monitored. Therefore, it is likely not only that they will be taught well but also that patients will be protected from serious errors. This appears to be the most efficient, least costly means of attaining an important goal—training new physicians.

The resident with whom Vivian Bearing frequently interacts is Jason Posner. These encounters demonstrate "the costs" to patients of the system of education typical in medicine. In this particular case, the problems are exacerbated because of a prior relationship between Jason and Vivian and by the radical change in social roles brought about by her serious illness. At the outset of their first encounter, Jason tells Vivian—whom he consistently addresses as "Professor Bearing"—that he had taken her course on seventeenth-century poetry. And he explains why: "You can't get into medical school unless you're well-rounded," and he had also made a bet with himself that he "could get an A in the three hardest courses on campus." In the past relationship, Vivian had the power; now Jason does.

In this first meeting, Jason conducts a medical history. Vivian tells him that "Dr. Kelekian has already done that." Jason is aware of this, but indicates that he needs to do it too, presumably as a part of his training. The entire interview is quite awkward, due no doubt in part to the past relationship between them and in part to Jason's inexperience. The latter is an unavoidable cost of any institution's training of new practitioners. Inexperience or insensitivity contributes to another of Jason's mishaps. As Jason prepares to do a pelvic examination on Vivian, he remembers that a woman must be present. So he goes in search of Susie. But two things about this stand out. First, he leaves Vivian uncomfortably positioned in the stirrups; and second, he describes the necessity of having another woman in the room as "some crazy clinical rule." The actual physical examination itself also shows Jason's lack of sensitivity. When he first feels the large mass growing in Vivian, he shouts, "Jesus!" We can be sure that is not something that a patient wants to hear from her physician! Jason's awkward interactions with Vivian may be due not only to inexperience and insensitivity but also to attitude. For later in the film he describes a course on bedside manner that he had in medical school as a "colossal waste of time for researchers." It would be an exaggeration to say that Vivian's suffering is exacerbated by Jason's inexperience; but it is accurate to say that it is irritating and uncomfortable. Speaking of which, we turn to "grand rounds."

Grand rounds consists of a visit from Dr. Kelekian and five residents, including Jason. Vivian is poked, prodded, and discussed in the third person as if she were not present. As she says, "They read me like a book. Once I did the teaching; now I am taught." This practice is clearly an integral part of medical training. Young physicians learn better how to identify symptoms, side-effects of drugs, and the like. And note that during grand rounds, Dr. Kelekian is playing two roles simultaneously: he is teaching residents while serving as Vivian's oncologist. But when he focuses on teaching, it is all but inevitable that he will speak about the patient in the third person.

Interestingly, Vivian herself seems to accept the utilitarian justification of training young physicians and the necessity of putting up with the accompanying irritations and discomforts. At the conclusion of grand rounds, she says, "At times, this obsessively detailed examination, this scrutiny seems to me a nefarious business. On the other hand, what is the alternative? Ignorance?" Vivian's verdict, then, is that training medical students and residents is justified even though it results in less-than-optimal experiences for patients.

The Trials of Professor Bearing

The film's verdict on research, however, may be less kind. At Vivian's initial meeting with Dr. Kelekian, she is told that she has "advanced metastatic ovarian cancer." Vivian's diagnosis is not accompanied with a prognosis, however. Whether this is standard practice may be difficult to ascertain. But in a landmark study on prognosis in medicine, Nicholas Christakis maintains that many physicians avoid giving prognoses for multiple reasons (Christakis 1999, pp. 92–98.). One reason is that such avoidance seems to be the simplest way to negotiate conflicts between the (role-related) obligations of maintaining hope and of being honest. A second reason is prognoses are regarded as arrogant and hubristic. After Dr. Kelekian gives Vivian her diagnosis, he immediately tells her that the most effective treatment modality for this type of cancer is a chemotherapeutic agent. He adds, "We are developing an experimental combination of drugs." This combination he refers to both as "treatment" and as "research." Kelekian tells Vivian that she will receive eight cycles of the drugs, and with each cycle she will be hospitalized as an inpatient. He discusses some of the likely side effects and then gives her the informed consent document. After reading the form in a perfunctory manner, she signs it. Viewers are not told what type of research protocol this is. It seems that it is not a phase III protocol, for that would be a randomized clinical trial (RCT); and in this case, Vivian is assigned directly to receive the experimental drugs (see Table 12.1 for a description of the different phases of drug trials). In a typical RCT, 50 percent of the subjects will be assigned to the experimental group (and will receive the drug under investigation), while the other half will be assigned to the control group (and receive either a placebo or the standard treatment). Because Kelekian and Jason obsess about levels of toxicity throughout the film, some might conclude that this is a phase I trial. But phase I trials have one principal purpose: to determine if and when the drugs being tested harm people. It is clearly a mistake to refer to a phase I trial as "treatment." So this is probably a phase II trial, done on a small number of patients to see if any benefits accrue. If there is truly no other treatment available for a given condition, then it may be accurate to say that a phase II trial is the best thing a health care provider has to offer. But to call it "treatment" is, at the very least, misleading.

It is also noteworthy that Dr. Kelekian does not discuss with Vivian the option of hospice care. As a researcher, it is clearly important for Dr. Kelekian to enroll eligible patients in his protocol. And this may be a protocol for which finding a sufficient number of subjects is difficult. If so, Dr. Kelekian's obligation as a researcher to produce reliable, generalizable knowledge may blind him to some of his therapeutic obligations; for

TABLE 12.1 *Types of clinical trials*

Type	Purpose
Phase I	To determine if, or at what point, the experimental drug or treatment is harmful to people.
Phase II	To determine if there is prima facie evidence that the experimental drug or treatment is beneficial to persons afflicted with the relevant illness (as preliminary animal studies led researchers to believe).
Phase III	To obtain definitive evidence of the effectiveness of the experimental drug or treatment by systematically comparing the outcomes of the control group with those of the experimental group.

exclusively palliative care is an entirely plausible option for patients with stage IV ovarian cancer, certainly one that should be discussed with them.

The scientific duty requires not only finding a sufficient number of subjects but also having as many of them as possible complete the regimen. Throughout the film, both Kelekian and Jason urge Vivian to persevere. At the outset Kelekian says to her, "We will of course be relying on your resolve to withstand some of the more pernicious side effects." And soon after that he says, "The important thing is for you to take the full dose of chemotherapy . . . The experimental phase has got to have the maximum dose to be of any use." This message is definitely received. Later in the film Vivian boasts, "I have survived eight treatments of Hexamethophosphacil and Vinplatin at the *full* dose, ladies and gentlemen. I have broken the record." And still later Jason remarks, "Eight cycles of Hex and Vin at full dose. Kelekian didn't think it was possible. I wish they could all get through at full throttle. Then we could really have some data." But with each cycle the side effects become more pronounced and Vivian's suffering increases. Such suffering should be bothersome to all researchers, even those who are not health care providers. For all researchers have what Merritt calls a "protective duty" (Merritt 2005, pp. 312–13). This is a general moral obligation to protect subjects' well-being in the face of risks incurred by participating in research. If the researchers are also physicians, they have an additional role-related obligation not to imperil the health of anyone.

This very conflict is demonstrated graphically in one scene. Vivian is between cycles, but arrives at the hospital in the middle of the night with a fever, a high pulse rate, and in great distress. After Jason provides Vivian with treatment, Susie says to him, "I think you need to talk to Kelekian about lowering the dose for the next cycle. It's too much for her like this." Jason's immediate retort is from the perspective of a researcher: "Lower the dose? No way. Full dose. She's tough." The focus here is not that the drug regimen is helping Vivian; rather, it is that more data are needed.

In another scene, Susie tells Vivian that she must go to the laboratory for an ultrasound. "They're concerned about a bowel obstruction." Vivian resists. She is adamant. "No more tests." But Susie persists, and Vivian eventually relents. It is not clear whether the ordering of this test is based only on Vivian's therapeutic needs or if it is connected with research. The question, presumably, is whether the same test would have been ordered were Vivian not a research subject.

Kindness

As Vivian's condition worsens, Susie does two things that one would expect Vivian's physician to do. First, Susie is truthful with Vivian about the "treatment's" lack of success. Vivian asks, "My cancer is not being cured, is it?" When Susie confirms this, Vivian adds, "They never expected it to be, did they?" Susie acknowledges this, saying, "They've learned a lot for their research. It was the best thing they had to give you, the strongest drugs. There just isn't a good treatment for what you have yet, for advanced ovarian. I'm sorry. They should have explained this." Vivian says that she knew. This suggests that Vivian's consent to participate in this research protocol was not informed. Or, more cautiously, if her consent was informed, it was not due to what Dr. Kelekian and the other researchers told her. It appears that they gave her more reason to believe that the drug regimen was curative than was warranted. What Susie does in this episode is confirm this point and convey to Vivian that her death is imminent. This is the first time in the film that the patient's prognosis is addressed.

The second thing that Susie does is raise the question about "code status." Most viewers of this film are apt to know that a hospitalized patient is by default "full code" unless a do-not-resuscitate (DNR) order has been written. If a patient is full code and her heart stops, she will receive chest compressions, drugs, and intubation as is necessary. Susie's discussion with Vivian about this is not very detailed; perhaps viewers can presume that Vivian is familiar with the standard procedures. In any case, Vivian says, "Let it stop." This is conveyed to Dr. Kelekian and a DNR order is written.

It is striking that Dr. Kelekian has discussed neither Vivian's prognosis nor her code status with her, given the severity of her illness and the imminence of her death. One can only speculate about his reasons. Many say that doctors are uncomfortable talking about death. But this seems unlikely in Kelekian's case. After all, he is an experienced oncologist who deals with dying patients regularly. It seems more likely that his role as a researcher led him, consciously or subconsciously, to avoid these issues. Awareness of the imminence of death might make it more likely that Vivian would stop her participation in the protocol. And sustaining her life a bit longer may provide more useful data. From the film's content, we cannot know Dr. Kelekian's motives or reasons. But given that his therapeutic obligations are not discharged fully, it is plausible to infer that he is more focused on his role-related obligations as a researcher.

Vivian's own observations suggest that she herself sees clearly that Jason and Kelekian are more focused on research than on patient care. After boasting about surviving eight cycles of the "treatment," Vivian notes, "Kelekian and Jason are simply delighted. I think they foresee celebrity status for themselves upon the appearance of the journal article they will no doubt write about me." Vivian quickly corrects herself; the article "will be about my ovaries." So if Vivian were under any illusions at the outset, they have long since disappeared. She sees the situation for what it is. But does it in any way disturb her?

A bit later, Vivian has a lengthy conversation with Jason about his interest in—or, rather, his fascination with—cancer research. When Jason leaves her room, Vivian observes, "So. The young doctor, like the senior scholar, prefers research to humanity." At several points in the film, Vivian has reflected about her interaction with students. She now regrets how she treated many of her students and sees the obvious parallel with her current situation. She goes on, "At the same time the senior scholar, in her pathetic state as a simpering victim, wishes the young doctor would take more interest in personal contact." So Vivian does long for more than being treated merely as a research subject. Such a longing explains, in part, the evolution of Vivian's relationship with Susie. For of all of the principal characters, only Susie treats Vivian with kindness and relates to her as a person. As they discuss Vivian's code status, they share popsicles and some lighthearted conversation. When Susie leaves, Vivian says, "Now is a time for simplicity. Now is a time for, dare I say it, kindness." As a research subject, she does not receive kindness. But is that inevitable?

The Therapeutic Misconception

When Susie brings up the topic of code status with Vivian, she hints that Kelekian and Jason might have a different view about the issue. Vivian presses Susie for an explanation about her differences with them. Susie explains, "Kelekian is a great researcher and everything . . . but they always . . . want to know more things." The suggestion is that acting on the desire to know—pursuing knowledge—is in conflict with doing what is best for the patient (at least sometimes).

If we reflect on the prominent character traits of Jason and Kelekian, we can see the potential conflict between scientific duties and therapeutic obligations in a different light. Jason has unbridled enthusiasm for cancer research. Such enthusiasm, no doubt, promotes the success of research and the growth of knowledge. Dr. Kelekian's most prominent trait is a kind of detachment, or objectivity. This too promotes successful research. But what do patients want from their attending physicians? Even though we reject the excessive paternalism of the past, patients presumably want their physicians to be compassionate, caring, and focused on their well-being. While these traits are not incompatible, there is a tension among them. Detachment and objectivity per se are certainly not at odds with caring. Indeed, one of the reasons that physicians are required not to treat members of their own family is that they lack objectivity; in that situation, there is too much caring and too little objectivity.

But the imbalance can go the other way too. Too much detachment can, at the very least, be perceived as too little caring. In the same way, enthusiasm for research is not incompatible with concern for the welfare of the patient. But at a certain point, the enthusiasm may blind the researcher to matters not directly relevant to the protocol. Throughout *Wit,* Jason's enthusiasm for the protocol and Kelekian's detachment compromise their ability to focus on Vivian's well-being.

To avoid misunderstanding, I should state clearly that human beings are capable of a wide range of emotional responses to others depending on the nature of their relationships to them. Note the different levels of emotional involvement that people have with family members and loved ones, with friends, with business associates, and with strangers. This is normal and demonstrates the human capacity for variable relationships. In these cases, however, the contrasting responses are typically directed toward different people. In the case of the physician-researcher, different responses must be directed toward the same person. Vivian Bearing is both Dr. Kelekian's patient and a subject in one of his research protocols. Still, this is not an insurmountable barrier. One does not have to engage in complicated psychological gymnastics to balance objectivity, enthusiasm, and caring. Indeed, as mentioned before, Merritt says that all researchers have both scientific duties and protective duties, and there is no reason to think that ordinary human beings cannot deal with both. Whether Kelekian or Jason achieve this balance is doubtful. Each seems far more focused on research than on care, and that probably makes Vivian's last days more difficult.

But there may be another problem here. Instead of focusing on the traits of the researchers, let us look at the situation from the perspective of the patient-subject. Dr. Kelekian is both Vivian's oncologist and someone conducting a clinical investigation. The Declaration of Helsinki, the World Medical Association's statement of "Ethical Principles for Medical Research Involving Human Subjects," specifically singles out those who combine medical research with treatment (Ezekiel et al. 2003, items 28 and 29, p. 32). This is what is known as *therapeutic research* (contrasted with nontherapeutic research). Of therapeutic research, the Declaration says, "The physician may combine medical research with medical care only to the extent that the research is justified by its potential prophylactic, diagnostic or therapeutic value. When medical research is combined with medical care, additional standards apply to protect patients who are research subjects."

The Declaration recognizes that special moral issues are raised when someone (such as Dr. Kelekian) has a dual relationship with the patient-subject. Two obvious issues come to mind. First, the patient is more likely to feel pressure to enroll in a protocol recommended by her attending physician. Thus outsiders appropriately wonder whether the subject's consent has been freely given. Second, patient-subjects are more likely to experience what is known as *therapeutic misconception,* mistaking what is research for established therapy (Appelbaum et al. 1987). There is certainly no indication in *Wit* that Vivian Bearing feels pressured by Dr. Kelekian to participate in the research. The picture of Vivian throughout is that she is quite capable of looking out for herself. But whether she is laboring under the therapeutic misconception is more difficult to say. As was noted earlier, in the informed consent process Dr. Kelekian says, "This treatment is the strongest thing we have to offer you." No doubt the actual consent form itself indicates that this is research and that the intervention is not proven to be effective. Unfortunately, Vivian's reading of the document is quite perfunctory.

These remarks presuppose the legitimacy of the distinction between therapeutic and nontherapeutic research. But this distinction has been challenged by Franklin Miller and Howard Brody (Miller and Brody 2003), and this challenge can provide the basis for a more fundamental objection. Miller and Brody distinguish between what they label the "similarity position" and the "difference position" (Miller and Brody 2003, p. 20). The former position holds that the ethics of clinical trials rests on the same moral considerations that underlie the ethics of therapeutic medicine. The latter view says that medical research and medical treatment are two distinct activities governed by different ethical principles.

The goal of clinical medicine is to provide optimal treatment for individual patients; the governing principles are beneficence and nonmaleficence. Clinical research is designed to answer scientific questions with the aim of producing generalizable knowledge; it is driven by a utilitarian purpose, the promotion of the welfare of future patients. In clinical medicine, the interests of the physician and the interests of the patient are in harmony; the goals of each are restoration of health and relief of suffering. But in clinical research, the interests of investigators and the interests of subjects may diverge. It is because of this latter point that prior independent review of research protocols is mandated (Miller and Brody 2003, p. 21).

With this framework in place, Miller and Brody discuss phase III RCTs to support the difference position (see Table 12.1). This is the final stage of testing investigational drugs, and subjects randomized to the experimental group may reasonably hope to benefit. Thus, such trials are often characterized as "therapeutic research." But, as Miller and Brody argue persuasively, there are distinct differences between the practice of clinical medicine and clinical trials. In clinical medicine, a physician would not decide which drug to administer by flipping a coin. Moreover, the physician would judge each case individually, not abide by some preestablished formula (Miller and Brody 2003, p. 22). So it is just a mistake to call these trials "therapeutic"; to do so makes it more likely that participants will suffer from the therapeutic misconception. Applying this to *Wit*, one is tempted to conclude that Dr. Kelekian misled Vivian by confusing research with therapy. But before drawing such a conclusion, two points are worth considering.

First, the differences between research and treatment highlighted above concern phase III RCTs. And Miller and Brody are certainly right to say that in the clinical setting a doctor would not give her patient a 50 percent chance of receiving what she thought was the best treatment available. But in *Wit* Vivian Bearing is not enrolled in a phase III RCT. As we saw, it seems most likely that it is a phase II trial; it definitely was not randomized. What difference does this make? In phase III trials, investigators have more evidence that the experimental drug is promising than they do at phase II. In typical phase III trials, however, the subject's chance of receiving the experimental drug is 50 percent. In many phase II trials, the subject's chance of receiving the experimental drug is 100 percent. Though it seems odd—indeed, counterintuitive—to say, perhaps some phase II trials could more accurately be described as "therapeutic" than could phase III trials. Two different variables seem relevant to using the term *therapeutic*: probability that the experimental drug is beneficial, and probability that the subject will receive the experimental drug. These variables can pull in opposite directions, and thus at least allow for the possibility of calling a phase II trial "therapeutic" without badly abusing the term. Curiously, if in recruiting a subject for such a phase II trial the researcher were to say (as Kelekian effectively does) that this is the "best" there is to offer, it would seem misleading. But if he were to say that there is "no evidence of anything better," that would be more honest.

The second reason for being reluctant to apply the Miller-Brody framework is not unique to *Wit*. Recall that the Declaration of Helsinki (2003) draws a sharp distinction between therapeutic and nontherapeutic research, and did so from the outset in 1964. The authors of the code seemed to have at least two reasons for doing this: (1) they seemed to think that there was more ethical "leeway" if investigators were conducting therapeutic research,[2] and (2) they thought that special moral problems could arise when physicians recruited their own patients as research subjects. We might be quite happy to dismiss the first of these. But the second consideration seems important. The possibilities of coercion and exploitation seem especially great when physicians are using their own patients as research subjects. Yet today it is doubtful that there would be an adequate number of research subjects if physicians did not enroll their own patients in protocols. The logic of the position developed by Miller and Brody suggests that either physicians should not recruit their own patients for research protocols at all (for it promotes therapeutic misconception) or they should in a dramatic manner announce that they are now changing roles (and then begin the recruitment process). While the latter seems more practical (in that it will make it more likely that there will be an adequate number of subjects), it also seems unfair. Vivian Bearing did not seek out Dr. Kelekian because he was a researcher; she sought an oncologist. To have one's attending physician suddenly switch hats can be disconcerting at best. We need not try to settle these issues here. Suffice it to say that *Wit* is an excellent teaching device about whether there is a legitimate distinction between therapeutic and nontherapeutic research, whether it is justifiable for physicians to recruit their own patients to participate in research, and if they do so whether obtaining freely given, fully informed consent is really feasible.

An Ambiguous Ending

The ending of *Wit* is appropriate, though not uplifting. Jason enters Vivian's room. Noting that she is unresponsive, he checks her vital signs. Detecting no pulse, he shouts, "Call a code!" He is apparently unaware that Dr. Kelekian has written a DNR order for Vivian. He picks up the telephone, calls the code, and then begins CPR. Susie enters and yells, "She's DNR!" Jason replies, "She's research!" The code team descends on the room. One member begins CPR, another prepares the defibrillator, and a third prepares to intubate Vivian. Checking the chart, Jason realizes his error. He screams, "I made a mistake!" Once members of the code team have assessed the situation, they chide Jason. "It's a doctor screw-up." "What is he, a resident?"

Clearly Vivian Bearing's last minutes as a patient are not easy. She is subjected, albeit briefly, to an unnecessary code. We do not know whether she suffers additionally during that time. But clearly this is not an optimal end to her case. What is the source of the problem? Two possibilities are suggested by the dialogue. When Jason says, "She's research!" the implication is that he wants to extend Vivian's life to get more data. But the code team's diagnosis appeals to Jason's inexperience (and, by implication, his incompetence): "What is he, a resident?" Each explanation appeals to one of the missions of the university hospital. It is in the business of caring for patients, training medical students and residents, and conducting medical research. Whether it is Jason's inexperience or his exuberance for research, Vivian's last dying moments do not pass as they should. *Wit* thus provides a clear illustration of how an institution's provision of patient care can be compromised by its commitment to teaching and research. But there is no clear message in the film that any of these missions should be abandoned.

QUESTIONS FOR CONSIDERATION

1. *Would you object to having residents, interns, or medical students being a part of the team that examines you in the hospital? How can this be handled in a way that is less alienating to the patient than is the case for Vivian in* Wit*?*

2. *How would you feel if you had a life-threatening medical problem and the physician whose care you were under asked you to be a participant in a research protocol that she was conducting? What questions would you ask? What factors would prompt you to agree to participate in the protocol? What factors would prompt you to decline to participate?*

3. *If you contracted an illness that was typically fatal, what would you want your doctor to tell you? Would you want your doctor to give you detailed statistics about death rates, no matter how grim those are? Would you want your doctor to tell you that there is hope, even if the statistics are horrible?*

ACKNOWLEDGMENT

I thank Sandra Shapshay for helpful comments and suggestions on an earlier version of this chapter.

NOTES

1. In this chapter, I shall use the terms *obligation*, *duty*, and *moral requirement* interchangeably; each refers to what an agent (morally) ought to do.

2. For example, in the first instantiations of the declaration, those who crafted it allowed some therapeutic research to be conducted without the fully informed consent of the patient-subjects if the doctor thought that was best; no such freedom was permitted for nontherapeutic research.

REFERENCES

Appelbaum, P., Roth, L., Lidz, C., Benson, P., and Winslade, W. 1987. False Hopes and Best Data: Consent to Research and the Therapeutic Misconception. *Hastings Center Report* 17 (2):20–24.

Christakis, N. 1999. *Death Foretold: Prophecy and Prognosis in Medical Care*. Chicago: University of Chicago Press.

The Declaration of Helsinki. 2003. In *Ethical and Regulatory Aspects of Clinical Research,* ed. E. J. Emanuel et al., 30–32. Baltimore: Johns Hopkins University Press.

Edson, M. 1999. *Wit.* New York: Dramatists Play Services.

McConnell, T., 1997. *Moral Issues in Health Care,* 2nd ed. Belmont, CA: Wadsworth Publishing.

Merritt, M. 2005. Moral Conflict in Clinical Trials. *Ethics* 115:306–30.

Miller, F., and Brody, H. 2003. Therapeutic Misconception in the Ethics of Clinical Trials. *Hastings Center Report* 33 (3):19–28.

Nichols, M. 2001. *Wit* [television program]. New York and Los Angeles: Home Box Office Films.

PART FOUR

Aging and the Good Death

THIRTEEN

"He Just Got Old"

Aging and Compassionate Care in *Dad*

Bradley J. Fisher and Sandra Shapshay

The film *Dad* (Goldberg 1989) is a story about intergenerational relations and what we can do as a family to protect, nurture, and even harm one another. The story revolves mostly around the relationships between three generations of men: the grandfather, Jake (played by Jack Lemmon), his son, John (played by Ted Danson), and the grandson, Billy (played by Ethan Hawke). The fragmented generations are united as a result of illnesses, first the heart attack of the mother, Bette (played by Olympia Dukakis), and then the bladder cancer of Jake.

When the characters are embroiled in the health care system, *Dad* raises some lesser-explored issues of patient and family rights in the context of medical treatment and care. These may be phrased in the form of questions: Who within a family has the right to know about the health condition of another, and who should control that information? What rights, if any, do family members have to conceal information about a patient's illness if they feel it is in that person's best interest? What rights do family members have with respect to advising medical personnel on how to present a diagnosis to a patient within that family?

Other questions raised by the film concern a non-rights-based realm of morality: the virtues and vices of family members and the imperfect moral obligations—moral duties which may be discharged in various ways and to varying degrees, without corresponding rights—of the young, especially, toward their elderly parents, to help maintain their physical, psychological, and social health. In addition, the film deals with the moral obligations of both medical personnel and family to help an older adult come to terms with physical decline and the end of life.

Many themes are interwoven in *Dad;* for instance, the reality of human frailty and fallibility, a familial love that both enables and disables, obligations of care within families, forgiveness, and what it means to be a man in American society, among many others. What we will focus on in this chapter, however, is arguably, the central theme of *Dad*, namely, deception, both the deception of others (mostly from benevolent motives) and the deception of oneself (predominantly to avoid painful truths and to find an elusive happiness). One of the main messages of *Dad* is to live true to one's deepest desires, goals and beliefs, or, in other words, authentically. Doing so will make for flourishing relationships with others, especially with one's family. Moreover, the film portrays involvement in a flourishing family as a central ingredient for individual meaning and happiness in life.

Paraphrased in this way, however, what we take to be the central message of the film may seem a cliché. Yet, when one vicariously experiences the existential journey that Jake, the eponymous "Dad," undertakes in the film—from coupon-clipping routine to donning outrageous leisure wear—one is invited to feel the profound importance of honesty, even when what one must be honest about seems unspeakably terrible: failure, terminal illness, dying, and irrevocable loss of people we love.

The Rebirth of Jake through the Reconnection of John

The film opens with a bucolic scene of a man in his prime, rousing himself in the early morning haze, to take care of his beautiful, well-managed farm, and, by extension, his lovely wife and four children. When the scene abruptly changes to an older man, Jake, being micromanaged by his wife, the juxtaposition leads the viewer to conclude that this once-so-capable farmer has now become infirm and needs his wife to infantilize him. Perhaps the opening sequence is a memory, one Jake recollects with wistful sentimentality? Or, perhaps it was his daydream? We viewers don't find out how to interpret the opening sequence until the end of the film—the idyllic scene serves as a crucial frame for the narrative.

The present-day action opens with Jake and Bette going through the motions of their typical day. Jake passively allows Bette to lay out clothes, to butter toast, and basically to direct the entire course of their day. In the bathroom, Jake moves very slowly and seems to have difficulty selecting his toothbrush from among the hairbrushes on the sink. One is left with the impression that Jake is either suffering from dementia, overmedication, or depression. He is the picture of learned helplessness. Later, at the grocery store, the first medical crisis hits: Bette has a heart attack and Jake seems not to even understand that she is ill. Even a response so basic as to call for help eludes him.

At this point, the family converges; we see John, a successful, type-A businessman being called away by his sister, Annie (played by Kathy Baker), from his high-powered job of mergers and corporate takeovers to fly out to Los Angeles. Mario, his brother-in-law (played by Kevin Spacey) picks him up and takes him first to the hospital to visit Bette. While hooked up to tubes and machines, his mother instructs John not to tell his father about the heart attack, but instead to say, "It's something went wrong with my insides. He'll understand that because I had the hysterectomy." It appears she is trying to come up with a comforting but ultimately misleading explanation on a level for a child. This is the first instance in the film where we see medical information being deceptively withheld by a family member, well intentioned or not, with the co-conspiracy of the two adult children. John warns his mother, "I think you should be worrying about yourself. You had a heart attack." In this way, John is fulfilling an important family responsibility by orienting Bette to reality and minimizing the likelihood of denial (though she continues to insist it was "gas").

Back at the house, John informs Annie that he can only stay for a few days. She updates John on Jake's state of mind saying, "He's scared, John, he's really, really frightened. I'm not sure he even understands what happened." When asked if Jake has seen his wife in the hospital, Annie says, "No, he was too scared. I didn't want to push it. I told him that she wasn't allowed to have visitors and he seemed okay with that." Both adult children view Jake as fragile and unable to handle stressful information and therefore conceal information and isolate him for his own protection. Are they morally justified in paternalizing and misleading their father?

John goes out back to visit his dad in the greenhouse. Jake looks up as John enters and greets him warmly, but not overly enthusiastically. The only affection shown between the two men is a "Good to see you" and a "You look good." When Jake asks about Bette, he offers his own understanding, "Something went wrong with her insides, huh?" and John simply replies, "Something like that." John returns to the kitchen and is given instructions by Annie. "The main thing for you while you're here is to keep everything on an even keel. Mom has a schedule and their life is essentially one long routine." All John can muster is a question, "When did he get so bad?" Annie reminds John that he has been away for a couple years and a lot can happen in that time. With an edge in his voice, John asks, "Why didn't you tell me." Annie fires back, "I told you. You didn't hear me." Annie sums up her understanding by saying, "Dad just got old." The general impression is that John has been uninvolved with his parents' lives (we later find out that he was embarrassed by his father) and is now shocked by the state of his father's deterioration.

Jake's learned helplessness is further illustrated later that evening when he can neither locate nor put on his pajamas. John helps his father put on the tops, but the physical contact is minimal and entirely instrumental. After getting settled in, John returns to Jake's bedroom to find him in his pajamas sitting on the edge of the bed looking down at the floor. John gently helps his father lie down and tucks him into bed. This is the first affectionate contact between these two men since John first arrived. The relationship appears caring but distant, though, John displays increasing concern for and tenderness toward his father when he goes to leave the bedroom, stops in the doorway, and returns to lie on the bed next to Jake to keep him company during the long night.

It is obvious that Jake has some mental disturbances, but what is the ethical responsibility of the adult children to intervene in a situation that has been managed by husband and wife for approximately fifty years? What responsibility or right do the children have to intrude on the mental health of an aged parent? John decides that he does have such a responsibility and begins the following morning by telling him that Bette is sick. Jake asks in a terrified voice, "It's not cancer is it? That cancer is a killer you know. Tell you, you have cancer you might as well pack your bags."

John reassures him by telling him the truth, "It was a heart attack. A serious one." John goes on to lay out a strategy for coping with the situation by coaching his father, "You're gonna have to learn to do a lot of things around the house by yourself. See, Mother's convinced herself that nobody can take care of you but her. We're gonna have to prove her wrong." John is trying to empower Jake and he responds enthusiastically by replying, "That's right, Johnny. I'm gonna learn how to do all of those things. You'll see. We'll fool her." It becomes a challenge and almost a game (fooling her). This simple dialogue between father and son is important because it shows that John does not underestimate his father's ability to comprehend the situation or to make a contribution toward lessening the stress on Bette. He is treating his father like an adult and as a partner in helping to manage Bette's health problem, and, at the same time, trying to pull his father out of his shell.

The next morning, Jake surprises John by laying out a sumptuous breakfast of cereal, fruit, and juices. This is the first significant sign that Jake is reengaging with life and showing initiative. The whole point of this sequence of events in the film is to portray a character that has been suppressed by life, and a dominant wife, and is now emerging from his learned helplessness and embracing a sense of efficacy. This initial transformation is made possible because of his wife's absence from the house and the encouragement and support of his son.

Over breakfast, Jake tells John he would like to visit Bette. John hesitates saying, "I'm not sure that's such a good idea. They want to limit the number of visitors." Here, John is stepping back from empowering his father by controlling his right to visit his wife and then coming up with a lame excuse. This time, however, Jake cuts through it by replying, "I'm her husband. I should see her. It's not right." Again, a renewed Jake is calmly standing his ground and advocating for his rights. Here is a man in his late seventies who has to ask his children for permission to see his wife. One wonders, how did the father became the child and the child the parent? Is this what happens when "one just gets old"?

After breakfast, as Jake carries dishes to the sink, he comments to John, "I think I could do these. I could do these dishes." John picks up on this and makes a set of very basic note cards that are color coded to particular chores. At first, the viewer may perceive John as infantilizing his father by creating such simplistic and "childish" step-by-step cards, but this is easily dismissed when Jake responds favorably, saying, "There's no way I can make a mistake as long as I follow these cards." It is a boost to Jake's confidence, and the viewer understands that John is trying to empower his father, to slowly rebuild the independence his father once enjoyed. What follows are a series of scenes, to upbeat jazzy music, in which John and Jake are shown doing a variety of household chores ending with a slow pan of a spotless house and zooming in on a shiny kitchen floor where John and Jake stand at one end, mops in hand, admiring their handiwork. John decides they have earned a night out.

Their night out winds up being a trip to the local bingo hall. At the concession stand, John asks Jake when he last went to bingo. Jake comments, "Three years ago. We just stopped doing the things we like." John tries to encourage his father saying, "You should remember the fun things you used to do and you should start doing them." Rather than resenting this advice, Jake embraces it and replies, "I'll make up a list of fun things and I'll do 'em." The impression is that this fun-loving Jake is the real person who has been suppressed over the years. Perhaps we're seeing a glimpse of that capable, energetic farmer from long, long ago.

The next scene shows Jake stepping out of the hospital elevator dressed in a suit and tie. Even Annie expresses delight by whispering to John, "I can't believe how good Dad looks. You've been terrific for him." John smiles but quickly replies, "He's been good for me too. It's been kind of fun." Jake is a renewed man, but so is his son who feels a tie to "family" that has been missing in his post-divorce life. This is when he informs a grateful Annie that he has changed his schedule and will stay until Bette returns home.

That night, John's son, Billy, arrives. His father greets him at the door and the two shake hands. In the kitchen, while Billy stuffs his face, they catch up on news. The words they use are the same formula used initially between Jake and John, "You look good." John adds, "I think you've grown." "Dad, you say that to me every time I see you and I stopped growing two years ago." The message is that this father and son have not been close and there is a strained truce between them. Billy observes that Jake is looking good, as the grandfather bustles around in the kitchen, preparing food for Billy, and John replies, "We've been spending a lot of time together." Billy takes on a sarcastic tone and comments, "Quality time, huh? They say that's good for parents and kids." There is an obvious barb in these words, but John sidesteps them and counters with, "Maybe you and I should spend some more time together." Billy holds up his hand, palm toward John as if holding him off and says, "Take it easy, Dad. Let's not get carried away."

Bette returns home and there is typical banter around the family table. Jake turns to Billy and comments, "I like that earring. Maybe I should get one of those." These simple aside comments can be overlooked, but the subtle message is that Jake is opening up to life, to new possibilities. He even gives a toast to his "bride." Jake is shown sitting with a beatific smile on his face as his eyes shine with tears. Annie turns to him with concern asking him what is wrong. "I'm just happy." We see the renewed Jake who embraces the return of his wife and the reunion of his family.

Cancer, Deception, and Jake's Fall

Just as we are drawn into the warmth of this family reunited, the story unfolds another layer as Jake discovers late that night that he is passing blood. The following scene flashes to the office of Dr. Santana (played by J. T. Walsh), who comes out of the examining room, leaving Jake to finish dressing. The doctor tells John that he suspects malignant growths in Jake's bladder, and it is serious enough to schedule exploratory surgery. Neither the doctor nor John reveals this information to Jake in the office. This concealment verges on a violation of the physician's ethical and legal obligations to his patient: to tell his *patient* his findings and to preserve the confidentiality of the patient's medical information, unless the patient authorizes him to share it with others. Current codes of medical ethics mandate both this disclosure of information and the preservation of physician-patient confidentiality. As yet, however, Dr. Santana has not made a firm diagnosis, and so this does not constitute a clear case of concealing vital information from his patient.

On the ride home, John lies, "If it were anything serious, Dad, they wouldn't have let you out of there today. They would have cut you right open and operated on the spot. I wouldn't be surprised at all if it were just a cyst." Although John has no professional obligation (as does Dr. Santana) to disclose the truth about Dr. Santana's suspicions, one might ask whether he has an obligation, as a son, to be truthful with his father, and not to paternalize him in this way. John advises, "I don't even think it's worth telling Mom about." Again, he is trying to control medical information that certainly Jake, and arguably Bette, has a right to know.

Here is an instance of what has been referred to by medical sociologists as *suspicion awareness* as Jake suspects something is wrong (and the doctor and John both know something is wrong). Suspicion awareness is one of four awareness states—suspicion awareness, closed awareness, mutual pretense, and open awareness—that can occur between the patient, the family, and the medical personnel (for an in-depth discussion of awareness states, see Glaser and Strauss 1965). In *suspicion awareness,* the patient asks questions about his or her condition but no one will confirm those suspicions and instead people try distraction techniques, changing the subject, or offering excuses (e.g., they need to run more tests). *Closed awareness* is when medical personnel and family may know an illness is serious but do not share that information with the patient. *Mutual pretense* is when everyone is aware that an illness is serious but they pretend as if it is not, going through the motions of a day without really acknowledging the significance of what is happening . . . or preparing for death. *Open awareness* is when there is open communication: The family, patient, and medical personnel can speak freely of the illness and the prognosis. Open awareness, is, on the one hand, harder, for issues are straightforwardly confronted, but it is, on the other hand, easier because people don't have to work at concealing and avoiding. It is an honest and open approach that allows the older adult to prepare for death, to tie up loose ends, to say good-byes, to fulfill whatever can and must be fulfilled in the time remaining.

In the movie *Dad*, we first are shown suspicion awareness because Jake knows something is not right (he did see the blood in the toilet) but no one will confirm how serious the situation may be. Bette is also suspicious, but John lies to her and convinces her that there is nothing serious going on.

Back at the house, Bette walks into John's room with a grim expression on her face. John knows instantly that Jake has told her. John continues to lie, saying, "It's nothing serious." Bette is unconvinced, replying, "If it weren't serious, you would have told me about it yourself." John justifies this by saying, "I was afraid you might get upset about nothing. That's why I didn't tell you. It's just a cyst. I'd tell you if there's anything wrong." Reluctantly, Bette accepts John's reassurance, but her look conveys a suspicion that not all has been revealed.

Here we have another instance of suspicion awareness, this time on the part of the mother. She is a forceful character and has been in charge of her household, and her husband, up until her heart attack. She tries to control everything. It is ironic that she does not like having information concealed from her but was willing to conceal medical information from her husband. All of this is well-intentioned, but it raises the issue of who has the right to know the health condition of an individual?

As for the confidentiality of the medical information, while no one but the patient (if competent) and the medical-care team has a *right* to know his or her medical information, most of us would probably agree that a well-functioning family would share this information openly among themselves, even in the absence of any explicit right of the family to know.

On the day of the surgery, John stands by the hospital bed preparing to leave; he seems uncomfortable waiting there for the start of the surgery. As he gathers up his coat, Jake mentions, "I see men now, they hug. We've never hugged." The two men hug, embracing tightly, and both men are able to verbalize their love for one another. The impression is that the bond they have rediscovered in the past couple weeks is now sealed forever. The significance of this scene is that here is a man confronting surgery who needs the support of a family member to help him cope with his fear. He well knows he could die on the table and needs some closure before surgery. While a surgery is not a dramatic event for the surgeon or the surgical technicians who have done many such procedures, for the patient it is a major life event. This suggests that both the family and hospital personnel need to be respectful of this and the anxiety that such events generate. It is too easy for medical personnel to view a patient as a procedure, and for family to give empty reassurances to deal with their own discomfort or fears. Family and medical personnel have an ethical obligation to be aware of and support the emotional well-being of the patient before and after a medical procedure.

Ethical Rule-Following versus Responsiveness to Particulars

The surgery is completed and Dr. Santana confirms the worst. It is a virulent form of bladder cancer, but Santana is confident he got it all. While he is optimistic, he is clinical and detached, what most might view as "professional." The question now arises: Should Dad be told the truth given his tremendous fear of cancer? Certainly, by current standards of medical ethics, with its emphasis on respect for patient autonomy, so long as the patient is legally competent, most writers on biomedical ethics believe that he has a right to be informed by his physician of his true condition (Beauchamp and Walters 2003, p. 111). One dissenting voice, however, is David C. Thomasma, who argued that "truth is a secondary good" and "[while] important, other primary values take precedence over the truth" (Thomasma 1994, p. 381). The values Thomasma cites are the patient's survival, and the relationship between the doctor and patient. In cases where the truth threatens the life of the patient or where the truth would threaten the ability of the patient to maintain any relationship with the doctor (both of which are distinct possibilities in the case of *Dad*), the truth may be withheld.

It is interesting, however, to note that even Thomasma, when applying his thinking to the scenario in question in the film, advocates for the disclosure of truth: "The movie *Dad* . . . had as its centerpiece the notion that Dad could not tolerate the idea of cancer. Once told, he went into a psychotic shock that ruptured standard relationships with the doctors, the hospital, and the family. However, because this diagnosis requires patient participation for chemotherapeutic interventions and the time is short, the truth must be faced directly" (Thomasma 1994, p. 379). Thus, even for a scholar who sees the truth as a secondary good, the threshold for withholding is, nonetheless, quite high.

The second distinct ethical issue raised is can another person, a family member, inform Dad instead? By contemporary medical-ethical standards, the physician is obligated to disclose the information to the patient in confidence, and only to let the family know the diagnosis if the patient authorizes this disclosure. In the film John asks the doctor to bend if not break the professional code of conduct by making a special request: "Whatever you do, don't mention cancer to my father. He's terribly anxious and frightened by that word. It's beyond anything rational." Dr. Santana responds in a tone that is slightly patronizing, "Come now, Mr. Tremont, you'd be surprised what these older people can take. Their children tend to underestimate them." John quickly responds, "I don't underestimate him, doctor. I just want to be the one to tell him." John is not asking that information be withheld, only that it be presented by someone close to Jake in a fashion that his father might be able to handle.

This request presents Dr. Santana with what seems to be a true moral dilemma. He has a professional and legal obligation to inform his patient, Jake, in confidence, unless Jake is incompetent or has authorized the disclosure to the family. But he also has a professional obligation to promote the overall health and well-being of his patient. John is informing him that the particularities of his father's psyche mean that the news should come first from the son, and not the doctor. But if Dr. Santana accedes to this request, then he would seem to fail in his obligation to inform the patient himself—after all, it is not clear what John will say, or whether John should even know the diagnosis in advance of Jake's hearing it. It seems that some ethically sound compromise might be worked out in this case. But the clash between the doctor's adherence to general ethical guidelines and a responsiveness to the particularities of the patient's situation is not mediated, to the detriment of the patient.

Back at the house, Bette confronts John saying, "It's cancer, isn't it?" John again denies this, "I told you, Mom, it's a cyst and they took it out." Bette insists on going to see her husband and the children have no choice but to comply (because she threatens to walk). Once again, we see the children trying to withhold information and even to block Bette from seeing her husband, just like they blocked Jake from visiting Bette in the hospital.

At the hospital, they find Jake lying in the bed whimpering in a highly agitated state. In a terrified voice, he whispers, "It's out there, it's out there," pointing toward the door. John confronts Dr. Santana out in the hall and the doctor explains, "This is standard with older people. They often go into delayed shock after minor surgery." He continues in a patronizing tone, "I'm sure it was frightening for you but what you have to understand is what we're seeing is senility." John protests, shouting, "He wasn't senile when he came in here." Dr. Santana says that they will not do any tests, but just wait for Jake to respond to the medicine. As Santana walks away, John asks, "Did you tell my father he had cancer?" Santana turns slowly and walks back toward John, "I have an ethical obligation to my patient. He had a right to know."

In the next scene, we see John in the office of the hospital administrator, Dr. Etheridge (played by Peter Goetz), telling him that he has lost confidence in Dr. Santana. Dr. Etheridge defends his colleague saying, "It seems he has been thorough and professional." John explains, "I asked him not to tell Dad about the cancer and he went ahead and did it anyway." Again, Etheridge defends this action, "That's always a difficult call for a doctor. He has to balance the will of the family members with the patient's right to know. I'm sure he had no choice." John does not buy this explanation countering with, "He had a choice. He could have listened to me. I know my father and what's happening to him right now is a direct result of Dr. Santana's poor judgment." While the doctor may have been "thorough and professional" he was not compassionate or considerate of the requests of the family.

In this ironic turn, the ethical obligation of a physician to be truthful with his patient, which is supposed to promote trust in the medical context and to respect patient autonomy, ends up backfiring, and sending the patient in this case, into a state of painful shock and withdrawal. The film seems here to present an object-lesson critique of the absolute rule-based morality that animates Dr. Santana's decision to inform Jake of his diagnosis himself. Ethical rules, it seems, can and do conflict, and thus, they cannot be absolute. Instead, the film urges us to view ethical rules or principles as only prima facie (or, at first sight, but defeasible) guides to conduct, requiring much, careful practical judgment and sensitivity to the particularities of a case to adjudicate between conflicting principles (Ross 1930). Or, more radically, this situation in *Dad* might lead us toward the view of moral particularism, which holds that true moral reasoning does not employ principles at all, but rather a context-sensitive appraisal of each situation on its own terms (Dancy 2004).

Whatever the meta-ethical lesson one might draw from this part of the film, Jake's "care" in the hospital becomes abysmal. In a dramatic scene, John wraps Jake up in a bedsheet and carries him out of the hospital. On the trip back home, John cradles his father in his arms and vows to care for him himself, rather than to consign him to a nursing home. Billy offers to stay and help, but John snaps, "I'll take care of him. He's my father." Billy retorts, "Well, he's my grandfather." "And I'm your father." Billy turns this aside saying, "Great, now that we know who everyone is can we please talk about what's best for this man?" Billy is bringing home the issue that the patient should be the center of concern, not the battle over who has control over caregiving duties. "I don't want you here right now, Billy. You don't have to see this." Billy protests, "I'm not a kid." In an irritated voice, John declares, "You're in the way here, don't you understand?" This scene dramatically raises the question of who has the right to be part of the support group within the family. Do the adult children have the ultimate right to control caregiving responsibilities, and should other family members be included and embraced for their willingness to take part in the process?

While John is well intentioned, it is obvious that his "zombielike" father will require extensive supervision and help with basic tasks of daily living. After some scary incidents, John returns Jake to the hospital. He is approached by Dr. Etheridge who tries to empathize with his situation: "It's very hard, I realize, for children to understand that their parents have gotten old." John replies with both sarcasm and bitterness, "I know what that means, to be old. It means most people would rather you were dead." Etheridge counters with, "Doctors are only human too. We can't solve every problem. We can't save every patient. We work in a system where old people tend to sometimes fall through the cracks." This is a not-too-veiled reference to the ease with which Santana wanted to dismiss Jake's condition as the onset of sudden dementia. Etheridge then offers to have another doctor look at Jake.

Compassionate Care

Enter Dr. Chad (played by Zakes Mokae), the anti-Santana. He talks to, not above, Annie and John, and he does not view Jake as "custodial." He explains his suspicions that Jake had a seizure and that he wants to get at its cause. John expresses his desire to move into the room in the ICU with Jake. A nurse immediately protests that this is a violation of hospital policy, but Etheridge responds to John's needs saying, "If it makes you more comfortable I think it's a good idea." The hospital personnel are now coming to see the pragmatic and ethical importance of particularities and are willing to break the rules to meet the family's needs and those of the patient.

John moves in and hangs up some family pictures. He is shown becoming a part of the medical team by taking on a variety of chores and helping the staff in their daily activities over the next three weeks. This series of scenes from the movie highlights the importance of the family's being involved and feeling they are making significant contributions to the well-being and recovery of a loved one. It illustrates the desire of family to take an active role in providing support and finding meaning in their own lives as caregivers. It also points out the suffering of family members who get pushed to the side as medical personnel tend to the physical needs of the patient, while excluding members of the patient's family.

Down in the hospital cafeteria, Annie asks John how long he can keep up his vigil. She points out that John is the only one who has not accepted that Jake is dying and asks why he can't let go. He explains:

> Maybe I want to be there to mark the end. To prove he was here. To prove I was his son. That man got up every day of his life and went to a job he didn't like. He just did it 'cause he was the father and that was the deal he made. Some part of that deal was that we'd care for him and watch over him when he got older. I screwed that up. I got embarrassed by him, by the way Mom dominated him, by the way he got old. Embarrassed that I had a marriage that failed, a job that didn't make sense, a son I'd barely recognize if I passed him on the street. Maybe this is more for me than for him. But I'm gonna be there when he dies. I'm gonna kiss him. And I'm gonna cover him, and I'm gonna mark the moment.

This soliloquy finally explains much of John's transformation. The family, perhaps more than any other institution, is the site of many unchosen obligations. John did not choose to owe his father such care, but his father sacrificed much for his sake. What Jake sacrificed, whether or not by necessity, was his authenticity, to work at a job he hated for "his whole life." Although he did not literally work at the factory every day of his life, Jake's spirit was indeed crushed by the mind-numbing routine; he became nothing but a worker, taking direction from others, and this carried over into his marriage with Bette as well.

Tied up with embarrassment of his father and of himself, for failing to be much of a husband or father, he tried to shirk this filial obligation. But the recognition of the "deal" and the imperative to reciprocate, as well as his deep love for the man, eventually hits home. John's declaration to his sister captures the essential importance of family involvement in major health events—the existential need for connection and closure.

The next morning, John wakes up on the cot to see his father sitting up holding the oxygen tube in his hands. "Where am I, Johnny?" he asks. "You're in the hospital, Dad," John replies. "I think I could have guessed that one," says Jake with a humor that will mark the remainder of his life. A nurse walks in saying, "He speaks." Again, with humor, Jake responds, "Yes, it's something he learned as a child." As John calls in the medical personnel, introducing each by name, the viewer is included in this celebration of Jake's reawakening as all present applaud and Jake, with more humor, tips an imaginary hat in acknowledgement of their congratulations. This scene is important to the broader discussion because it illustrates that the medical personnel have become almost like "family" and genuinely care about Jake as a person, not just as an "interesting case." The smiles and hugs demonstrate the bond John has forged with the medical personnel and they with him. Both the medical personnel and the family benefit when they work together; it is the human and compassionate side of medical care. Medical professionals are not just treating a patient but also they have an obligation to be responsive to the family members who are drawn into the medical event, and the family has to be responsive to the needs of the staff in return.

Dr. Chad first offers a medical explanation saying that Jake may have been so fearful of cancer that his brain "froze up" and stopped producing some essential chemical or enzyme. Then he smiles and leans toward John saying, "If we were back home, we'd say that it was not that at all, but rather it was your love and caring that called your father back from where he'd gone." With this simple folk explanation, Dr. Chad acknowledges the love and sacrifice of the son and elevates that effort to one of great significance to the father's recovery. Doing so does not distance the family but recognizes the importance of family involvement in recovery from any illness. The whole family comes to visit Jake, and it is a tearful reunion with everyone hugging and kissing. It is the picture of a family unified and joyous (just like the dreamlike sequences of the farmer working and playing with his family in harmony).

Authentic Living

In a following scene, Jake and John and Billy drive to Venice Beach. Jake explains, "Your mother and I are starting a new life together, Johnny. We need some new clothes." When asked what Bette will say about this, Jake replies, "She'll probably laugh and call me crazy, but she'll laugh. We haven't had enough laughter in our house for the past ten years." This renewed Jake, who began emerging when John first showed up in Los Angeles, is now coming full forward. It brings up the issue of the role of family members as important supports for mental well-being in older adults. In Venice, they buy all sorts of wild outfits for Jake's "jogging on the beach" or "watching baseball games at home." The three men put on a fashion show back at the house and Annie and Bette get drawn into the humorous antics. At one point, Bette shouts through shrieks of hysterical laughter, "I pissed my pants. Tell 'em to stop. I'm dying." Jake replies, "I've never heard of anyone dying from laughter, Bette, but wouldn't that be nice?" He goes over to touch her cheeks and kiss her. This is the first indication that Jake is beginning to come to terms with death and dying.

Viewers will, no doubt, laugh and delight at the antics of this seventy-eight-year-old man as he plays his one-hole golf course out back, does his old man pushups, takes Bette on a mission to meet all the neighbors, and pesters Bette with his renewed interest in sex. He tells Bette, "We gotta get over the fear we're old fogies and stop worrying what people think." He is trying to pull Bette into the joy he is bringing into his everyday life. Bette is scared because she doesn't recognize this Jake, but John defends his father saying, "I think this is the real Jake Tremont. He's just been hiding for fifty years." Here John is serving as an advocate for his father, and also trying to help Bette accept, rather than resist or fear, the reemerged Jake.

When Bette opens up to Jake, she explains, "I'm scared, Jake. I don't know who you are anymore. I don't recognize you. Was it so terrible with me?" Jake responds gently with an edge of sadness, "We just got off the track a little. A lot. I'm asking you to remember the life that you wanted to have. You took it all on by yourself and I let you. You were so good. I'm asking you to let go a little, open up. Not just to me, but to the world. We used to have such good times together. We used to dance. You were a wonderful dancer. I'd like to dance again with you before I die." Bette responds to this last comment, "Don't talk about dying." Jake smiles, saying, "Dying's not a sin. Not living is." He touches her cheek and she reaches toward him leading to a tight embrace and kiss. Then Bette raises her right arm into the dance position and the two begin a slow waltz as the camera pulls away and we see them slowly turning from above. This scene is very significant as touch once again indicates a turning point, Jake's acceptance of death, his refusal to live apathetically, and the willingness of Bette to give herself over to the joy that Jake is trying to recreate in their marriage.

As this story has done a couple of times before, it takes another unexpected turn. In Doctor Chad's office, the doctor hesitates and Jake encourages him to be frank. "The cancer is back. It's spread. It's in the lymph system." When Jake asks how long he has, the doctor hesitates but Jake insists, "You can tell me the truth." The simple reply is "not long." Jake takes the news somberly as he looks out the window with a slightly trembling lip.

We normally think of compassionate care at the end of life as involving what others give to the dying individual. Actually, compassionate care can go both ways. The dying person can show compassion by helping achieve closure for those he or she is leaving behind. He can assist, for example, in his "bed and body work," by accepting it with gratitude and as much goodwill as possible. This mutually beneficial compassion is shown in one of the closing scenes when John comes to visit his dad in the hospital. Jake tells John that he feels he should be having deep thoughts, but keeps coming back to the sixth game of the 1947 World Series. Rather than dismissing his father's unusual train of thought, John encourages him to tell the story. The story revolves around a hit by Joe DiMaggio that had "home run all over it." At the last possible moment, a second stringer center fielder jumps up and reaches over the rail to snag the ball preventing the home run. Jake explains the significance of this memory as a life lesson: "In America, anything is possible if you show up for work."

This disclosure and John's response are important for two reasons. First, John is listening and this opens up a dialogue for Jake to explore his memories and pass on something of value to his son (we see John do this with his own son earlier in the movie: "Be forgiving.") and to experience a moment of generativity. *Generativity* involves guidance offered by relatively older individuals to those who are younger. While Erik Erikson (1959/1980, 1968) saw this effort to forge generational continuity as occurring in the stage prior to old age, research has shown that "purposeful action oriented toward some meaningful goal" (Fisher 1995, p. 241) extends well into later life.

Jake's disclosure is important for a second reason, namely, that it shows the value of family members as partners in the dying process as they help the individual in his or her struggle to die with dignity. This open communication allows Jake to confess his regrets to John, "Sometimes I wish I'd held you more when you were a kid. I wish I'd kissed you more." With this disclosure, John is able to reassure Jake that he had been a good father and Jake, in return tells John, "You know how much I love you." John gets up on the bed to lay by the side of his father, unasked, to hug Jake and allow his father to provide him comfort even as he provides comfort to Jake. It is a scene of love, of respect, of a life that did not always go well but ended well, a time of closure for both father and son.

In the final scene, which occurs after the death of Jake, Billy gives his dad a nod and they both separate from the crowd to go out to the greenhouse, where they put on a couple of Jake's favorite wild jackets. Billy picks up an orchid and brings it over to a table, where he stands next to it with John. In a tearful voice, he says, "Grandpa, we just wanted to take some time and say good-bye our way. I guess it's your way. And this seemed the right place to do it 'cause there's so much of you in here. So much that's alive and growing. Grandpa, I love you and miss you already. Dad and I are here and we're together." Father and son embrace and cry and the viewer is left with the impression that just like with Jake and John, the gap between these two characters has been permanently bridged.

Conclusion

One of the fascinations of the *Dad* narrative is that, for a film set in the United States and that deals with families in their attempt to cope with illness and dying, religion is never mentioned. This lacuna is highly suggestive. Many people find tremendous comfort and strength, in facing death and loss, through religious belief and ritual. The characters in *Dad* do not turn toward comforting thoughts of heaven, an eternal soul, or God's plan. The world of *Dad* is, by default, and only implicitly, agnostic. It is an unspoken assumption in the film that modern medicine is what stands between them and the scientific, cold reality of death.

The coping mechanism used by many of the characters in *Dad* to deal with this harsh reality is deception. Rather than open communication about illness and prognosis, many withhold information to protect others, especially those who are closer to death. The evasion from the truth, however, represents in the film a general fleeing from life. As Martin Heidegger wrote in the seminal work of early existentialism, *Being and Time* (originally published in 1927), a common part of ordinary social life is to "flee" from death: "This evasive concealment in the face of death dominates everydayness so stubbornly, that in Being with one another, the 'neighbors' often still keep talking the 'dying person' into the belief that he will escape death and soon return to the tranquillized everydayness of the world of his concern. Such 'solicitude' is meant to 'console' him" (Heidegger 1927/1962, p. 297).

Unlike, say, an apple, which grows, ripens, and disintegrates according to an inexorable plan, a human being's life does not have a defined trajectory; rather, it is characterized by myriad possibility. For Heidegger, the authentic person "lives toward death," that is, keeps the final endpoint of human life in mind throughout life, and this way is constituted in part by a certain anxiety. This is anxiety "in the face of that potentiality-for-Being which is one's ownmost . . . that in the face of which one has anxiety is Being-in-the-world itself" (Heidegger 1962, p. 295).

An authentic way of being, characterized by anxiety over the nature of one's multiple possibilities for being, while difficult to maintain in Western culture, should not be paralyzing. Rather, "being toward death" should serve as a spur to active, conscious, meaningful living, where the full value of one's life is seized every day, and the value of others' to our lives is adequately appreciated.

Ultimately, the frame of this film—the parallel fantasy world Jake inhabited on a farm in Cape May, New Jersey—might just present a challenge to the viewers to question which fantasy realm we might be inhabiting, albeit in a less extreme way. The film reveals to us, through an oftentimes painful, emotional engagement with narrative, what existentialist philosophers such as Heidegger have tried to convince readers of discursively: keep death in mind throughout life; do not flee into a hazy, inauthentic fantasy life; rather, construct an honest life, built on honest relationships with family, and ultimately liberating truths, and make of one's actual life, something rich and beautiful.

QUESTIONS FOR CONSIDERATION

1. *The* Dad *narrative portrays the difficulty of achieving open communication about illness and death in one family. Is the family in* Dad

typical of how families deal with these issues, in your experience? What can families do to be more prepared for major health events that may affect the independence of older members of the family?

2. Do the adult children have the ultimate right to control caregiving responsibilities? Should other family members (and even friends) be included and embraced for their willingness to take part in the process? And, if so, should there be an age criterion to allow a family member to participate in caregiving duties?

3. Compare and contrast the virtues and vices of Dr. Chad and Dr. Santana in the film. Although the film lauds Dr. Chad's willingness to break hospital policies to fit the particularities of a situation, do you think this is a good trait for a physician to possess?

4. What sort of ethical compromise might have been worked out between Dr. Santana and John with respect to disclosing the diagnosis of cancer to Jake? Is it ever right to conceal medical information from a family member and, if so, under what circumstances?

REFERENCES

Beauchamp, T., and Walters, L., eds. 2003. *Contemporary Issues in Bioethics,* 6th ed. Belmont, CA: Wadsworth.

Dancy, J. 2004. *Ethics without Principles.* Oxford: Clarendon Press.

Erikson, E. 1968. *Identity: Youth and Crisis.* New York: Norton.

———. 1980. *Identity and the Life Cycle.* New York: Norton. (Originally published in 1959)

Fisher, B. J. 1995. Successful Aging, Life Satisfaction, and Generativity in Later Life. *International Journal of Aging and Human Development* 41 (3):239–50.

Glaser, B. G., and Strauss, A. 1965. *Awareness of Dying.* Chicago: Aldine.

Goldberg, G. D. 1989. *Dad* [motion picture]. Los Angeles: Amblin Entertainment.

Heidegger, M. 1962. *Being and Time,* trans. J. Macquarrie and E. Robinson. San Francisco: Harper & Row. (Originally published 1927)

Ross, W. D. 1930. *The Right and the Good.* Oxford: Clarendon Press.

Thomasma, D. C. 1994. Telling the Truth to Patients: A Clinical Ethics Exploration. *Cambridge Quarterly of Healthcare Ethics* 3:375–82.

FOURTEEN

False Images

Reframing the End-of-Life Portrayal of Disability in *Million Dollar Baby*

Zana Marie Lutfiyya, Karen D. Schwartz, and Nancy Hansen

In this chapter, we examine the depiction of euthanasia in the film *Million Dollar Baby* (Eastwood 2004) by analyzing the film's reinforcement of the associations between disability and death. We use this portrayal to open a philosophical dialogue about the reality of disability, how we know what we know about disability, and how misleading and dangerous it can be to turn the experience of disability into an end-of-life issue.

Much praise and many accolades have been heaped on Clint Eastwood's 2004 film *Million Dollar Baby*, culminating in its being awarded Best Picture by the Academy of Motion Picture Arts and Sciences. The movie tells the story of boxer Maggie Fitzgerald, who, notwithstanding her gender and a late start in the sport, trains diligently and gets a chance at a title fight. During this championship bout, however, she is viciously attacked from behind and sustains a career-ending spinal cord injury. The last section of the film portrays someone broken and defeated, struggling to end her life. With this surprising twist of story-telling, the movie wades into the murky philosophical waters of bioethics and the controversy surrounding the right to die. It also finds itself, whether by accident or by design, in the middle of a heated debate about what it means to live (or die) with a disability.

What Is Euthanasia?

Discussions about bioethical issues have gained prominence in our modern world for several reasons. First, because modern medicine has advanced to the point of being able to eliminate many causes of disability and disease and, second, because certain technological advancements have made it possible to keep people alive from conditions that might have killed them in the past. Even though people are now living longer and disability is becoming more common with advanced age, a disabled life is still devalued. Thus our thoughts turn, inevitably, to how we would deal with illness and disability should we find ourselves faced with such a situation in the future. One of the major dilemmas in our society is the issue of euthanasia; should a person have the legal and moral right to ask for assistance in ending his or her life?

The word *euthanasia* is derived from the Greek root meaning "good death." Sanders and Chaloner (2007) defined the term as the "deliberate intervention or omission with the express intention of hastening or ending an individual's life, to relive intractable pain or suffering" (p. 42). Sometimes the words "active" and "passive" are used in conjunction with the term *euthanasia.* Active euthanasia "describes the deliberate and active intervention to end a person's life" (Sanders and Chaloner 2007, p. 42). Passive euthanasia occurs "when an individual is allowed to die. The death is deliberate and intended and brought about by an omission" (Sanders and Chaloner 2007, p. 42). In addition, other terms have been used to describe related concepts. The term *voluntary euthanasia* connotes that a competent individual has made a request to be killed. When an individual is killed after expressing a wish to the contrary, this is termed *involuntary euthanasia* and is considered murder. The term *assisted suicide* is used to describe the actions of a person when providing the means for another individual to commit suicide. When a physician is the person providing this assistance, the act is known as *physician-assisted suicide.*

In the film *Million Dollar Baby*, only the voluntary type of euthanasia is focused on. Before we begin to discuss the portrayal of euthanasia in the film and what this means to people with disabilities and to the field of disability studies, we must first briefly review some of the major arguments in favor of and against allowing an individual to choose death.

These arguments will give us a springboard for understanding the philosophical debates that will follow.

Arguments in Favor of Euthanasia

As the meaning of the word "euthanasia"—a "good death"—suggests, proponents advocate euthanasia as a means of ending an individual's pain and suffering. These proponents assume that people who would choose to die are necessarily suffering and in pain and that their only alternative is death. There is also a strong belief in our society in patient autonomy and the right of patients to make choices about their care. This conviction is now enshrined in the legal systems of both Canada and the United States, which allow patients to refuse medical treatments, even if such a choice might lead to their death (Derse 2005). The watershed legal decision in these matters in the United States was the case of *In re Quinlan*, in which the New Jersey Supreme Court ruled that the Constitution of the United States provided a "right to privacy." This right allowed a father to have ventilation support to his comatose daughter discontinued, culminating in her eventual death.

Advocates in favor of euthanasia encourage the right to die "with dignity." Indeed, the law in Oregon permitting physician-assisted suicide is actually called the Death with Dignity Act. The very name of the act implies that the right to choose death is a way of dignifying the end-of-life experience. "Some studies suggest that 'loss of dignity' is one of the most common reasons physicians cite when they agreed to their patients' request for euthanasia or some form of assisted suicide" (Chochinov et al. 2004, p. 134).

The right to die has generated much debate about the meaning of the phrase "quality of life." When medical decisions are made concerning a course of treatment, the continuation of treatment, or whether to treat at all, quality of life discussions inevitably follow. When we can say that a person has little or no quality of life, we can take a certain comfort in our decision to end that life. But in doing so, we have to acknowledge that underlying these conversations are (1) subjective values about what quality of life means and (2) assumptions about the consistency of quality of life over time (Carr, Gibson, and Robinson 2001).

Finally, there is always a concern about financial cost. Health care is expensive. There are only so many dollars to go around, and how much money do we want to spend on people who are ill, disabled, suffering, dependent, and a burden? Wouldn't it be more prudent to spend those scarce resources on healthier, younger, and more able-bodied members of society? Euthanasia is far less expensive than continuing to support life at any cost.

Arguments against Euthanasia

Some members of society feel that there are significant religious reasons for rejecting euthanasia. If one believes in the sanctity of human life, then there is no "good" reason to perform euthanasia no matter how merciful the intent behind it. There are also doctors and health care professionals who feel that to kill or to assist in killing a patient goes against the values of medicine. These include the "fundamental tenet of medicine: to heal and not to harm" (Steinbock 2005, p. 236).

Cohn and Lynn present an interesting discussion of the pressures vulnerable people might feel toward choosing euthanasia. They say: "For many, no reasonably desirable choices may exist. Then, physician-assisted suicide may not merely be a choice, one option among others; rather it may become a coercive offer . . . ending one's own life could come to be perceived as an obligation, that is, a societally endorsed course of action that is the only way to avoid suffering, indignity, and impoverishment" (Cohn and Lynn 2002, p. 241). They go on to suggest that "personal circumstances and societal expectations do often shape individual desires, but what one believes he or she should do is not necessarily the same as what an individual really wants" (p. 241).

Finally, but perhaps most critically, studies have shown that opening the door to euthanasia can close the door to excellent end-of-life care (Chochinov 2002; Chochinov et al. 2002, 2004; Cohn and Lynn 2002; Curry, Schwartz, Gruman, and Blank 2002). It is much simpler to end a life than to plan for holistic, dignified, end-of-life scenarios that value each and every patient, regardless of societal values and prejudices. Tied to this notion is the acknowledgment that good end-of-life care is not practiced by the majority of physicians and health care professionals and is not adequately taught in medical school curricula (Curry et al. 2002). Therefore, doctors who have a deficiency in end-of-life care knowledge have a greater propensity to turn to euthanasia as an appropriate care solution (Curry et al. 2002; Hendin 2004). In contrast, doctors who are well versed in end-of-life medicine are able to ease suffering and raise patient dignity through means other than death. "When the preservation of dignity becomes the clear goal of palliation, care options expand well beyond the symptom management paradigm . . . systematically broaching these issues within discussions of end-of-life care could allow patients to make more informed choices, achieve better palliation of symptoms, and have more opportunity to work on issues of closure" (Chochinov 2002, p. 2254).

The Portrayal of Euthanasia in *Million Dollar Baby*

Maggie Fitzgerald grew up, as the narrator of the film tells us, "knowing one thing. She was trash." She describes how she feels about boxing. "The problem is, this is the only thing I ever felt good about doin'. If I'm too old for this then I got nothing." To reach her goal, she seeks the help of an old trainer, Frankie Dunn, owner of the Hit Pit Gym. At first, he refuses to help Maggie because he doesn't, as a rule, train "girls."

Eventually Maggie convinces Frankie to take her on, and she begins to advance through the boxing ranks and to win fights, ultimately earning a shot at the title fight with a million dollars on the line. Her opponent, Billie "the Blue Bear," is known as unbeatable, tough, and dirty. Partway through the bout, after the bell has rung and Maggie turns to go back to her corner, "Blue Bear" hits her from behind and Maggie falls against the stool that has been set out for her. In the process, she hits her neck with a sickening crack and is rushed to the hospital. There she learns that she has sustained an injury to her spinal cord and her future shifts from one of physical prowess to one of physical disability.

Maggie's world as she has known it ends after her injury, and she is convinced that she does not want to live without boxing. Boxing alone defined her and made her whole. Maggie becomes determined to die. "I can't be like this, Frankie. Not after what I done . . . People chanted my name . . . they were chantin' for me. I was in magazines. You think I ever dreamed that would happen? . . . Don't let 'em keep taking it away from me. Don't let me lie here till I can't hear those people chantin' no more." Because she is paralyzed, she cannot end her own life, though she does try to do so at one point by biting her tongue in an effort to bleed to death. Undaunted in her mission, she asks Frankie to help her do what she herself cannot accomplish. And Frankie, out of love for Maggie, eventually agrees to help. "All right. I'm gonna disconnect your air machine and you're gonna go to sleep. Then I'll give you a shot and you'll stay asleep."

Wolfensberger writes about social devaluation and its link to societal perceptions about certain people and groups of people within society. He discusses the various influences on an observer that help shape perceptions and may, in turn, lead to social devaluation. These influences include (1) the observer's own characteristics and experiences, (2) characteristics in the observer's physical environment, (3) characteristics of the observer's social environment, including values and norms, and (4) what is actually observed (i.e., the object of potential devaluation; Wolfensberger 1998). How Maggie is portrayed during the period after the accident is very important. The imagery that director Clint Eastwood uses conveys a specific message that links disability with death.

Our society's values and norms often exclude and devalue differences, including the difference of disability. Therefore, the moviegoer's perceptions about death and disability are only partially influenced by what he or she actually sees in the film. They are also influenced by other messages within society about the nature of disability. "Unfortunately, cure, death and tragedy have been a part of every era's representations of disability in cinema and in culture in general" (Darke 1997). For example, images of disability revealed in the film such as Maggie's grimly institutional room, her hospital bed, and her wheelchair are highly devalued in our society. It is likely that movie viewers would be either unconsciously or consciously aware of their own preconceived notions of a life "condemned" to living as Maggie will after the accident. Moviegoers may well put themselves in Maggie's position and might dread the notion of being "confined" to a bed or wheelchair.

Longmore (2003) argues that on screen, characters with disabilities are often presented in a negative light. "Among the most persistent is the association of disability with malevolence. Deformity of body symbolizes deformity of soul. Physical handicaps are made the emblems of evil" (p. 133). Longmore also suggests that these representations of disability "express to varying degrees the notion that disability involves the loss of an essential part of one's humanity . . . the individual is perceived as more or less subhuman" (Longmore 2003, p. 135).

Like *Million Dollar Baby*, the movie *Whose Life Is It Anyway?* (Badham 1981) portrays an individual with a spinal cord injury who wants to die. Longmore describes the "unacknowledged" theme of the movie; it is "the horror of a presumed 'vegetable-like' existence following severe disablement . . . Disability again means the loss of one's humanity. The witty, combative central character in *Whose Life Is It Anyway?* refers to himself as a 'vegetable' and says that he is 'not a man anymore' " (Longmore 2003, p. 136). Similarly, how the preaccident Maggie is juxtaposed against the postaccident Maggie feeds into societal perceptions and misconceptions about what it is like to have a disability and what disability is.

Several scenes in *Million Dollar Baby* image Maggie as a professional fighter. When she is training, Maggie's body is clearly portrayed as a lean, fit, conditioned machine. Her perfectly defined abdominal muscles are evident as she skips rope. Her muscled and toned limbs are clearly visible and impressive. When she boxes, her long hair is carefully braided, not a hair out of place. Her body glows with health and vitality, willing and able to take on all challengers. As she begins to mount win after win, we see her adoring fans and hear their roar of approval as she knocks out contender after contender. Maggie Fitzgerald is on top of the world.

After the accident, Maggie is imaged in a very different way. First, she is in a hospital. When nothing more can be done for her there, she is moved to the Serenity Glen Rehabilitation Center. She is shown, primarily, lying in a hospital-style bed, in an institutional room, wearing a hospital gown. On only two occasions is she sitting up in a wheelchair and dressed, but she is never taken outside her room. When we first see her out of bed as she is transferred into her wheelchair, Scrap says, "It took several hours every day to get her ready for the wheelchair," perhaps implying it was not time well spent. And if she was assisted into her chair daily, we see no evidence of it.

We do see quite distinctly, however, the image of her physical decay. Bedsores and the gangrene she develops result in the loss of her leg. After her operation, Maggie's "deterioration" is plainly evident. She is never out of bed or dressed. She never smiles. Her hair is loose and tangled. Gone are the fancy braids of the beloved fighter. Her eyes are sunken, ringed in black. Her lips are chapped. Her skin looks white and pasty. She is, in short, the image of death.

Watching the film, we share her despondency. She can no longer fight. She has lost the will to live. Who would want to live a life of paralysis, relying on a respirator to take a breath? Of course, she wants to die, we empathize. Who wouldn't, in her situation? Life has nothing to offer her, and she is competent to make the decision to die. If she were able, she could kill herself, no questions asked. Frankie is right to help her die because Maggie feels worthless and is convinced she has nothing to live for.

But wait a minute! She is paralyzed and does need help to breathe. In fact, she has significant and complex needs. But is she near death? Is she suffering and in pain, with an incurable illness? Must we assume she has lost all dignity and has no quality of life? Is she merely a worthless, dependent burden on society? Now let's look at Maggie again, through a new lens.

The "Reality" of Disability

We argue that people with and without disabilities view and experience the world differently. One reality may be to wake up every day, walk the dog, and drive the car to work, with no thought to the effort of traveling through time and space. Another reality may be to rely on others to provide transport, walk with the aid of a cane, and require considerable time and effort to move through space. The two realities are diverse, but each describes an everyday lived experience. When it comes to ethical issues of life and death, the difficulty begins when those who have little knowledge or understanding of the experience of disability make decisions, assumptions, and judgments about quality of life, life worth living, pain and suffering, dignity, and death of those who do.

In North American society, disability has traditionally been defined as a deficit, defect, or problem that resides within an individual. It is treated as a condition in need of a remedy or cure, placing it within the realm of medical and rehabilitation professionals to manage. And if remedy or cure cannot be realized, rehabilitation management will enable the individual to be made to fit into society—the able-bodied and able-minded world (Longmore 2003). Disability has not generally been understood as a difference that society can, in fact, accommodate. We have built stairs, designed narrow doorways, placed sinks and light switches too high, demanded doors be pulled open, often with rounded knobs. Our kids stare at difference, trying to understand it. Yet when they ask us why, we hush their questions, ignore their curiosity, and, in doing so, attach a shame to difference. We fail to explain that people can be different but still have value.

Our society defines disability in several ways. These definitions allow us to treat people with disabilities accordingly. Disability is a tragedy, and those with disabilities carry the stigma of inferiority. We see people with disabilities as burdensome, lacking in autonomy and dignity. We pity the disabled and fear that we, too, might become afflicted. In our fear and ignorance, we discriminate and isolate, resentful of those who dare challenge our comfortable norms and ways of being. As a result of our ingrained feelings and beliefs, we devalue people with disabilities. Such devaluation can and does lead to the casting of devalued people into undesirable roles such as (1) the "alien" or "other," (2) the subhuman or nonhuman (especially with the use of the term *vegetative* to describe certain mental states of being), (3) the "sick, ill or diseased organism," and (4) those related to death or death imaging (Wolfensberger 1998, pp. 14–16). The portrayal of Maggie Fitzgerald in the film *Million Dollar Baby* is a good example of imaging a person with a disability as someone near death or embodying death.

How Do We Know What We Know about Disability?

The next question that we must look at is this: how do we know what we know about disability? All of these descriptions and characterizations paint a grim picture of living life with a disability. How has this reality been created and perpetuated? The answer is multifaceted and involves, in part, the combination of a number of beliefs, ideas, and theories over the course of history.

From the earliest periods, disability was seen as the result of an act of God, a punishment for wrongdoing. Deuteronomy 28:15 warns that "if you do not carefully follow his commands and decrees . . . all these curses will come upon you and overtake you: the Lord will afflict you with madness, blindness and confusion of mind" (28–29). Barnes argues that "biblical text is replete with references to impairment as the consequences of wrongdoing" (Barnes 1997, p. 15). Wilson traces this back to classical Greece and Aristotle's conception of the "normal/abnormal" dichotomy: "In *Nicomachean Ethics* Aristotle takes his argument to its (il)logical conclusion, identifying the norm (or mean) with moral virtue and the abnormal with vice. Thus physical 'deformity' becomes moral flaw, exposing Aristotle's binary configuration for what it really is—a social hierarchy" (Wilson 2000, p. 153). St. Augustine claimed, "impairment was 'a punishment for the fall of Adam and other sins' " and that Martin Luther "proclaimed he saw the Devil in a disabled child; he recommended killing them" (Barnes 1997, p. 17).

By the mid-nineteenth century, disability had become inexorably intertwined with medicine: "The emergence of a medical model in the modern era redefined disability as a biological insufficiency that could be ameliorated by what we now call professional intervention. It came to be believed that treatment could cure, or at least correct, most disabilities or their functional concomitants enough for handicapped individuals to conduct themselves in a socially acceptable manner" (Longmore 2003, p. 150). In addition, early and misinformed research in genetics and heredity led to charges that disability was genetically created (Goddard 1912).

The rise of statistics and its application to human populations helped create the categories of "normal" and "abnormal," labels with which we are very familiar today. As Davis says, "an important consequence of the idea of the norm is that it divides the total population into standard and non-standard subpopulations" (Davis 1997, p. 14). He goes on to suggest that "normalcy is constructed to create the 'problem' of the disabled person," thus "when we think of bodies, in a society where the concept of the norm is operative, then people with disabilities will be thought of as deviants (Davis 1997, p. 13).

Disability Studies: Challenging the Discourse

How can we challenge this traditional discourse of disability? The first step is to acknowledge that disability needn't be and isn't what it has traditionally been. Darke, who writes about disability and cinema, says, "It is, in reality, a misnomer to talk of the stereotypes of disability imagery; the stranglehold that able-bodied people have over the definition of disability makes their representations of us, 'the disabled', more akin to being archetypal in conception. Disability, to the nondisabled society and image maker, is a world-wide and eternal truth that is for them so obviously correct that it cannot be challenged" (Darke 1997, p. 13).

Let's look for a moment at the "other" reality—life for people with disabilities. Let's examine some societal stereotypes or misconceptions about disability and how these feed into the notion "that disability reduces quality of life to a degree that justifies an exceptional response—that compels medical and mental health professionals, when confronted by disabled persons requesting suicide assistance, to deviate from the conventional standard of suicide prevention applied to physically unimpaired suicidal individuals" (Gill 2000, p. 528).

One of the original premises of the right-to-die debate is the notion that bringing about death will end pain and suffering. In the general end-of-life context, it has been recognized that doctors have not been successful in managing pain for patients with terminal illness (Curry et al. 2002; Arnold 2004; Derse 2005). However, are people with disabilities suffering and in pain solely as a result of having a disability? Although societal perceptions of disability include pain and suffering, this is not necessarily the experience of disability. "Society often identifies the cause of suffering as a permanent sickness, creating only a semblance of life within the individual, or as an imprisonment from which the individual seeks to be freed at any cost" (Miller 1993, p. 50). Although some people may be in pain, we cannot assume that this is always the case. The film *Million Dollar Baby* portrays Maggie as suffering, and she clearly looks sick with her pale skin, dark, sunken eyes and parched lips. However, she is not ill. This depiction is sending us a message, not so much about Maggie, but about disability, one that reinforces the traditional disability discourse but not the disability experience. Many people who are quadriplegic like Maggie lead full lives and are contributing members of society. They do not see themselves as sick, nor do they conceptualize themselves to be at the end of life.

Another issue in the argument in favor of voluntary euthanasia is the supposed right to choose. Some would argue that Maggie is simply making the choice to die and that she has every right to make this voluntary decision. However, we suggest that a number of things are preventing her from making an informed choice. Depression is a common issue for people in Maggie's situation. Good care would ensure that individuals going through this difficult time have access to psychiatric counseling, physical and occupational therapies, and information about the services and supports available in the community to help in this complex transition process. So too would talking with others who have lived through these types of experiences. "Without being offered the choice of independent living alternatives and counselling, with special emphasis on psychological issues facing persons with disabilities, the right to assisted suicide is no right at all; it is the inevitable manifestation of society's prejudice" (Miller 1993, p. 55). Unfortunately, the film shows only Maggie lying in bed in her impersonal room at the rehabilitation center bereft of music, television, or personal touches of any kind. The closest she gets to the outside world is looking though a window. She is the embodiment of the disability stereotype. She would be far better served by being informed of alternatives to death. In this way, she could become truly autonomous.

The notion of dignity is another theme that is presented as a leading concern in support of euthanasia. Society's basic presumption is that people like Maggie cannot possibly have any dignity in life, and therefore dignity can only be achieved by choosing death. This presumption of loss of dignity comes from a perceived loss of control and from being dependent on others, especially in matters of personal care. In our society, to be unable to independently deal with issues such as personal hygiene is seen as the ultimate form of degradation and humiliation. Longmore quotes Stephen Darke on these "devaluating attitudes of our society that tell sick or disabled people they lack dignity because they need assistance with basic activities of daily living, and would be better off dead" (Longmore 2003, p. 189). Indeed, "disability is considered antithetical to dignity" (Miller 1993, p. 50), but if we saw dependence as a fact of life that most of us will have to face at some point and realized that people have an inherent dignity in their "humanness" (Bogdan and Taylor 1998, pp. 242–61) that supersedes their inability to shower or use the washroom without assistance, we would come to understand that dependence bears no relation to dignity at all. We suggest that Maggie would be much more dignified if she were dressed, in her chair and engaging in some sort of meaningful activity, rather than simply lying in bed. It is not the disability that takes away Maggie's dignity; it is the way in which her image is treated in the film.

The final issue to address is the notion of quality of life. A number of authors have provided excellent examples that highlight the importance of viewing disability from a disabled perspective, rather than from the traditional, nondisabled perspective. One story (Kaufert and Koch 2003) tells of two clinicians who were presenting a case study on end-of-life decision-making for a man with amyotrophic lateral sclerosis (also known as Lou Gehrig's disease) who had decided to discontinue using his ventilator. The presentation "emphasized their presumption that the course of his illness necessarily would result in a deteriorating life quality that was progressively bleak" (Kaufert and Koch 2003, pp. 2–3). Some audience members, themselves users of mechanical ventilation, strongly disagreed with the assumption that "life on ventilation . . . necessarily reflected a diminished quality and minimal sustainability." Thus, "what to the clinicians was a textbook case of 'end-of-life' decision making was, for their audience, a story in which a life was ended as a result of failures of information and assistance" (Kaufert and Koch 2003, p. 4). Similarly, Maggie's disability need, and, indeed, ought, not to be treated as an end-of-life issue. Rather, it should be an exploration of a different kind of life and a reaffirmation of her value and worth.

Toombs writes from the experiences of someone living with multiple sclerosis. She discusses the "prevailing cultural attitudes" of "health, independence, physical appearance" and the "strong cultural message that we should be able to stand on our own two feet, look after ourselves. Dependence on others is perceived as weakness" (Toombs 2004, p. 193). She emphasizes feelings of shame at being a "burden" on other people, and says that "so ingrained are these societal attitudes that the incurably ill may unwittingly feel that, by killing themselves, they are acting unselfishly, in the best interests of others and, furthermore, that they are, in some sense, obligated to do so" (Toombs 2004, p. 194). After her accident, Maggie reassures Frankie that when her family finally arrives to see her, it will relieve some of the burden he shoulders.

Researchers (Nantais and Kuczewski 2004) have shown that caregivers and other third parties often believe that individuals with a disability have a much lower quality of life than the individuals believe. Other researchers have indicated that when nondisabled people imagine life with a spinal cord injury, they see themselves as significantly worse off than do people who actually have a spinal cord injury. In response to the statement, "I feel that I am a person of worth," 95 percent of disabled respondents answered in the affirmative whereas only 55 percent of nondisabled respondents imagining life with a disability agreed (Wolbring 2003).

The term "quality of life" is value laden and highly subjective. Yet we continue to cling to the notion that others know better than people with disabilities themselves about how valuable or worthwhile their lives actually are. Through its imagery, *Million Dollar Baby* reinforces the societal perception that people who are disabled have no quality of life. In portraying Maggie's life as worthless, the film ignores any positive steps she might have taken toward adapting to her new life.

Conclusion

The traditional disability discourse has been built on largely medicalized notions of disability as a defect or deficit that lies within the person. Furthermore, this discourse reinforces the shared belief that the individual has an obligation to attempt to remedy this defect or deficit or at least to ameliorate the condition to fit into the nondisabled world.

To begin a new discourse on disability it is necessary to bring out the voices and experiences of people with disabilities. Michel Foucault calls these voices "subjugated knowledge" and holds that "it is through the re-emergence of these low-ranking knowledges, these unqualified, even directly disqualified knowledges . . . that criticism performs its work" (Foucault 1980, pp. 80–82). The first step, however, is recognizing the importance of listening to and accepting a type of knowledge that is different from the one we've always known. We look forward to the time when society hears the voices of people with disabilities and pauses before assuming that disability is, in and of itself, an end-of-life issue. And while negative imaging of disability and the issue of euthanasia in the film *Million Dollar Baby* are disappointing, the film becomes a useful tool in opening up the dialogue we need to have to recognize, once and for all, that disability is not a fate worse than death.

QUESTIONS FOR CONSIDERATION

1. *What role do you think imagery plays in shaping and communicating already held assumptions or beliefs?*

2. *If imagery has relevance, what are some ways in which people with different disabilities are portrayed?*

3. *What effect might the portrayal of those with disabilities have on the treatment they receive, how people interact with them, and on how assumptions, beliefs, and stereotypes are created and maintained?*

4. *If a disabled person experiences untreatable pain, or if a disabled person, like Maggie, makes a truly informed decision to die, should such a person be allowed assistance in dying?*

ACKNOWLEDGMENTS

The preparation of this chapter was supported by the Canadian Institutes of Health Research New Emerging Team Grant on End of Life Care and Vulnerable Populations held by Harvey M. Chochinov, Deborah Stienstra, Joseph M. Kaufert, and Zana M. Lutfiyya.

REFERENCES

Arnold, E. M. 2004. Factors that Influence Consideration of Hastening Death among People with Life-Threatening Illnesses. *Health and Social Work* 29: 17–25.

Badham, J. 1981. *Whose Life Is It Anyway?* [motion picture]. Los Angeles: Metro-Goldwyn-Mayer.

Barnes, C. 1997. A Legacy of Oppression: A History of Disability in Western Culture. In *Disability Studies: Past, Present and Future,* ed. L. Barton and M. Oliver, 3–24. Leeds: The Disability Press.

Bogdan, R., and Taylor, S. J. 1998. The Social Construction of Humanness: Relationships with People with Severe Retardation. In *Introduction to Qualitative Research Methods: A Guidebook and Resource* (3rd. ed), ed. S. J. Taylor and R. Bogdan, 242–58. New York: Wiley.

Carr, A. J., Gibson, B., and Robinson, P. G. 2001. Is Quality of Life Determined by Expectations or Experience? *British Medical Journal* 322:1240–43.

Chochinov, H. M. 2002. Dignity-Conserving Care: A New Model for Palliative Care. *JAMA* 287:2253–60.

Chochinov, H. M., Hack, T., Hassard, T., Kristjanson, L. J., et al. 2004. Dignity and Psychotherapeutic Considerations in End-of-Life Care. *Journal of Palliative Care* 20:134–41.

Chochinov, H. M., Hack, T., McClement, S., Kristjanson, L., and Harlos, M. 2002. Dignity in the Terminally Ill: A Developing Empirical Model. *Social Science and Medicine* 54:433–43.

Cohn, F., and Lynn, J. 2002. Vulnerable People. In *The Case against Assisted Suicide,* ed. K. Foley and H. Hendin, 238–60. Baltimore: Johns Hopkins University Press.

Curry, L., Schwartz, H. I., Gruman, C., and Blank, K. 2002. Could Adequate Palliative Care Obviate Assisted Suicide? *Death Studies* 26:757–74.

Darke, P. 1997. Everywhere: Disability on Film. In *Framed: Interrogating Disability in the Media,* ed. A. Pointon and C. Davies, 10–15. London: British Film Institute.

Davis, L. J. 1997. Constructing Normalcy. In *The Disability Studies Reader,* ed. L. J. Davis, 9–28. New York: Routledge.

Derse, A. R. 2005. Limitation of Treatment at the End-of-life: Withholding and Withdrawal. *Clinics in Geriatric Medicine* 21:223–38.

Eastwood, C. 2004. *Million Dollar Baby* [motion picture]. Burbank, CA: Warner Bros. Pictures.

Foucault, M. 1980. Two Lectures. In *Power/Knowledge: Selected Interviews and Other Writings 1972–1977,* ed. C. Gordon, 78–108. New York: Pantheon Books.

Gill, C. J. 2000. Health Professionals, Disability, and Assisted Suicide. *Psychology, Public Policy, and Law* 6:526–45.

Goddard, H. H. 1912. *The Kallikak Family: A Study in the Heredity of Feeble-Mindedness.* New York: Macmillan.

Hendin, H. 2004. The Case against Physician-Assisted Suicide: For the Right to End-of-Life Care. *Psychiatric Times* 21:1–10.

Kaufert, J., and Koch, T. 2003. Disability or End-of-Life: Competing Narratives in Bioethics. *Journal of Theoretical Medicine and Ethics* 24:259–69.

Longmore, P. K. 2003. *Why I Burned My Book and Other Essays on Disability.* Philadelphia: Temple University Press.

Miller, P. S. 1993. The Impact of Assisted Suicide on Persons with Disabilities: Is It a Right without Freedom? *Issues in Law and Medicine* 9:47–61.

Nantais, D., and Kuczewski, M. 2004. Quality of Life: The Contested Rhetoric of Resource Allocation and End-of-Life Decision Making. *Journal of Medicine and Philosophy* 29:651–64.

Sanders, K., and Chaloner, C. 2007. Voluntary Euthanasia: Ethical Concepts and Definitions. *Nursing Standard* 21:41–44.

Steinbock, B. 2005. The Case for Physician Assisted Suicide: Not (Yet) Proven. *Journal of Medical Ethics* 31:235–41.

Toombs, K. 2004. Living and Dying with Dignity: Reflections on Lived Experience. *Journal of Palliative Care* 20:193–200.

Wilson, J. C. 2000. Making Disability Visible: How Disability Studies Might Transform the Medical and Science Writing Classroom. *Technical Communication Quarterly* 9:149–61.

Wolbring, G. (n.d.) *Science and Technology and the Triple D (Disease, Disability, Defect).* At www.bioethicsanddisability.org/nbic.html.

Wolfensberger, W. 1998. *A Brief Introduction to Social Role Valorization: A High-Order Concept for Addressing the Plight of Societally Devalued People, and for Structuring Human Services*, 3rd ed. Syracuse, NY: Training Institute for Human Service Planning, Leadership and Change Agentry (Syracuse University).

FIFTEEN

"I Can't Be Like This, Frankie, Not After What I've Done"

Million Dollar Baby and the Value of Human Lives

Helen Frowe

A common objection to the view that euthanasia is morally permissible is its alleged implication that the lives of the terminally ill or severely disabled are not worth living. Some of its opponents claim that one can believe euthanasia to be permissible only if one believes that the lives of the disabled lack value. This objection is understandable, because it might seem that one can advocate ending a person's life only if one believes that the life is not worth living. However, this objection stems from a misconception of the underlying rationale for euthanasia. In this chapter I argue, through a careful consideration of the film *Million Dollar Baby* (Eastwood 2004), that those who support euthanasia need not make any assumptions about the worthlessness of a life to claim that its deliberate termination is sometimes permissible.[1]

In *Million Dollar Baby*, boxer Maggie Fitzgerald asks her trainer, Frankie Dunn, to end her life after an illegal punch leaves her paralyzed from the neck down. Maggie does not want to live as what she perceives to be a shadow of her former self. After much soul-searching, Frankie, who is Catholic, agrees, injecting Maggie with enough adrenaline to kill her in an act that his priest claims will leave him "lost somewhere so deep" he'll never find himself again. Critics of the film allege that Maggie's rejection of a life as a quadriplegic reinforces the view that a disabled life is worse than no life at all (see chapter 14 of this volume for an example of this line of reasoning). Associations such as the disabled rights group Not Dead Yet object that *Million Dollar Baby* perpetrates the view that the lives of the disabled are worth less than those of the able-bodied.[2] Such propaganda, they claim, erodes the sense of self-worth of disabled people and puts pressure on individuals to relieve their families of the "burden" of caring for them. I will argue that while *Million Dollar Baby* may have negatively affected feelings of self-worth among disabled people, such effects do not follow from a proper philosophical understanding of the film.

I argue that *Million Dollar Baby* does not endorse the view that disabled lives in general are not worth living. By considering the nature of the value of human life, I aim to show that advocates of euthanasia are not committed to the claim that human life can fail to retain intrinsic value. Frankie, certainly, still believes Maggie's life to have value, despite his eventual complicity in ending her life. To illustrate how this is possible, I draw various distinctions, some perhaps unfamiliar, that are ultimately necessary to fully understand and resolve these contentious issues.

Derivative and Ultimate Value

What Sort of Value?

Things can possess many types of value. The most straightforward form is *instrumental* value, in which a given thing (money, for example) is valued because of the effects it can bring about, like the acquisition of a car or laptop. In contrast, things may have *noninstrumental* value, often called *intrinsic* value.

Intrinsic value can be further divided into two categories: derivative and ultimate value. The former describes something that has worth because it forms part of a valuable whole. It derives its value from being part of something with ultimate value, which indicates things that have value in themselves and not from their contribution to something else (Raz 1986). For example, a pet can have derivative intrinsic value, because its worth is derived from its being an essential part of a certain relationship with a human. This relationship in turn has derivative value because it contributes to the well-being of the human concerned, and the well-being of the human concerned is taken to have ultimate value (Raz 1986, pp. 179–81).

It is useful to mention here the idea of *absolute value*. When we talk of something's being absolute we normally mean that is not relative, that is to say, it is not dependent on other considerations. Absolute moral laws, for example, are those that should never be broken, regardless of the consequences of such adherence. For something to have absolute value, then, is for it to have value irrespective of the circumstances in which it appears.

This is not true of things that have ultimate value, like friendship. Friendship does not have absolute value, for considerations of friendship do not always triumph over competing considerations, like those of justice. For example, even if it will compromise the friendship between Sally and Jane if Sally were to turn Jane into the police; if Sally knows, for example, that Jane has committed a terrible crime for which she deserves punishment, that is just what Sally, it seems, ought to do.

Does human life, however, have *absolute value*, such that no matter what the circumstances it should not be destroyed? Only someone who endorses total pacifism would claim that human life has absolute value in the sense I have described. Such a claim renders impermissible killings that we normally think are morally acceptable, such as the killing of enemy soldiers during wartime or of an aggressor in self-defense.

I suggest that there are two senses in which a person can have a life, and thus two ways in which a life can have value. We can talk of Maggie having a life purely in terms of her biological existence: her simply being "alive" in the medical sense of the term. But there is another sense in which we use the word *life*. We use it to mean the things that a person has experienced or done—*how* they have lived rather than just *that* they have lived.[3] I will argue that a person's biographical life has ultimate intrinsic value, whereas biological life has only derivative intrinsic value, conditional on whether it contributes to a valuable biographical existence. The question of who is in a position to judge whether biological life makes such a contribution will be discussed below.

Being alive is valuable because it allows us to participate in the things that have value for us. I will argue that if being alive fails to contribute to (or in is in fact detrimental to) an individual's biographical life, the person's biological life ceases to have value. However, the position for which I will argue can also make room for the view that biological life has both derivative *and* ultimate value. I will show that even if one takes biological life to have ultimate value that persists when derivative value has ended, this is still compatible with a belief in the permissibility of euthanasia. As

I mentioned above, to show that a value is ultimate is not to show that it is absolute.

John Finnis, a prolific opponent of euthanasia, argues that an individual who requests euthanasia "will be proceeding on one or both of two philosophically and morally erroneous judgements: (i) that human life in certain conditions or circumstances retains no intrinsic value or dignity; and/or (ii) that the world would be a better place if one's life were intentionally terminated" (Finnis 1995, pp. 33–34).

How plausible is this claim that any choice of euthanasia must invoke at least one of these judgments? Couldn't an argument for euthanasia rely on (1) a judgment that the subsisting value in an individual's life is outweighed by the disvalue and (2) that the individual has persistently asked to be killed? Maggie is not forced to judge either that the world would be better off without her or that her life has no value, as Finnis claims. She need only make the weaker claim that there is insufficient value in her life to make continued existence desirable for her. The logic of Finnis's dialectic would seem to be that if one chooses option A, one must believe that there is no value in option B. If I wish my life to be ended, I must believe that there is no value whatsoever in staying alive. This claim is simply false. I must believe only that there is more value in option A to rationally reject option B.

It is a mistake, therefore, to claim that to terminate a life is to pronounce it lacking in intrinsic value. Frankie does not acquiesce to Maggie's request to kill her because he has decided, on reflection, that her life is worthless. There is, however, a difficulty specific to the euthanasia issue of trying to explain how one can claim both that some people's lives are not worth living, and yet that their lives still have value. The first claim seems to be what motivates the case for euthanasia. But not many people wish to be committed to the claim that the biological life of a disabled person has no value. This would seem to be particularly true from the perspective of the disabled person herself, who, even in the event of requesting euthanasia, would probably object to her life's being treated as worthless.

Many opponents of euthanasia argue that deliberately terminating a life is always a violation of the intrinsic value of individuals (Finnis 1995, p. 33). But as we have seen, there are two ways in which we can interpret the word *intrinsic*. To apply the derivative sense of intrinsic value to human biological life in Maggie's case would be to claim that Maggie's biological life is valuable insofar as it facilitates her partaking of the things that make her biographical life meaningful, thus implying that a meaningful human life—rather than a biological human life—is of ultimate value. But I do not think that this is the sense of intrinsic to which Finnis is referring when he talks about biological life. Rather, Finnis's claim that the value is "still subsisting" irrespective of a person's condition implies that he has in mind ultimate intrinsic value. Finnis holds that the value of Maggie's biological life is not derived from the contribution it makes to something else but rather it is valued for its own sake. This is consistent with his claims and general stance on euthanasia. However, even a belief that biological human life has ultimate intrinsic value can be reconciled with a belief in the permissibility of euthanasia. I discuss this claim below.

Biographical Value

My account of the permissibility of euthanasia rests on the two distinct types of intrinsic value that I outlined above. Different factors determine the value of Maggie's biographical and biological lives. Her biographical life has ultimate intrinsic value, and it has this value because of her ability to set herself goals and pursue them. The value of Maggie's biological life, however, is derived from how well it allows her to pursue these goals.

Various philosophers have argued that any theory of individual well-being must recognize that such well-being will be largely dependent on how successful people are in pursuing their goals in life. For a rational human being to have a valuable life, it must be shaped by her decisions about that life (Scanlon 1998, pp. 142–43). By reflecting her choices, her life becomes something with which she is engaged, rather than something that she passively experiences.

Maggie's passion in life is boxing. To do well in this field is the only end she seems to have. Lying in the hospital, she tells Frankie, "I got what I needed, I got it all." I have suggested that the value of a person's biological life derives from its contribution to her biographical life. This value, then, can diminish and even cease if it no longer enables an individual to partake in the things that make their biographical life valuable. Maggie's being alive no longer fulfils this criterion.

Maggie's background is such that in some form or another she has been fighting all her life. It might seem, then, that to have her refuse to continue to struggle after her injury is to contradict the ambition and determination that had been so prominent in her character up to the point of her injury. But Maggie's relentless pursuit of what she wants is wholly in keeping with her character earlier in the film. She treats her desire to die with the same single-minded tenacity that she approached the various class, gender, and economic obstacles that should have prevented her success in the ring.

It might be objected that Maggie could acquire new goals and that to deny this is to deny that quadriplegic people can have worthwhile aims. The film's suggestion that as a quadriplegic person, Maggie has no reason to adopt goals other than her own demise could be interpreted as implying that no quadriplegic person can have such reasons. Such an interpretation, however, ignores the fact that the film shows only that once *Maggie* has become quadriplegic, she has no reason to adopt new goals. The only goal Maggie has is to excel at her chosen sport. Maggie describes boxing as "the only thing I ever felt good doing," telling Frankie that "if I'm too old for this then I got nothing." But to show that Maggie no longer has any goals is not to argue that nobody in her position can have goals. *Million Dollar Baby* is not suggesting that quadriplegic people cannot have valuable biographical lives. On the contrary, someone in Maggie's position who developed new interests could have just as valuable a biographical existence as anyone else. But it is clear in the film that Maggie, given her medical position, cannot. Deprived of the ability to pursue the only goal she cares about, her biographical life has ceased to have meaning for her.

I would not contest the claim that in theory a person can be mistaken about the value of her biographical life. It may not be true that such value can be judged only from the first-person perspective. Somebody can have a valuable life even if they fail to recognize it as such.[4] But it seems to me that the value of one's biographical life is inextricably entwined with the meaning and pleasure that a person derives from that life. Rarely will it be the case that the value of a biographical life will persist despite the total failure, on the part of the person whose life it is, to recognize its value. The things that contribute to my valuable biographical life are important because they matter to me (Scanlon 1998, p. 142). If Maggie is permanently deprived of the means to fulfil the only end that she cares about, the detrimental effect that this will have on her well-being, and the value of her biographical life, is substantial.

Biological Value

Finnis might grant that biographical life can cease to have value. He could point out that all that the opponent of euthanasia need show is that biological value is retained at all times, and that this value is such that it is always wrong intentionally to end human lives (Finnis 1995). But advocates of euthanasia do not need to deny that biological life has ultimate value, merely that it has absolute value. Many things are of ultimate value (knowledge, friendship, and pleasure, for example), but this does not mean that they can never be compromised in favor of something else with such value. And if opponents of euthanasia want to allow that killing can ever be permissible (e.g., in a just war, in self-defense), they had better think so too. But suppose that Finnis even goes so far as to grant us that there is no logical inconsistency in accepting both that human life has ultimate value and that euthanasia is permissible. What he might still deny is that the best account of the value of life implies this permissibility.

In *Cruzan v. Director, Missouri Department of Health* (1990), Nancy Cruzan's parents attempted to gain permission to allow medical staff to cease treatment of their daughter, who had been irreversibly injured in a car crash. Their request was rejected by U.S. Supreme Court Justice William Rehnquist. In the absence of convincing proof that Nancy Cruzan would have favored the cessation of treatment, the court ruled that the wishes of her parents could be overridden because the state has an interest in preserving life for its own sake (McMahan 2002, pp. 464–72). "We think a State may properly decline to make judgements about the 'quality' of life that a particular individual may enjoy, and simply assert an unqualified interest in the preservation of human life to be weighed against the constitutionally protected interests of the individual" (Rehnquist, 1990).

The basis of Rehnquist and also of fellow justice Antonin Scalia's claims appears to be that the lives of individuals are so valuable that the state may protect this value even in the face of competing considerations, such as the best interests of those individuals. This is consistent with the claim that the best account of the value of life is not compatible with euthanasia in most (or perhaps all) circumstances. To explain why such an account is mistaken, we must look in more depth at the origins of the value of human life.

The Sanctity of Life

The Source of Human Value

Even if believing in both the intrinsic value of human life and the permissibility of euthanasia can be shown to be coherent, this does not in itself show that human life really is intrinsically valuable. Arguments for the intrinsic value of life must themselves be examined. Much of the debate surrounding *Million Dollar Baby* focuses on a perceived lack of regard for the sanctity of life. But what does this well-worn phrase "sanctity of life" actually mean?

An answer to this question will require some thought about what it is to be a human, and the characteristics that putatively set us aside in a morally significant way from other forms of life. It will be sufficient for the purposes of this essay to have a rough understanding of personhood as involving something like autonomy, broadly conceived to include ideas like rationality, self-awareness, reflection, and so forth.[5] This is consistent with what both those who argue for and against euthanasia generally take to be the defining factors of humanity. Rather than analyzing the factors themselves, I will consider the plausibility of the claims based on them.

Finnis suggests that one's humanity lies in "one's capacity to live the life, not of a carrot or a cat, but [of] a human being . . . for human metabolism, human awareness, feelings, imagination, memory, responsiveness and sexuality, and human wondering, relating and communicating, deliberating, choosing and acting. To lose one's life is to lose all these capacities" (Finnis 1995, p. 31).

The abilities to deliberate and choose are picked out by John Harris, a supporter of euthanasia, as necessary conditions for valuing one's own existence. Deliberation involves comparing different possibilities, which seems integral to assigning value to something. And there seems little point in deliberation alone without the ability to choose on the basis of what one's deliberations reveal. Harris thus cites the abilities to deliberate and choose as the hallmarks of personhood and as what give persons value: Humans are valuable because we can deliberate and decide, because we have autonomy (Harris 1995, pp. 36–45).

The autonomy-based objection to euthanasia goes as follows. It is always wrong to intentionally end human life, because human life is of a special, more valuable sort than the life of a cat or a carrot (Finnis 1995). Cats and carrots cannot value existence, because they cannot contemplate nonexistence. So the kinds of ethical issues that arise when dealing with ending human life are simply not relevant to other life-forms. But any human who requests euthanasia, competently and as the result of an informed deliberation, is necessarily also the type of being who fulfils the criteria for having a valuable life, and as such this is a life to be preserved rather than ended.[6]

The critics of euthanasia would seem to have neatly defended their view. Autonomy makes people valuable—it makes human life sacred. Killing a person who is capable of such autonomy, therefore, violates the sanctity of life and acts as a denial of human worth. Because advocates of euthanasia would require the consent of a patient like Maggie to make euthanasia permissible, they are effectively requiring that patients exhibit the very feature that their opponents claim makes euthanasia impermissible.

Autonomy and Euthanasia

There is a difference between showing that human life can be particularly valuable because we have the necessary capacity for rational deliberation and showing that these capacities are sufficient for human life's being valuable. Even if being able to exercise autonomy is necessary for a good life, this capacity by itself may not be enough to constitute a good life.[7] And even if human value does stem from our autonomy, it is not obvious that ending a life is a violation of that value.

Maggie's consent is regarded as crucial by both opponents and supporters of euthanasia.[8] Both sides of the debate view autonomy as something to be valued, but differ in how they approach it. Those who support euthanasia often do so because of the importance they place on an individual's interest in controlling how his or her life goes. But what is it about Maggie's autonomy that critics of euthanasia value? What is it that autonomy allows her to do? It seems that any answer ought to include the fact that autonomy enables Maggie to make decisions about her life and to prioritize her interests and determine the values that are important to her. If this feature "autonomy" is so valuable, what justification can an opponent of euthanasia offer for disregarding it so completely when it is exercised? Why may we ignore Maggie's autonomous request that her life be ended? Maggie is not deprived of her rational abilities, and to insist that disabled people who seek their own deaths must be in some way misguided or confused is no less mistaken, or offensive, than the assumption that disabled lives are always less happy or fulfilled that those of the able-bodied.

Opponents of euthanasia are likely to reply that while they allow that we ought generally to respect autonomous decisions, this is not true in cases where an autonomous life is being destroyed. The power of one's autonomy to alter other people's (i.e., doctors', family members') reasons for action does not extend this far. Restricting that power's scope is more plausible than, and morally preferable to, allowing an unrestricted view of autonomy. Having no limits on what autonomy can allow us to do would, for example, leave people free to enter into slavery contracts. These unwelcome consequences of an unrestricted view of autonomy are certainly a persuasive point against such a position.

There may still be good reasons for arguing for a restricted view of autonomous powers that nonetheless encompasses the power to authorize others to end one's life. Selling oneself into slavery is to agree (albeit autonomously) to have one's autonomy permanently disregarded for the rest of one's life. John Stuart Mill (1806–1873), in his famous *On Liberty*, argues that slavery contracts should be prohibited because they constitute the alienation of one's freedom. One cannot invoke the importance of freedom to justify allowing an action that will comprehensively undermine that freedom.

Mill believes that this proviso applies equally to bringing about one's own death (Mill 1869/1974, pp. 172–73). I think that this is a mistake. There is a difference between having one's autonomy permanently disregarded or violated and having it eliminated. Asking to have one's life ended is to agree to the permanent elimination of one's autonomy. One cannot violate the autonomy of a person who has ceased to exist. That this is an important difference will, I think, be illustrated by an analysis of how we ought to value autonomy.

The different ways in which we can value something are the source of much debate in moral philosophy (Swanton 1995; Baron, Pettit, and Slote 1997). By reconsidering the way in which we value autonomy, I believe we can avoid any unpalatable implications about the ability of disabled individuals to make rational choices. There seem to be two plausible ways in which we can show that we value autonomy: by either protecting it or respecting it. Finnis's belief that we should not, in general, intentionally destroy human life is suggestive of the "protective view" that, because autonomy is to be valued, it is wrong to deliberately reduce the number of autonomous agents. The second, contrasting, view is that the value of autonomy demands that we respect it by adhering to the wishes of autonomous individuals regarding certain aspects of their lives, including when and how they end.

Clearly, the second view is much more compatible with voluntary euthanasia than the first. Here we respect a value by refusing to contravene it, even if this decreases the overall amount of the value in the world. If we believe that violating a person's autonomy means disrespecting it, rather than failing to protect it, then we can see why slavery violates autonomy, whereas euthanasia does not. It is not the case that the only way to show that we value autonomy is by insisting on keeping autonomous agents alive as long as possible. Frankie's actions in *Million Dollar Baby* suggest that he shares the view that respect for Maggie's autonomy demands that he respect her wishes, even if ultimately this results in the elimination of her autonomy altogether.

Conclusion

The best account of the value of life is that biological existence derives its value from its contribution to biographical existence. Thus, biological value can diminish and even cease under certain conditions. However, I have argued that a defender of euthanasia need not be committed to the view that human life can cease to be valuable. I have shown that it is coherent to hold that biological life has ultimate, persistent value irrespective of its contribution to biographical life, while also believing that euthanasia is still permissible. The allegation that in depicting voluntary euthanasia *Million Dollar Baby* perpetrates the view that disabled lives lack value has been shown to be false. It is not permissible to kill Maggie because, as a quadriplegic, her life lacks value. It is permissible to kill Maggie because the things that give *her* life value are no longer accessible to her, and she consistently asks that her life be ended. Philosophical reflection on the film reveals that there is no suggestion therein that this will apply to the lives of *all* quadriplegic people.

If the value of human life stems from our capacity to make autonomous decisions about the ends that we set ourselves, then the appropriate attitude toward this value is that we respect it by acquiescing to Maggie's request. That she can be mistaken about the value of her life is something for which I have allowed, arguing that respect for autonomy demands that we adhere to her wishes even if we believe her judgment incorrect. However, I have disputed the likelihood of such an error, because the value of her life is heavily dependent on Maggie's own judgment of that value.

QUESTIONS FOR CONSIDERATION

1. *If we grant the author's main argument that the value of Maggie's biological life derives from its contribution to her biographical life, and we assume that Maggie's own assessment of her biographical life is crucial in determining whether her life has value, are there any grounds on which to claim that Maggie is mistaken about the value of her life, and thus, should not be killed, despite her consistently expressed wishes to die?*

2. *Frowe discusses two ways in which the value of autonomy is seen to make demands on those considering voluntary euthanasia: the "protective view"—which holds that it is wrong deliberately to diminish the number of autonomous agents—and the "respective view" which holds that we properly respect autonomy by adhering to the wishes of autonomous individuals. Which view seems better to capture the value of autonomy, and why?*

3. *The authors of Chapter 14 claims that the imagery of* Million Dollar Baby *perpetuates the stereotype that severely disabled lives lack value and are not worth living. Does Frowe's argument convince you that the film, when understood through a properly philosophical lens, does not entail such a conclusion? Why or why not?*

1. The arguments advanced in this chapter are intended to apply only to voluntary euthanasia, because this is the sort of euthanasia dealt with in this film. Nonvoluntary euthanasia may require additional, or different, justification, or might be unjustified even if voluntary euthanasia is justified.

2. In her discussion of *Million Dollar Baby* on the Not Dead Yet Web site, W. C. Cleigh (n.d.) objects to the film on the grounds that "it diminishes us all to assume that any life is valueless." Similarly, disability rights lawyer Harriet McBryde Johnson argues that Peter Singer's argument for the permissibility of euthanasia rests on the "unexamined assumption" that "disabled people are inherently 'worse off,' that we 'suffer,' that we have lesser 'prospects of a happy life.' Because of this all-too-common prejudice, and his rare courage in taking it to its logical conclusion, catastrophe looms" (McBryde Johnson 2003).

3. Ronald Dworkin employs the terms *zoe* and *bios* to distinguish biological and biographical life, respectively (Dworkin 1993, pp. 82–83).

4. Arguably, Alejandro Amenábar's film *The Sea Inside* portrays Ramón Sampedro as someone who fails to recognize that he enjoys considerable well-being and is thus mistaken in his judgment that he would be better off dead. But it does not follow from this that we should refuse his request. A demand that we respect autonomy, even when we believe it to be badly exercised, might require that we adhere to the individual's wishes. See chapter 20 of this volume for a full discussion of *The Sea Inside.*

5. Some philosophers distinguish between humanity and personhood. However, I will take Finnis and Harris to be referring to the same concept but with different labels, because the dialogue between them suggests that this is what they also assume.

6. This issue is further complicated by the introduction of "living wills," in which individuals give instructions that are to be followed in the event of their ceasing to be autonomous. But I do not have sufficient space to discuss this additional dimension here.

7. There is also a distinction to be drawn between things that are good in themselves and things that facilitate those goods. Finnis (1995) rightly argues that to lose one's life is to lose all the capacities that are the basis of one's humanity (i.e., to lose the capacities that serve as necessary conditions for one's having goals, friendships, knowledge, and so on). But this does not entail that one's life itself must therefore be a basic good or part of one's humanity. However, for the sake of this chapter I am allowing for the possibility that even mere biological life can have value in order to demonstrate how this view is compatible with euthanasia.

8. Few supporters of euthanasia would allow that merely asking to be killed is

sufficient for euthanasia. Rather, it is regarded as a necessary condition in cases in which such consent is possible.

REFERENCES

Amenábar, A. 2004. *Mar Adentro* [English title *The Sea Inside;* motion picture]. Madrid: Sogecine.

Baron, M., Pettit, P., and Slote, M. 1997. *Three Methods of Ethics.* Cambridge, MA: Blackwell Publishers.

Cleigh, W. C. Why We Protest. At www.notdeadyet.org/docs/oscars05protest/cleighwhy protest0305.html.

Cruzan v. Director, Missouri Department of Health. 1990. 88-1503, 497 U.S. 261.

Dworkin, R. 1993. *Life's Dominion.* London: HarperCollins.

Eastwood, C. 2004. *Million Dollar Baby* [motion picture]. Burbank, CA: Warner Bros. Pictures.

Finnis, J. 1995. The Philosophical Case against Euthanasia. In *Euthanasia Examined: Ethical, Clinical and Legal Perspectives,* ed. J. Keown, 23–35. Cambridge: Cambridge University Press.

Harris, J. 1995. The Philosophical Case against the Philosophical Case against Euthanasia. In *Euthanasia Examined: Ethical, Clinical and Legal Perspectives,* ed. J. Keown, 36–45. Cambridge: Cambridge University Press.

McBryde Johnson, H. 2003. Unspeakable Conversations. *New York Times Magazine.* February 16.

McMahan, J. 2002. *The Ethics of Killing: Problems at the Margins of Life.* Oxford and New York: Oxford University Press.

Mill, J. S. 1974. *On Liberty,* ed. G. Himmelfarb. London: Penguin. (Originally published 1869)

Raz, J. 1986. *The Morality of Freedom.* New York: Oxford University Press.

Rehnquist, W. 1994. Majority Opinion in *Cruzan v. Director Missouri Department of Health.* In *Killing and Letting Die,* ed. A. Norcross and B. Steinbock, 79–87. New York: Fordham University Press.

Scanlon, T. M. 1998. *What We Owe to Each Other.* Cambridge, MA: Harvard University Press.

Swanton, C. 1995. Profile of the Virtues. *Pacific Philosophical Quarterly* 76: 42–72.

SIXTEEN

Providing *Critical Care* for a *Big Fish* at the End of Life

How Sydney Lumet and Tim Burton Can Help Us Avoid Becoming the Next Terri Schiavo

Kenneth Richman

Watching the outlandish interplay among the forces of science, money, and compassion (love) in *Critical Care* (Lumet 1997; based on Dooling 1996) helps focus our attention on some basic issues in bioethics: what is the relationship between scientific knowledge and caring for individual patients? Do we want our health care providers to love us? Who should choose what happens to us at the end of our lives, and on what basis should they choose? Can a living will protect us from the sort of battle that arose around the fictional Mr. Potter and the real-life Terri Schiavo? Drawing on Kantian themes, in this chapter I promote an understanding of patient-centered care based on respect for individual preferences. I recommend that we understand our lives as stories that we tell through our actions and suggest that this way of thinking sits comfortably with our actual ways of thinking about ourselves and others. I illustrate these notions by drawing on *Critical Care* and on *Big Fish* (Burton 2004), in which the father needs help to see how the story of his life ends. Once his son is able to participate in completing the narrative of his father's life, the older man is able to accept a death that could be the end of *his* life, an extension of the story he has shaped with his own choices. The chapter concludes with suggestions for constructing medical advance directives to support patient-centered care consistent with the patient's own life narrative.

Raphael

In *Critical Care*, we meet three patients on the ninth-floor intensive care unit of Memorial Hospital. The first patient is an older woman who at first seems only somewhat confused. We eventually learn that she has a dementia that causes her responses to questions—any questions at all—to alternate between "pizza" and "Eisenhower."

The second patient is Raphael, a young man with such severe kidney failure that he can no longer take in any liquids even though his blood is becoming increasingly toxic. He has rejected two donor kidneys, leaving no obvious course of treatment. Raphael has bouts of delirium in which his doctors appear to him as a taunting devil (played by Wallace Shawn) in a white lab coat. When not hallucinating, Raphael consistently expresses a desire for his life to end. In an early scene, Nurse Stella (played by Helen Mirren) replies to Raphael, "I can put that in your chart, but I don't think it will do any good." She instructs him to make his request to the doctors when they do their rounds.

The scene in which the doctors come to Raphael's bedside is remarkable in several respects. The color palette is cold and sterile, suggesting a high-technology laboratory rather than a place where anyone could be truly comfortable. (The only place in the hospital that seems the least bit hospitable is the office of the bumbling, alcoholic old-timer Dr. Butz, played by Albert Brooks.) The camera centers on a senior physician called simply Hofstader (played by Philip Bosco). His title is absent even on his white coat. With Hofstader is a gaggle of residents—recent medical school graduates completing the next stage of their training. But no one, not even Hofstader, is looking at the patient. Even the viewer is looking over Raphael to see Hofstader, where the real action is.

The exchange that occurs over the patient is about the patient, or at least about the patient's body, but it completely fails to reflect the fact that the patient is in the room. Dr. Ernst, the film's protagonist (played by James Spader) is the only one who hears Raphael repeat his plea for an end to his suffering. Even when Dr. Ernst speaks up to report Raphael's request, Hofstader reacts without addressing or even taking notice of Raphael. He dismisses the patient's request as a symptom that need not be taken seriously. The young doctors-in-training take notes while Stella looks down and shakes her head behind the group. The scene is so plausible, so cold, and so cruel that it is at once appalling and funny.

So what is going wrong? The message of the scene seems to be about the role of the patient in today's medical system. To put the lesson in context we must look at the intellectual background fueling the emphasis on informed consent before we can tell a story about how it ends up exacerbating Raphael's troubles.

The Traditional Concept of Autonomy

In the contemporary Anglo-American medical environment, health care professionals are told that patients have the right to decide what happens to them. Patients exercise this right by saying "yes" or "no" to individual treatment options in a process called *informed consent*. Proper informed consent requires the making of a free and rational decision (a logical application of individual preferences to individual decisions without influence or coercion by others).

It is standard to trace the intellectual roots of our concept of autonomy to the enlightenment philosopher Immanuel Kant (1724–1804). For Kant, autonomous choice requires that we be able to consider the decision in a rational way. For an enlightenment understanding of rationality, this means thinking about whether some action may be chosen by everyone—that is, whether the thinking behind the action can be accepted as a law.

A straightforward Kantian understanding of autonomy is thus very literal. The word *autonomy* means self-rule (from the Greek roots *auto*, for self, and *nomos*, for law). Rational action is action based on reasons; in rational action those reasons are applied consistently. If we give ourselves laws, we are the source of laws. We are, in Kantian terms, sovereign beings, where *sovereign* is another word for *autonomous*. This lawgiving also serves as the basis of the Kantian claim that autonomous individuals are ends in themselves, sources of value in the world. In Kant's system, rationality forms the basis not only of autonomy in general but also of morality. We see this in the first formulation of Kant's categorical imperative, which demands that I act only in such a way that I could will the maxim of my action to be a universal law (Kant 1785/1959, 39). Where an action is based on reasons that could not be universalized, or is simply not based on reasons at all, that action is neither autonomous nor ethically laudable.

Nearly two hundred years after Kant, the American philosopher John Rawls used Kant's ideas to formulate his own definition of autonomy: "acting autonomously is acting from principles that we would consent to as free and equal rational beings . . . these principles are objective. They are the principles that we would want everyone (including ourselves) to follow were we to take up together the appropriate general point of view" (Rawls 1971, p. 516). To be objective in the sense used here is to be intersubjective—to be accessible by others. The connection between rationality and objectivity entails that if I am unable to embrace your decision as one I would make in your situation, at least one of us is not approaching the situation rationally.

Note that lack of rationality is not the only way in which autonomy could fail. The failure could also be due to lack of freedom or lack of equality. Indeed, coercion, in which patients experience pressure from health care providers, family members, or others, is a common way for patient freedom to become compromised. Coercion is frequently the result of inequality of understanding, inequality of control over the situation at hand, inequality of social position, or all of the above.[1]

In the medical context, it is a commonplace that patients have a right to exercise autonomy. What this means is that they have a right to make rational, consistent, independent decisions about their care. Such a right comes with a responsibility on the part of health care professionals to respect patients' autonomous decisions and to help patients avoid coercion. However, it is not permissible to demand that patients exercise autonomy if they cannot do so or wish not to do so.

Health care providers are deeply influenced by the traditional concept even if they do not know about Kant or Rawls and even if they have never had a formal course in ethics. It is simply part of our culture. The ideas trickle down, so to speak, from philosophy classrooms to other environments, and philosophy is used to assess ideas that trickle from the broader culture into the academic consciousness.

Raphael and the Traditional Concept of Autonomy

Valuing autonomy brings us a long way toward promoting respect for persons and their choices. However, the traditional conception of autonomy has two sharp edges for cutting patients. One edge cuts patients loose. Health care providers who believe that patients are making inappropriate choices can use autonomy as an excuse not to spend time advocating the patient's interests, in effect abandoning the patient. The other edge of the traditional concept cuts patients out. This happens when a patient is viewed (correctly or incorrectly) as incompetent and, as a result, is left out of the decision-making process entirely.

The move of cutting the patient out can be as simple as what we see in Hofstader's reply to Raphael. Raphael makes a request that seems irrational to Hofstader, so the doctor simply continues to treat Raphael as an object to be acted on rather than as a person capable of making choices about his life. He makes no effort to explain decisions to Raphael, to ask whether anything could be done to make Raphael more comfortable, to understand his perspective, or even to distract the patient from his desire to die.

We could also say that Hofstader fails to treat Raphael with respect or that he fails to honor Raphael's dignity. Respect and dignity are important concepts that contribute to a full discussion of Raphael's predicament, but here I want to focus primarily on autonomy.

Patient autonomy looks like an obvious thing to value, but when we stick to the traditional concept of autonomy, we too often get trouble. Because the ideal of free, rational choice is so difficult to realize, patients get cut loose, get cut out, or give up.

As one might expect, this is not a new point. Every aspect of the ideal of informed consent has been subject to scrutiny by bioethicists.[2] The traditional concept of autonomy is problematic in health care settings for a variety of reasons. One important objection is that people simply are not rational in the ways required for autonomy in the traditional sense. This is true of all people most of the time, and it is especially true of people when they are ill. Illness generally makes people less rational and more open to coercion—that is, less free. One way that illness makes patients less free is that it puts them in unequal relationships with health care providers who have the knowledge and authority to do what the patient needs and is unable to do for herself. All of this makes autonomous action as traditionally conceived an impossible ideal. Indeed, we might even say that embracing it as an ideal for patients is dangerous. It seems to have done Raphael no good.

When patients are incompetent to make autonomous decisions, paternalism (also called parentalism or maternalism) comes in. Paternalism is the practice of making decisions for another with the aim of serving the other's best interests.[3] Hofstader was not simply being mean to Raphael; he just thought he was in a better position than Raphael to determine what was rational to choose for Raphael's own good.

It would be relatively easy to practice paternalism responsibly if the good of the patient were indeed an objective matter accessible through rational contemplation of the facts. For instance, one might hold the view that what is good for patients is whatever supports the proper function of their bodies, and that what constitutes biological good functioning for a human body is grounded in observable, objective evidence. However, there are reasons to think that there may be a variety of different goods for people when we think of them not just as organisms, but also as persons (Richman 2004; Richman and Budson 2000).

For instance, some people like being thin more than eating rich foods; others like eating rich foods more than they like being thin. Some people desperately want to become parents; others desperately want to avoid becoming parents. To do a good job of being paternalistic for a whole person (and not just for the person's body as a biological organism) often requires knowing something that is not available in a textbook, captured by computer models of patient bodies, or concluded by sitting and thinking rationally about things. The question is: what do we need to know? An answer is suggested by a theme that recurs throughout *Critical Care*: it might have something to do with love.

If You Love Me: What Should We Do for Mr. Potter?

Hofstader is presented as a stereotypical practitioner of scientific medicine. The scientific movement in health care is increasingly identified with evidence-based medicine, which promotes using quantitative research data from many patients to predict the probability that a treatment will succeed in a particular patient. We learn more about Hofstader's approach when Dr. Ernst is informed that he may be invited to work for Hofstader next year and is summoned for a tour of Hofstader's lab. Hofstader explains: "Seeing patients is a waste of a doctor's time. We're trying to correct that problem. We like to think of patients as information that can be digitized. Then we can build computer models for surgeons to practice on that are identical with any patient."

While at the lab, we meet Poindexter (played by James Lally), a nurse who has his own version of Hofstader's technical approach to medicine. Poindexter explains how it is that none of his patients have ever died while he was on duty: "Just a matter of carefully monitoring the patients and then adjusting the medication accordingly. There is no longer any condition that is truly terminal, just patients we choose not to maintain."

Hofstader and Poindexter are hard-core representatives of the scientific approach, oblivious to the richness of patient preferences and experience. The film presents this approach as amazing but clearly inhumane, and it offers as a contrast the idea of love. For instance, eventually the jaded but compassionate nurse Stella is able to act in the face of the scientific juggernaut to promote Raphael's preferences. As she surreptitiously allows him to die, she whispers in his ear: "I love you," and love becomes a motif woven throughout *Critical Care.*

I have discussed only two of the three patients introduced in *Critical Care*. The third is Mr. Potter, who is referred to most often as "Bed Five" or "Bed Five, Nine ICU." Bed Five has been unconscious for months. His health care providers hold no expectation that Bed Five will ever regain consciousness; he is judged to be in a persistent vegetative state, exhibiting involuntary hand movements but no cognitive life or experiences. His two daughters disagree on the matter. One wants all treatment to stop; the other insists that his hand movements are purposeful attempts to communicate.

Dr. Ernst is in charge of Bed Five's care, under the supervision of Dr. Butz. Bed Five has received an absurd array of medical treatments. For instance, although he can't see, he has had cataract surgery. According to his medical record, he was moved to the ninth floor for "a change of scenery." (Ernst asks, rhetorically, "Do the insurance forms go to Medicare, or to Amnesty International?") To meet the patient's nutritional needs, Dr.

Butz has ordered a gastrostomy (a feeding tube inserted through the abdomen). Ernst is uncomfortable with this decision on the basis that Bed Five is unlikely to derive benefit from further treatment. On one side, Dr. Ernst wants to avoid wasting resources through unwarranted assaults on the body in bed five. On another side, he has a duty to respect the orders of the befuddled but oddly wise Dr. Butz. And then there is the beautiful daughter who is suing the hospital to get her father's treatment stopped and who has lured Dr. Ernst into a compromising position. That daughter is opposed by her half sister, who claims that Bed Five is merely "convalescing."

Because of the lawsuits, Poindexter is assigned to the ninth-floor intensive care unit to ensure that Bed Five does not die at a moment that might be legally inopportune for the hospital. Taking in all of the available data, Poindexter notes the tapping movements Mr. Potter makes with his hands. Learning that Bed Five was a signalman in the Navy, Poindexter tries to interpret the tapping using Morse code. It seems that Bed Five's tapping repeats code for the phrase "if you love me." Poindexter excitedly explains this finding to Dr. Ernst: "I asked him if he was sending Morse code. He tapped out 'if you love me.' . . . I asked him if he could hear me. He tapped out 'if you love me.' " These responses not only make sense, they appear to be sophisticated, even poetic replies to Poindexter's questions.

Ernst explains that it is common for patients in vegetative states to exhibit a limited set of behaviors that they repeat over and over, and takes Poindexter to visit the Eisenhower pizza woman. ("Who's your favorite president?" "Eisenhower." "Good, good. And what is your favorite food?" "Pizza." . . . "Who empties your bedpan for you?" "Eisenhower." "What is your doctor's last name?" "Pizza.") We are left with a renewed sense that a simplistic reliance on observable data can be very misleading indeed.

It is natural to interpret human movements as flowing from intentions and meanings. This fact is behind some important thoughts in philosophy of mind and the science of artificial intelligence (Dennett 1987, 1991). Even hard-nosed Poindexter was taken in by what seemed to be evidence that Mr. Potter was attempting to communicate. In a real-life parallel to the movie, Terri Schiavo's parents had the same very natural reaction.

Although Poindexter's interpretation of the tapping data was diffused and defused by the comparison with the behavior of the patient in the next bed, the phrase "if you love me" continues to haunt Dr. Ernst. At one point, while Ernst is considering whether to take the initiative to withdraw Mr. Potter's treatment, he finds that a nun (played by Anne Bancroft, dressed in an exaggerated white habit) has suddenly appeared across the bed from him. The viewer understands that this is a mirage, a vision, from a change in lighting. (The same technique is used to mark Raphael's visions of the devil: blue light for the angelic nun; red for the other side.) Dr. Ernst talks to the nun about his uncertainty concerning what to do for the patient lying before them hooked up to numerous tubes, wires, and machines. She speaks to him in a calm, kind voice: "Listen to your heart. Think of this man as your father and love him, comfort him." Eventually, Dr. Ernst utters the phrase: "if you love me." The nun replies: "And what if you did love him? How would you act towards him? What would you do for him?" Dr. Ernst's answer: "I don't know."

A Love Story: The "Narrative" Concept of Patient Autonomy

Dr. Ernst's honest answer is a good beginning. Near the end of the film, Ernst offers a passionate monologue in which he expresses his deep frustration to the other characters. "We should care," he implores, both about Mr. Potter himself and about a health care system that is failing. *Critical Care* is not an instructional video on medical ethics, however, and we get very little insight into how to implement caring beyond pacing earnestly about the patient lounge.

In this section, I offer a way of thinking about how to "care" for patients. The model of caring I will offer is different from the ethics of care associated with feminist ethics.[4] It is, however, very well suited to the overall project of this volume in that it draws on a central characteristic of film: narrative, establishing a story.

Here's the idea: the caring way to treat people is to promote their ability to live a life that continues their life narrative, the story that they have established for themselves. How do you act toward someone if you love that person? You embrace that person's story, promote that person's ability to live according to her values, to continue a coherent life narrative. We can help others live out their own life narratives. When we know those close to us, we can sense when a decision "fits," just as we can sense when a film or television script includes something "out of character" for a familiar persona.

One virtue of this notion of caring as promoting an individual's life narrative is that it preserves some attractive elements of the traditional concept of autonomy. Recall that the traditional concept tells us that an action is autonomous when it is independent and based on reasons applied consistently. We made note of how people are often inconsistent and dependent, and how this causes difficulties when clinicians seek to apply the value of respect for patient autonomy. But the traditional concept does capture some things that we do and should value when patients make decisions. For instance, although we cannot expect patients to make decisions without influence from others, we do want patients to make choices that reflect their own core values, choices that allow them to live their own lives and not live for someone else. (The reader might note that when coercion or other factors result in a person living life for someone else instead of for herself, this violates the second formulation of Kant's categorical imperative: treat humanity, whether in yourself or in others, always as an end in itself and never as a means only.)

Although we cannot demand complete rationality, it does seem right to treat inconsistency as a sign of trouble. When a friend who always plays it safe suddenly turns up on a motorcycle without a helmet, we wonder if he's okay. We might say: "he's not himself."

We question unexpected behavior because, despite the fact that people are inconsistent and subject to all kinds of influence by others, a radical change in the way someone acts generally indicates a problem, or at least requires an explanation. Strange behavior does not seem autonomous. This idea is captured in the widely accepted dictum that consent is informed when it is consistent with an individual's previous decisions. So the idea that consistency is a sign of autonomy has strong appeal despite the problems that come with the traditional conception. The narrative conception of autonomy that we are entertaining here softens up some of the sharp edges of the concept in ways that help our thinking about how to assess patient choices and how to decide what a patient would have chosen for himself.

On the narrative conception, to be autonomous is to live a life story that seems like one's own. Rather than assessing each choice individually to see whether it was rational and independent, as demanded by the traditional conception, the narrative conception looks at choices in context. "To say that a person's life is narrative in character . . . is at least in part to claim that no time-slice (if you will) is fully intelligible—or even definable—outside of the context of the life in which it occurs" (Schechtman 1996, p. 97). An individual's life narrative can be understood as a sort of trajectory, like that of a football. Footballs pass through the air in predictable ways; one part of the trajectory determines the next, and the whole makes sense together.

Of course, trajectories can change, as can lives. When this happens, we look for a reason. Where a reason can be given, the change can be understood and accepted. The trajectory of a person's life may also have some blips and rough spots that don't quite fit in. As with experimental error in science, this doesn't mean that we need to throw out the rest of the data.

I recommend the narrative conception of autonomy as an improvement over the traditional concept, but not because it gives clear answers in all circumstances. Applying the narrative conception of autonomy poses a variety of challenges. For instance, what do we do if a patient expresses preferences that seem contrary to her life narrative as we understand it? As with the traditional concept of autonomy, this might be taken as evidence that the patient is not competent. But the narrative conception is an improvement over the traditional one because it recognizes that a life narrative requires only coherence, not strict consistency. A coherent series of decisions and actions allows for gradual change; where change is sudden and radical those who care for the person (in various senses of "care") have a responsibility to demand reasons that can be woven into the story of the person's life. It is when no such reasons can be given that we worry about the person's competence. The same applies, *mutatis mutandis*, to decisions made by a proxy decision-maker.

Some changes in values or behavior may seem to make sense to the individual but seem incoherent to others. Given the fact that people are very good at providing post hoc reasons for irrational decisions, the narrative conception requires that a competent person's narrative make sense to a thoughtful and knowledgeable observer and not just to the individual. This demand tethers life narratives to reality; although everyone's narrative will include false memories and delusions, narratives that are sufficiently unrelated to the way the world is will not make sense to others and will fail to provide guidance or ground decisions about our obligations to others (Schechtman 1996, p. 119).[5]

Coherence could be elucidated in a variety of ways. For instance, it could be treated as an aesthetic concept or as a sort of logical property holding among the set of an individual's experiences. I haven't the space in this short essay to develop any one such elucidation, which would need to provide an account of when two components or time slices can be parts of the same narrative. Whatever the details, the ways in which we judge whether two parts of a person's life (two total psychological states, two judgments, two sets of values, etc.) can be understood as parts of the same life narrative will be a lot like the ways in which we judge whether two physical states can be parts of the history of the same physical object. Chairs, buildings, and our own bodies change in ways that are predictable in various degrees. If we don't see someone for a long time, we expect their bodies to change in various ways. Where the face we see at one time is too different from the face we see at a later time, our intuitions will tell us that they are not the same person's face. We have similar intuitions about life narratives.[6]

Several philosophers and bioethicists have considered how a narrative conception of personal identity can help us to understand how to address end-of-life decisions.[7] The discussion has focused on whether an individual's previous choices, perhaps as specified in a living will, have authority for someone whose life may have changed so dramatically that her previous reasons no longer apply. (Indeed, a central issue is whether such a human being even counts as the same person as the person before such changes.) My approach here does not come out of that specific concern. Instead, it comes rather out of worries about how to capture what seems reasonable and right about the tradition of valuing patient autonomy while letting go of the problems it introduces for patients and for those who have the responsibility of caring for patients at end of life.

A guiding value for end-of-life care is preserving patient autonomy or extending it when it is diminished or lost. In the United States, this value is codified in the Patient Self-Determination Act, the law that made sure that patients are aware of medical advance directives, including living wills and proxy documents (documents that name a decision-maker to stand proxy for a person when she is unable to decide for herself). Autonomy is best extended by applying the patient's preferences, by continuing the patient's own life story when the patient is not able to choose.

Fishing for the End of Our Story

Very few of us have adopted rules for how we want to die; none of us has a record of previous deaths that others can use to judge whether our choices in the face of death show consistent application of reasons across multiple instances. This is a major drawback for the traditional concept when a patient or her proxy needs to decide what to do when faced with situations like those of Raphael and Mr. Potter. The narrative concept of autonomy, on the other hand, allows us to recognize that all life stories end. The question becomes how to work out a coherent ending to a particular patient's narrative.

Furthermore, as bioethicist Mark G. Kuczewski notes: "It is always possible that more than one choice is compatible with the person's self-conception . . . This is actually good news for the narrative theorist, because it emphasizes that surrogate decision making is not about guessing the unique choice that a patient would make if he could suddenly express a preference" (Kuczewski 1999, par. 11). This is another way in which the narrative approach to end-of-life decisions sets up more realistic expectations than does the traditional approach.

Big Fish offers a beautiful, if complicated, example of how the idea of a life narrative can be applied at the end of life. Based on Daniel Wallace's (1999) book of the same name, *Big Fish* introduces us to Edward Bloom, an older gentleman with a habit for telling fantastical stories about his life. (Albert Finney plays the elder Edward Bloom; Ewan McGregor plays out the "mythic" adventures of the younger Edward Bloom on the screen.) Hearing the same stories again and again, his son William (played by Billy Crudup) eventually comes to abhor them. William resents the way the stories take center stage, leaving him in the wings. After Edward uses his toast at William's wedding to tell a long story about himself, the two don't talk for three years. Then William is called to his father's deathbed.

Returning to his parents' home, he tries to use the opportunity to make sense of his father. What is behind all of these stories? Why can't his father simply tell things as they really happened? Going through his father's papers to help his mother prepare, William comes across something he never thought he'd see: evidence that some of the most outlandish stories might have some basis in reality.

The situation here is multilayered. Edward Bloom's stories are over the top, but telling the stories is absolutely central to his identity. This makes Edward's stories different; while all of us tell the stories of our lives in words and action, very few life narratives feature the act of story telling as prominently as Edward's does, and most of us care a lot more than he does about whether our life narratives have at least the appearance of being true. However, these differences may be more a matter of degree than a matter of kind. Telling stories is not just something some people do; we are all engaged in living our life stories. Physician-bioethicist Jason Karlawish puts it thus: "the elegance of narrative is that we practice it whether we wish to or not" (Karlawish 1996, p. 396).

The opening credits are still progressing when we hear a voice-over of William explaining what we are about to see: "In telling the story of my father's life, it is impossible to separate fact from fiction, the man from the myth. The best I can do is to tell it the way he told me. It doesn't always make sense, and most of it never happened. But that's what kind of story this is." From his kind and accepting tone, we know that this is William looking back after making peace with his father. What is interesting about this line is that it seems true of most of our life stories. William doesn't give up on the idea that there is truth, that there is a matter of fact about what happened in his father's life. He does, however, come to understand that a precise adherence to literal fact is not required for a life story to have authority, to give meaning to a life. We see, as well, that such stories can and should help guide proxy decision-making.

Edward and William are alone at the hospital at Edward's last hour, as shown in Figure 16.1. The father needs his son to help him see how his own story ends. At first, William doesn't get the significance of what is being asked of him: "I don't know that story, Dad," William says. "You never told me that one . . . I need your help . . . Tell me how it starts." Edward responds: "Like this." So William begins the story of his father's death with the literal facts: the two of them are in the hospital early one morning. William quickly comes to understand that he is helping his father to integrate these last moments into the broader tale of his life, and he makes use of the characters from his father's other stories.

When the story comes to an end, William concludes: "And that's how it happens." His father responds with his last words, through which he lovingly accepts this great gift from his son: "Yeah. Exactly." The father's

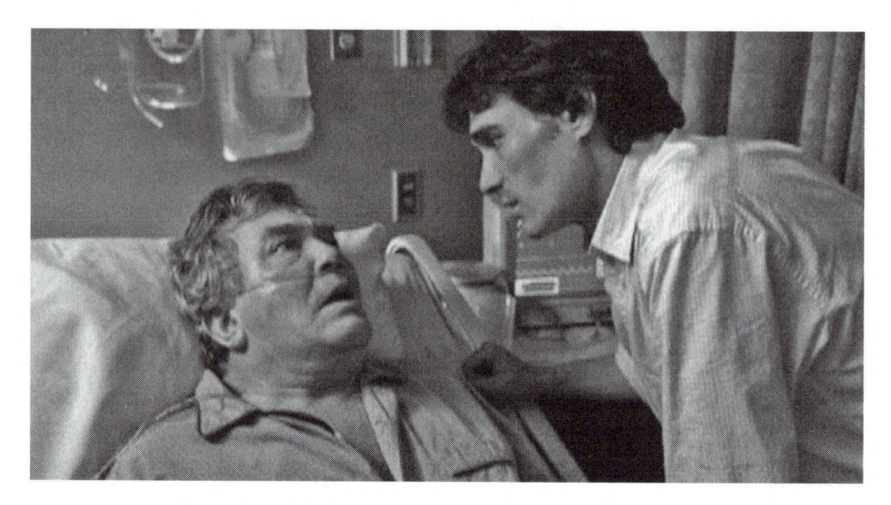

FIGURE 16.1 Father, played by Albert Finney, and son, played by Billy Crudup, share an emotional moment as the father faces the end of his life. *Source*: Columbia Pictures.

stories help father and son work together to create a meaningful end-of-life narrative, even if it is a big fish tale.

It is not entirely a fish tale, however. As it turns out, the actual event bears greater resemblance to the story than William had ever imagined.

It becomes the responsibility of another character in the film to consider how to extend Edward's stories and bring his life narrative to a conclusion. The fact that Edward needed help with this does not mean that his life's end—his death narrative—was not autonomous, or at least an extension of his autonomous choices. Nearly all of us rely on others to carry out our lives. Of course, our imagined lives do not always match the stories we have told in our actual day-to-day choices. Even so, as we live our life stories, we set trajectories for our lives in a way that bears a close family resemblance to the traditional concepts of being self-legislating, auto-nomos.

I have described the traditional understanding of autonomy and recommended a modified conception as a way to hold on to the most compelling aspects of the tradition while sidestepping some of the traps laid for those charged with caring for those who are unable to choose for themselves. Elsewhere (Richman 2004), I have explored these issues using the concept of practical identities, roles that we adopt in our lives that structure our choices. The concept of narrative autonomy offers another tool for the same job, the job of thinking through how to judge when to take requests seriously when they come from patients (such as Raphael) whose judgment is impaired, and how to determine what ought to be done for patients (such as Mr. Potter in bed five) who can no longer even express preferences. The narrative concept is more forgiving of reality and human foibles than the traditional theory. It demands only that a choice cohere with the patient's life narrative, not that it be strictly, logically consistent with all or even most of the patient's other choices.

What Does It Mean for You? Autonomy and Medical Advance Directives

End-of-life issues were front and center in the American consciousness during the winter of 2004–2005, when difficult decisions were being made about what to do for Terri Schiavo, a woman who lived in a persistent vegetative state for several years before her feeding tube was removed after a protracted legal battle. One difficulty facing those involved was that the patient did not have an advance directive specifying her preferences. (The term *advance directive* refers both to documents naming a proxy decision-maker and to living wills, which state preferences more specifically.) Another difficulty in the Terri Schiavo case was disagreement about the facts of the case, in particular whether the patient had any awareness or mental life at all.

Several models of living wills are available. Following passage of the Patient Self-Determination Act in 1990, sample living wills were entered into state law. Hospitals and other institutions that, pursuant to the act, are required to provide advance directives generally distribute the sample adopted by their state legislature.[8]

Standard living will forms tend to offer limited outlets for expressing preferences. They tend to offer minimal descriptions of situations in which decisions might need to be made for the person, making it difficult for people to imagine what that might be like, what variations might arise, or how such a situation would feel to them. A common living will question might ask: "If you have a terminal condition, are expected to live less than six weeks and your heart stops, do you want CPR?" The available responses are typically "yes," "no," and "unsure." We might say that this way of eliciting preferences shows the influence of the traditional concept of autonomy, in which an individual exercises freedom by considering each decision by itself, considering what reasons can be given for each action.

The standard sort of living will provides clear answers to questions, but these answers are likely to miss information important to extending the individual's life narrative. The approach supported here is summed up well by Jeffrey Blustein: "proxy decision-makers are to act as continuers of the life stories of those who have lost narrative capacity" (Blustein 1999, p. 20). To do this, proxies need living wills that include answers to different sorts of questions. The following questions could be used in a living will that reflects a narrative concept of autonomy: "How do you envision the end of your life? Where and with whom do you imagine spending your last days?" I recommend that readers consider creating advance directives that combine narrative questions with the more specific standard ones to improve the chances of a meaningful end of life that reflects, coheres with, and completes the life that has been lived.

QUESTIONS FOR CONSIDERATION

1. *Was it appropriate for Nurse Stella to say "I love you" to Raphael as he died? When she withdrew his treatment, was her action really an act of love?*

2. *Do health care professionals and proxies have a duty to respect and extend a patient's life story no matter what that story is like? Are there life narratives that ought not to be respected? If so, what makes the difference?*

3. *Do all lives tell a coherent story? Is it possible to live a life that is so incoherent as to fail to have a narrative? What would such a life look like?*

ACKNOWLEDGMENT

I dedicate this chapter to my father. May he continue to live a long, storied life.

NOTES

1. Susan Sherwin uses the term *empowerment* to explain some of these issues. See Sherwin 1992, chapter 11.

2. For more extended objections to the traditional concept of autonomy, see Pellegrino and Thomasma 1988; Karlawish 1996; Schneider 1998; O'Neill 2002; Richman 2004, chapter 4. It may well be that I am joining these others in objecting to a straw man (perhaps a straw Kant). That is, I might be arguing against a position that no one has held. If so, I hope it is yet worth the reading to draw out the alternative offered.

3. Paternalism draws the most attention when an action is taken that is contrary to a patient's expressed wishes. However, this type of conflict is not a necessary feature of paternalism in my definition.

4. Feminist ethics of care emphasizes connections and relationships between individuals. Although such relationships would certainly enhance the provision of care, the model of caring I advocate here could be applied without the kind of connection between patient and decision-maker promoted by the ethics of care.

5. For a discussion of the "reality constraint" on life narratives, see Schechtman 1996, esp. pp 119–20; Blustein 1999, par 15.

6. There are also facts about human psychology that can help us predict how an individual's narrative may change. For instance, if we know that people tend to adjust to and even value life with certain types of disabilities, it may be appropriate to practice paternalism during that transition rather than to try to extend the individual's narrative as previously lived. I am not treating these situations more fully because my focus is primarily on efforts to extend autonomy when that is determined to be appropriate.

7. See, e.g., Kuczewski 1994; Karlawish 1996; Rich 1997; Blustein 1999; Kuczewski 1999.

8. Some bioethicists and activists have developed alternative approaches, including the Values History developed by Doukas and McCullough (1991) and variations of a "will to live," promoted by pro-life activists and by disability rights groups.

REFERENCES

Blustein, J. 1999. Choosing for Others as Continuing a Life Story: The Problem of Personal Identity Revisited. *Journal of Law, Medicine and Ethics* 1:20–31.

Burton, T. 2004. *Big Fish* [motion picture]. Culver City, CA: Columbia Pictures Corporation.

Dennett, D. C. 1987. *The Intentional Stance*. Cambridge, MA: MIT Press.

———. 1991. Real Patterns. *Journal of Philosophy* LXXXVII:27–51.

Dooling, R. 1996. *Critical Care*. New York: Picador.

Doukas, D. J., and McCullough, L. B. 1991. The Values History: The Evaluation of the Patient's Values and Advance Directives. *Journal of Family Practice* 32 (2):145–54.

Kant, I. 1959. *Foundations of the Metaphysics of Morals*, trans. L. W. Beck. Indianapolis, IN: Bobbs-Merrill. (Originally published 1785)

Karlawish, J. H. T. 1996. Shared Decision Making in Critical Care: A Clinical Reality and an Ethical Necessity. *American Journal of Critical Care* 5 (6):391.

Kuczewski, M.G. 1994. Whose Will Is It, Anyway? A Discussion of Advance Directives, Personal Identity, and Consensus in Medical Ethics. *Bioethics* 8 (1):27–48.

———. 1999. Narrative Views of Personal Identity and Substituted Judgment in Surrogate Decision Making, *Journal of Law, Medicine and Ethics* 27 (1):32.

Lumet, S. 1997. *Critical Care* [motion picture]. Los Angeles: Live Entertainment.

O'Neill, O. 2002. *Autonomy and Trust in Bioethics*. Cambridge: Cambridge University Press.

Pellegrino, E. D., and Thomasma, D. C. 1988. *For the Patient's Good: The Restoration of Beneficence in Health Care*. New York: Oxford University Press.

Rawls, J. 1971. *A Theory of Justice*. Cambridge, MA: Harvard University Press.

Rich, B.A. 1997. Prospective Autonomy and Critical Interests: A Narrative Defense of the Moral Authority of Advance Directives. *Cambridge Quarterly of Healthcare Ethics*. 6:138–47.

Richman, K. A. 2004. *Ethics and the Metaphysics of Medicine: Reflections on Health and Beneficence*. Cambridge, MA: MIT Press.

Richman, K. A., and Budson, A. E. 2000. Health of Organisms and Health of Persons: An Embedded Instrumentalist Approach. *Theoretical Medicine and Bioethics* 21 (4):339–52.

Schechtman, M. 1996. *The Constitution of Selves*. Ithaca, NY: Cornell University Press.

Schneider, C. E. 1998. *The Practice of Autonomy: Patients, Doctors and Medical Decisions*. New York: Oxford University Press.

Sherwin, S. 1992. *No Longer Patient: Feminist Ethics and Health Care*. Philadelphia: Temple University Press.

Wallace, D. 1999. *Big Fish: A Novel of Mythic Proportions*. New York: Penguin.

SEVENTEEN

The Thanatoria of *Soylent Green*

On Reconciling the Good Life with the Good Death

Matthew Burstein

I've lived too long.

SOL ROTH, *Soylent Green*

Does dying have its own aesthetic? Can one choose death well? These are peculiar, perhaps macabre, questions to ask. Yet at the time I write this, there is much death in the news: man-made and natural disasters, plagues, war, famine, and the like take lives in very public, and very horrifying, ways. Surely there are better ways to die than drowning in a flood or being torn asunder by one's neighbor in the streets.[1] Of course, things could be worse: the planet could be so overpopulated and so polluted that all the people of the world live in squalid, overcrowded conditions under a repressive, exploitative, and violent government that operates in cahoots with the single corporation that provides artificial foodstuffs to the populace. Forget the strife between supporters of organic farms and "slow foods" on the one hand and factory farms and fast food on the other; we're talking about nutrient-rich crackers as the sole source of nutrition for the vast majority of humanity. If New York City seems crowded with a population of eight million, imagine a future where it shelters forty million souls.

This latter, rather worse New York, is depicted in Richard Fleischer's 1973 science fiction film *Soylent Green*. In *Soylent Green*'s dystopian future, unlike our present, people are able to choose death in a manner that abides by their aesthetic sensibilities. Indeed, there is an institution that provides them with the means of fulfilling such desires, which I call the *thanatorium*.[2] What are we to make of such an institution, and what would we say about it if it existed under conditions rather more conducive to human flourishing? In this chapter, I argue that the thanatorium has the potential to be a salutary institution, and, moreover, that it is rather more compatible with a standard conception of human agency than current alternatives offered to us by various medical, religious, and moral institutions.

Setting the Scene: Nonfiction, News, and Death

In recent years, debates about the "end of life" have become front page news in the United States. Indeed, 2005 may have marked a watershed in end-of-life spectacles. After Terri Schiavo spent fifteen years connected to life-support systems, clinging to the merest of lives through the aid of modern medical technologies, a media deathwatch grew up around her—fueled by endless sparring between Schiavo's parents and her husband as well as some of the year's most shameful appropriation of human life for purposes of political pandering. In mid-March of 2005, Schiavo's feeding tube was removed, and she died approximately two weeks later of "marked dehydration."[3] During this period, the media bombarded audiences with views about what was going on in Florida: was it murder or compassion? Those suggesting the latter claimed that Schiavo's persistent vegetative state was irreversible and that she was living an undignified, merely biological life. Those opposing frequently—though not exclusively—claimed that life was the ultimate gift, and that euthanasia in this case, as well as more generally, should be seen as an affront to human dignity and the sanctity of life.

When we look at accounts of personhood and the kinds of lives that are good, we tend to think in terms of agency. That is, we think in terms of how we are masters of our lives: autonomous decision-makers, self-motivated and -determined agents who act in light of rational consideration of our good, to control of our living conditions, and the like. This model of personhood as a kind of mastery has been useful, and it informs many of our attitudes about ourselves and the world; however, the model seems to break down at a point when we try to make sense of our lives when we become seriously ill or debilitated (see other chapters in this volume, including those on *Million Dollar Baby*, for more treatment of this issue). Once we are faced with the kind of conditions that rob us of the kind of mastery—over body or mind or life—it appears that we are unlikely to get any guidance from a model that presupposes precisely this sort of control. A standard attitude taken toward end-of-life issues within this model of agency involves expressing a preference for being "unplugged" over languishing in a persistent vegetative state. Because a life without agency is not worth living, as the reasoning goes, it is rational to refuse some care that extends a less-than-agentive life.

Although this is a traditional interpretation of what the mastery model requires, it is not mastery; this is acquiescence. In the face of the end of life, those taking this approach to the mastery model take it that the model is no longer apt, and so it is now time to, as it were, stop fighting the human fight. The difficulty in seeing beyond these options comes from having arranged our other institutions in a way that obscures the wisdom of the model at the end of life.

The dominant philosophical conception of our lives is marked by choice and action, but the dominant conception of our deaths is marked by resignation and surrender.[4] This is an unsatisfying and vexing set of attitudes, in that it presumes that there can—or perhaps should—be no agency in death. Were we genuinely incapable of being agents in the face of death, then a "hybrid" model of agency that delineates different sets of virtues in light of differing outcomes (a flourishing life or a proper recognition of our finitude in the face of death). After all, one might reasonably suggest that the agency model aims at the living of life, and so, when our activities can no longer aim at living, a new model which understands our humanity and our finitude is required.

Such a hybrid model gains traction only if we cannot properly treat a view of one's death as properly within one's view of life. Yet, we already do treat one's death as loaded with various choices that are to be made as continuous with one's actions in life: we may choose to be cremated or buried in a particular place (perhaps next to someone we love), volunteer to be organ donors, allocate the resources of our estate, and the like. These are not done haphazardly, but rather are undertaken in a considered fashion as an expression of our agency in death. We already express preferences about the end of our lives, and these preferences reflect our moral and aesthetic judgments about what we value. It is a bit of moral gerrymandering to say that these are perfectly normal elements of our agency, but when it comes to, say, choosing how we die, *then* we must acquiesce.

The medicalization of death brings the conflict between these attitudes into starker relief. The advances of Western science have transformed the hospital from a place where the poor went to die into a place where people go to get healed; the aseptic and antiseptic tools and methods of the hospital are entirely appropriate in treating disease because, after all, such tools reduce the spread of disease. But the practice of medicine is one in which the physician has various powers over a patient (e.g., access to facilities and the power of prescription) that diminish a patient's ability to have mastery over the conditions of her life. The treatment of a patient as an object, as a problem set, may well be of central importance to medicine; the problem is that this treatment and the medical institutions that have been constructed around it conflict with the mastery model of agency.

It is telling that the discussions about possible alternatives to "letting nature take its course" center on the idea of what is called physician-assisted suicide. Whether or not arguments that physician-assisted suicide violates the Hippocratic Oath succeed, they do point to the peculiarity of assigning the role of death's gatekeeper to the profession charged with saving lives. Clearly, scientists and physicians do many important things well when it comes to the science of life and health; however, we should ask why the end of life is their province as well.[5] We would do well to leave Hygia and Thanatos to their respective provinces.[6]

The standard framing of the debate about the permissibility of physician-assisted suicide inaptly poses the "pro" and "con" as being the fundamental philosophical divide; instead, both positions share the same problematic aesthetic of acquiescence and passivity, but disagree about where to locate the proper passivity (in the face of "Nature" or "the Physician"). Yet, what other option is there? Consider a contrast case from February 2005. Just weeks before Schiavo's ultimate demise, there was another noteworthy news item regarding end-of-life issues: the suicide of Hunter S. Thompson. After a lifetime of "living out loud"[7] —though not necessarily to the cartoonish excesses of his writings—Thompson found himself incapable of living a life that reflected his sense that life was to be lived vigorously. The period before his suicide was marked by painful injuries and surgeries that limited his mobility and undercut his ability to participate in his usually robust lifestyle.[8] Thompson's suicide note, entitled "Football Season Is Over," reads:

> No More Games. No More Bombs. No More Walking. No More Fun. No More Swimming. 67. That is 17 years past 50. 17 more than I needed or wanted. Boring. I am always bitchy. No Fun—for anybody. 67. You are getting Greedy. Act your old age. Relax—This won't hurt."
>
> (BONE 2005)

While I do not want to defend Thompson's choice specifically, we can see in his suicide an aesthetic choice that reflects a certain view about the nature of agency. What makes a person's life worth living is not mere existence; it is rather, the ability for that person to live her life in light of her view of the good. We need not conceive of the end of a life well lived as one that ends only when the body has absolutely nothing left to give. Instead, it is worth considering the possibility that a rational agent could "choose death" even though his or her body could function well for decades *if* that body is incapable of fulfilling core aspects of the agent's view of the good.

We may recover such an account from the mastery model of agency. After all, if the hallmark of agency is this power to shape one's life—one's self and one's environment—there seems to be a kind of cruelty in requiring (either formally through law or informally through social sanction) that a life dedicated to the moral and aesthetic values of the mastery model be capped by occupying a body that is incapable of achieving the agent's view of the good.

These reflections about the limitations of the mastery model in the face of an agent's decreased capacity to achieve her good leads us to some rather unpleasant conclusions. Are we condemned to the choice between an indolence unto death, the medical surrender of physician-assisted suicide and the frequently lonely death of suicide when we are faced with a body that is incapable of achieving the good? At first blush, it would seem so: we must wait for "nature to take its course" or for "the exercising of God's will" through our bodies; or we must request help from socially sanctioned authorities; or, as a last resort, we seem driven to exercise our independence in a catch-as-catch-can fashion by committing suicide.

These appearances are illusory, however. There is room for an institution—both in the broad sense of a social practice (e.g., marriage) and in the more narrow sense of an establishment (e.g., the Supreme Court)—that empowers people to choose the time, manner, and circumstances of their death when they are faced with conditions that undercut their capacities for agency and self-mastery. I call this institution the "thanatorium" in this chapter; it is an institution that gives death a proper place in the life well lived. The question, though, is how to describe such an institution that clearly does not exist and, in many ways, cuts against many taboos regarding the end of life.

Setting the Scene: Fiction, Film, and the Thanatorium

The science fiction classic *Soylent Green* is a text ripe for examination of the problem at hand. New York City, circa 2022, is a portrait of dystopia: it is overpopulated, has scarce resources, and is run by a corrupt, repressive government that protects its own privilege—hardly the conditions for human flourishing. As a result of the consumption-driven consumer lifestyle enjoyed in the late twentieth and early twenty-first centuries, the environment is severely polluted, living conditions are horrendously overcrowded, and "real" food sufficiently scarce that people receive nourishment from various-colored chips produced by the Soylent Corporation. By 2022, we have "lived" ourselves into dystopia. The masses live in squalid housing projects that have limited access to water and electricity. When they protest their decrepit conditions, the citizens are met with violence by the government; not only do the riot squads wield weapons but also giant trucks scoop up protesters and dump them into a holding bin in the truck's bed. This degradation of humanity isn't total, of course; there is a class of elites who run the society and who do not suffer such indignities. For the elites, traditional foodstuffs, alcohol, and well-appointed housing are available. Indeed, for the elites there is the benefit of "furniture": attractive women who, along with their "services," are included with the housing and can be exchanged. For everyone else, fruits and vegetables are mere history, as are many other elements of the natural world that we take for granted: beautiful vistas, clean air and water, and wild animals.

This society that provides so little for its citizens readily provides an institution that assists suicide—a thanatorium, if you will.[9] Our introduction to the thanatorium comes when Sol Roth (played by Edward G. Robinson) chooses to end it all. When Roth enters the thanatorium, he encounters an environment that is clean, peaceful, and orderly—in stark contrast to the world outside. Roth is greeted by a friendly face and is asked to specify various preferences regarding music, colors, and preferred scenery. At every turn, Roth is treated with warmth and tenderness; when he arrives in the room where his "ceremony" will be held, he is greeted by two people in long, white, and vaguely priestly gowns. These people help Roth undress and get comfortable on the altarlike bed. Shortly thereafter, Roth's bed is rolled into a large room. The lights dim, Beethoven's *Pastoral* Symphony begins to play and motion pictures depicting nature scenes appear on a large screen: woods, a sunset, a river, aquatic life, and the like. Roth is visibly moved by all this. After a brief discussion with Detective Robert Thorn (played by Charlton Heston)—one that reveals the truth so horrible that Roth cannot continue living with the burden of such knowledge—Roth passes on quietly under lights glowing orange (his favorite color). In stark contrast to the brutal conditions of the lives outside the thanatoria, the deaths are serene, sensuous, and under the control of the person wishing to die.

The richness of *Soylent Green* comes from this contrast; on the one hand, its dystopia would be a terrible place to live. On the other hand, it might be a much better place to die than, for example, the sterile and alienating hospital room of contemporary life.[10] Instead of dying in the laboratory environment of the hospital surrounded by medical technicians, one dies surrounded by the comforts of favored, sensuous experiences. The film's thanatoria let us see how dying well can be the capstone of a life lived well: much as we learn to live well when we accept our nature as human agents, we die well when we embrace our finitude by choosing death. By accepting death as natural, we can reshape our practices and institutions such that the good death is possible; we can become agents even in our own deaths, rather than merely passive victims of the dying process.

The film's thanatoria allow us to envision the good death in a way that critiques the current surrender approaches to the end of life. Rather than being something that is to be struggled against at all costs—social, financial, and emotional—death can (and perhaps ought to) be seen as something that needs to be integrated into our account of living well. In essence I propose that we may ferry ourselves to the afterlife on our own terms, and, thereby, we may preserve the mastery model of agency until we die well.[11]

Moving beyond the Screen

Let me turn now to articulating, if only tentatively, a strategy that would allow the traditional account of personal agency to recover some of its usefulness in the face of end-of-life issues.[12] The medicalization of the end of life has served to usurp our agency, even as it makes promises of "respecting the autonomy" of patients. What autonomy there is in such circumstances is unclear, as the patient is both highly vulnerable and dependent on the physician, who has specialized knowledge, access to facilities, and powers of prescription. Moreover, the patient is legally barred from these last two forms of power. When combined with the necessary treatment of a patient as a mere "sick body" to be examined and intervened on, there is precious little room for mastery in one's life. Could an institution like the thanatorium solve this problem?

The Idea of the Thanatorium

The idea of the thanatorium—or at least the notion of an institutionalized public facility for choosing to die—is not unique to *Soylent Green*, and its use in fiction has varied wildly in tone (though seemingly never in endorsement). The animated television series *Futurama* (Groening 1999–2003) depicted New New York (New York City in the year 3000 C.E.) as a future that combines the utopian hopes and dystopian fears common to science fiction. One element of the New New York cityscape is the "suicide booth"—America's favorite brand being Stop 'n' Drop—where, for the price of 25 cents, one can choose between a "quick and painless" or a "slow and horrible" death. Suicide booths are available on street corners in much the same way telephone booths were before the widespread adoption of the cellular phone. Where the thanatorium of *Soylent Green* is used to horrify the audience, the suicide booths of *Futurama* are put to humorous ends.

Yet the idea of a public space for suicides made its appearance even before the twentieth century. In the 1895 short story by Robert Chambers, "The Repairer of Reputations" (Chambers 1895), the repeal of legal prohibitions on suicide "bore its final fruit in the month of April 1920, when the first Government Lethal Chamber was opened on Washington Square."[13] Opened with much official fanfare, the governor of New York announces that there is "a painless death await[ing] him who can no longer bear the sorrows of this life. If death is welcome, let him seek it here."[14] Unlike the banality of *Futurama*'s suicide booth, the Government Lethal Chamber is an ornately decorated place of great moment:

> The block, which had formerly consisted of a lot of shabby old buildings, used as cafes and restaurants for foreigners, had been acquired by the government in the winter of 1913. The French and Italian cafes and restaurants were torn down; the whole block enclosed by a gilded iron railing, and converted into a lovely garden, with lawns, flowers, and fountains. In the centre of the garden stood a small, white building, severely classical in architecture, and surrounded by thickets of flowers. Six Ionic columns supported the roof, and the single door was of bronze. A splendid marble group of "the Fates" stood before the door, the work of a young American sculptor, Boris Yvain, who had died in Paris when only twenty-three years old.

Whereas *Soylent Green* envisions the thanatorium as the ultimate objectification of the general population, here it is conceived of as a part of urban "renewal." Even this partly salutary picture is a part of cultural criticism. None of these depictions are particularly favorable to the institution that I've called the thanatorium. Rather, they use the thanatorium as a device for criticizing a society that insufficiently values human life. My first task, then, is to extricate the institution from the context in which it has been placed. Doing so will require showing how such an institution is both compatible with the mastery model of agency, and, moreover, dictated by the conflict between the mastery model and the end of life. I turn to this task now.

Rehabilitating the Thanatorium

The mastery model is marked by the agent's determinations of valuable ends and their pursuit; to be an agent is to have an understanding of the good life and to act in ways that reflect this understanding. There are two components to the mastery model, one metaphysical and one aesthetic. Metaphysically, the mastery model defines agents in terms of their capability to control; agency is the ability of the agent to order her environment in such a way that she may achieve her ends. This model assumes that certain intellectual and kinesthetic resources and competencies are in place. The model presupposes that a person who is incapable of controlling her body or her environment to enable her to act in light of her beliefs is likewise incapable of voluntary action. The model of agency is one that centers on calm, sober, sane, competent, and rational persons who are capable of using their bodies appropriately.

However, this model of agency is not merely a metaphysical view; it isn't merely a view about what kinds of intellectual and practical resources an organism must (aspire to) have to be an agent. Beyond being an account of the metaphysics of agency, this model brings with it a set of aesthetic judgments about what sort of resources are good and what sort of uses of them are desirable. The mastery model's implicit aesthetic is one in which what is valued is the kind of competency ascribed by the model's metaphysics. The metaphysics of the mastery model aren't value neutral; they don't provide an account of a kind of thing without weighing in on its merit.[15] Instead, they have, embedded within them, assumptions about what makes an agent's life worth living. For better or for worse, the life worth living is one in which a person has a relatively high degree of control over his or her destiny. What is at stake in our conception of person is not only the capacity for responsibility but also the manner in which those choices reflect a conception of one's own flourishing.

This conception of flourishing is as much aesthetic as moral. Inquiries into the relationship between freedom of the will and moral agency are inquiries into the kind of things that agents are. The picture of humans as agents who make choices in a certain fashion—a fashion that reflects the mastery model—brings with it a collection of values favoring activity and control over passivity and resignation. The thing that makes us free—that makes us more than mere wantons—is the control we come to exhibit over our environments, our bodies, and our thoughts.

Acknowledging these facts allows us to see that the thanatorium can function as a salutary rather than a sinister institution. The thanatorium can serve to empower people in precisely the ways that the mastery model accounts for: it allows an individual to act in a way that is self-determined in light of their aesthetic judgments about the limits of human lives. Further, it facilitates both the metaphysical and the aesthetic parts of the mastery model. With regard to metaphysics, it makes it possible for people to have the death they desire. In the absence of the thanatorium, people who choose to die are forced to do so in ways that may be problematic; the means of death must be painful or violent or, at best, improvised (e.g., carbon monoxide poisoning achieved by sitting in a car in a garage). With an institution like the thanatorium, one may choose the time, location, and mode of death—that is, control it—while protecting loved ones from the horror of discovering the corpse by surprise.

The importance of the thanatorium to a mastery model of agency isn't just metaphysical. The aesthetic message of a properly implemented thanatorium reclaims death from the passivity required of the medical subject. That is, the existence of the thanatorium can express the value of mastery to a life; it could serve as a celebration of a life marked by agency up to its very end. In contrast, the medical subject is a problem for the physician to solve, a sick body to be acted on and treated. Rather than affirming life, the injunction against suicide (physician-assisted or otherwise) in the face of debilitating, terminal illness is an injunction against the mastery model of agency.[16] This injunction denies that what matters most is agency and affirms the values of passivity and resignation. Notice, though, that the movement for physician-assisted suicide is guilty of the same problematic aesthetic. While the movement that "affirms life" (at whatever cost) requires passivity and resignation in the face of death, the movement to medicalize the end of life requires passivity and resignation in the face of the medical authorities: One must get the physician's approval to end one's life, and one must secure the methods from the pharmacist who controls the relevant medications.[17] In both cases, the aesthetics of the end of life run precisely contrary to the values we endorse in every other part of our lives under the mastery model. The implementation of an institution such as the thanatorium would be an alternative that allows persons (at least, those who so choose) to maintain mastery of their deaths; thanatoria empower agents to choose death well.

Are We Talking about the Same Film?

The main objection to the line of reasoning that I have been pushing is that the thanatoria really represent a further form of degradation and devaluation of humans found in the movie's society at large; they provide no "empowerment" whatsoever. Ultimately, the people using thanatoria are the raw materials for *Soylent Green*'s eponymous foodstuff. The thanatoria are useful because they trim the excess (and excessively miserable) population, and they provide the grim raw materials for the survival of the remainder of the population; hence, the thanatoria are essentially exploitative. In this way, the thanatoria represent yet another manifestation of a culture of death that, in its core, devalues human life. My response to this objection is to acknowledge that this is an artifact of the film, but that it is inessential to the notion of thanatoria. In fact, providing an account of the good death within our view of the good life can allow us to hold concerns about exploitation and the disvalue of persons at bay.

The Concern

The horror of *Soylent Green* comes from a few different directions, but the ones relevant to my discussion involve that the vast majority of people live squalid lives. The need for thanatoria in *Soylent Green*'s world comes directly from the terrible living conditions of the populace. The hook of the movie is that life is sufficiently unlivable—resources are so scarce, living spaces so overcrowded—that choosing death is a relatively unproblematic activity. Choosing death is commonplace, and an institution exists to help fulfill the needs of people for whom suffering is objectively the nature of their existence. Even worse, the corpses from the thanatoria are processed by the Soylent Corporation into Soylent Green. This is a paradigm of the "culture of death."

The thanatoria of *Soylent Green* are both emblematic of and crucial to the culture's ultimate exploitation of human life. The lives of the majority are ones of deprivation, and so death seems to offer greater comfort than life. Moreover, the thanatoria, by their very existence, serve to legitimize this sort of reasoning; they offer an inviting environment that is clean, orderly, and full of the promise of sensual fulfillment that is unmatched by the realities of everyday life. Ultimately, this invitation to "enjoy one last, wondrous experience" is duplicitous in the same way that the mousetrap is; whereas the mousetrap offers the promise of nourishment and delivers death, the thanatorium's offer of respite conceals the horrible fact that one is about to become the Soylent Corporation's most popular foodstuff.

All of this suggests that *Soylent Green*'s thanatoria are not candidate institutions for serving human autonomy, self-mastery, and, thus, the good life. Rather, they are precisely the kinds of institutions we would expect from a society that *de*values human life. It is not accidental that such places exist within the context of a society that exploits persons to the point where even their corpses are to be treated as mere resources; not even death frees these people from exploitation. The thanatorium undercuts the aesthetic of the mastery model precisely because it provides yet another way to steal control from agents. The power of these people to make a decision about the way they end their lives is embedded within a troubling social environment that robs them of just about all possibility for mastery. The fact that committing suicide is the only way in which these people can genuinely express their agency only exacerbates the film's horrific reality.

A similar concern arises out of the suggestion that the "life worth living is one in which persons have a relatively high control over their destiny." Rather than worry, as I have so far, that the thanatorium is a symptom of a society with disordered values, one could be concerned that the thanatorium itself could infect a society and thereby create a disordering of values. In particular, I have in mind the concerns that have been raised in other contexts by activists among the sensory- and mobility-impaired populations: that we could quickly slide from having "diminished capacities" from the perspective of the mastery model to being of diminished (or little or no) value. Talk of an ideal human (well, agent) form combined with an institution that facilitates the deaths of those who may not meet such an ideal smacks rather more of an experiment in morally odious eugenics than it does a proposal for celebrating our agency.

A Defense of the Thanatorium

It would be foolish to deny the grim reality of *Soylent Green*; the duplicity of the thanatorium there is central to the film's horror. However, for this critique to be an analysis of the institution of the thanatorium per se, it will have to hold across different background conditions. That is, we can all agree that the thanatoria of *Soylent Green* are morally indefensible, and we can agree that they are indefensible for the same reason: they are one final insult to the agents in the film. Would they be equally indefensible given an entirely different set of background conditions?

One reason to think not is that the set up of *Soylent Green* is one in which precisely the kind of agency I've been concerned with virtually does not exist. Between the scarcity of resources, repressive governmental regimes, and corporations literally feeding people to one another, there is little room for a person to make considered, rational choices about how to act in ways that reflect a conception of agency. However, if the conditions are such that we have the ability to make these choices—to master our lives—it is possible to see that building up an institution around voluntarily ending one's life could enhance our agency by allowing us to decide the time, manner, and place of our own demise. A life that was actually spent pursuing and exercising agency—a life lived fully in light of the mastery model—would be served well by an institution that further facilitated a person's ability to shape her life. Much as the thanatorium functions as the ultimate symbol of misery in *Soylent Green*, it could serve as the ultimate symbol of mastery in a properly ordered world.

With a background of practices that enhance, encourage, or facilitate the mastery of agents, the absence of the thanatorium and the perpetuation of our current practices would, in fact, be perverse. Consider what such a world might be like: on the one hand, all of our institutions would aim at the sustenance of agency. On the other, the end of life is marked by the options I began this chapter considering: seeking medical permission to die, waiting for nature to take its course, and committing suicide in an isolated fashion.[18] Having spent a lifetime cultivating one's sense of self in light of one's agency, a person would (or could, given that some deaths would be quite sudden) be forced to face death in a way that snatches all that away. Much like poor Charlie Brown, whose determination, focus, and efforts are frustrated by Lucy's snatching away the football just as he is about to kick it (and contrary to all her promises to abstain from such snatching), society would pull away that which we value just at the time it could serve to be most useful and comforting (i.e., in the face of our mortality).

But what about the concern that the view I'm espousing can make a quick slide into, say, institutionalized pressure to off those we view as having "diminished capacities"? This concern is worth some discussion, as it has been a feature of the previous century that institutions were created to shape humanity to fit a certain ideal—frequently under the guise of "scientific" or "medical" progress. I have in mind here both the eugenics programs of the Nazis as well as the state of Virginia's policies that prohibited miscegenation and allowed the state to involuntarily sterilize the "mentally feeble" (among others). Both Germany and the United States provide examples of how we ought to be suspicious of efforts to make us all "measure up" to an ideal.

There is an important way in which these concerns may not challenge the analysis that I've provided. The question I've raised is whether, given an individual's valuing of her abilities and future, it is rational for her to choose her own death. Judgments about the value of human lives generally or of the lives of specific agents is not even on the table; rather, the concern is about the way in which being an agent requires a conception of one's self as an agent. What I propose here is that the mastery model of agency requires us to understand that there can be conditions under which an agent can choose death well (i.e., over a life not worth living)—and that our current "death" institutions cannot reasonably accommodate this fact. Understood this way, we can see that what we are talking about is the morality of which model a rational agent chooses for herself. If we change the situation to discuss those who aren't competent (or rational) or choosing for others, then we're changing the moral terrain in significant ways; deciding for others, especially those who, like Terri Schiavo, are utterly incapable of deciding for themselves and have left an ambiguous record of their rational desires, requires a different kind of reasoning than Hunter Thompson's deciding that he could no longer *be* Hunter Thompson.[19]

Conclusion

In contrast to the two major approaches to end-of-life issues (i.e., permitting or prohibiting physician-assisted suicide), embracing the thanatorium as an institution facilitates rather than frustrates the view of agents as having a certain mastery of their environment and of themselves. Rather than being left to acquiesce to nature or beseech a physician, we would have an institution that would allow us to choose death—and to choose it well. My arguments here have been focused at the intersection of moral theory and, for lack of a better term, aesthetics; while the former should be obvious, the latter is more surprising—or, rather, *seems* so insofar as we may not attend to our preferences regarding our deaths and the institutions that subsequently come into play (e.g., wakes, funerals, wills, etc.). Perhaps one might not want to *die*, but, given that one *will*, it is rational to prefer one death over another. The question I have posed here is whether there is a better way for humanity to honor the conception of persons as agents even in the face of our own finitude—is there a way for us to avoid "letting nature take its course" *and* treating death as the province of medicine's therapeutic (and objectifying) glance? The answer, it seems, is "yes"—if we have an institution like the thanatorium, we can facilitate agents choosing death well and, thereby, enhance their agency with regard to their lives.

A lingering concern one might have about the view I've sketched here is that it involves a "liberal atomism" of sorts; that is, that I've committed myself to a view that takes us to be isolated agents who should be allowed to do as they please. However, this worry is misguided, though it is also understandable given the necessary brevity of my remarks. My goal here is the creation of an essentially *social* space for accommodating our deaths. To choose death well may require that one take careful stock of one's obligations to others—and the essentially social orientation of the thanatorium can serve to highlight this sociality of the self. The thanatorium need not be envisioned as a private place; it is, rather, a more public institution. (How we implement such institutions is a knotty problem that, alas, must be left for another occasion.)

This concern revisits a recurring motif of this chapter, namely, that the institution of the thanatorium itself might be only as good or as bad as the surrounding society and other institutions: in *Soylent Green*, the thanatoria are immoral; in a society with a "liberal atomism" as its metaphysic, they might serve to further isolate individuals; in a collectivist society, the thanatorium could serve as a community's final farewell. I have spoken about the background conditions under which an institutionalized approach to thanatoria could be seen in a positive light. Having institutions—social practices or formal bodies—assist persons in their chosen death can play an important role in recovering agency in the face of debilitation; this assistance ought not to be the province of Hygia, of the physician, but rather is the chore of Charon—ferrying the dead to their final rest.

QUESTIONS FOR CONSIDERATION

1. *Is Burstein correct in suggesting that an aesthetic dimension is essential to the "metaphysics of mastery" account of agency? If so, how might one fill out such an account, especially in the light of the ways in which social norms (gender, race, class, sexuality, etc.) complicate matters? If not, what alternative aesthetics are compatible with this account of agency?*

2. *A key claim in this argument is that, in framing the debate about whether physician-assisted suicide should be permitted, the standard approach to end-of-life issues inaptly poses the "pro" and "con" as being the fundamental philosophical divide; instead, both positions share the same problematic aesthetic of acquiescence and passivity but disagree about where to locate the proper passivity (in the face of "Nature" or "the Physician"). How might those defending the standard approach to this debate respond to this charge?*

3. Soylent Green *is a disturbing, dystopian view of the future, and it seems odd to find an ideal for humanity in such a film. What is the relationship (epistemically or metaphysically) between the aesthetically repellent and the morally good?*

ACKNOWLEDGMENTS

I thank Nathaniel Goldberg, Elisa Hurley, Eran Klein, Adam Burstein, Martin Rice, Michael Cox, and Sandra Shapshay for their support and comments on various drafts of this chapter. I am deeply indebted to Kier Olsen DeVries; many of my ideas in this chapter are the result of a series of conversations we had about finitude, mastery, and bioethics, and, though we may disagree about these issues, this chapter would not have been without the inspiration of her moral wisdom.

This chapter is dedicated to the memory of close friend, confidant, conspirator, and comrade Geoff Hartman, who died far too young on June 7, 2007, as I was completing revisions on this chapter; my world is a dimmer place in his absence.

NOTES

1. In November 2006, Mohammed Halim, a forty-six-year-old schoolteacher in the Afghan city of Ghazni, was disemboweled and then drawn and quartered (with motorbikes rather than horses) and his "remains were put on display as a warning to others against defying Taleban [*sic*] orders to stop educating girls." Kim Sengupta, "Disembowelled and Murdered for Teaching Girls," *New Zealand Herald*, November 30, 2006. www.nzherald.co.nz/section/story.cfm? c_id=2&ObjectID=10413099.

2. There is some question as to the origin of the term *thanatorium*. The term itself does not appear in *Soylent Green*, and I was unable to track down any alternative sources for its origins.

3. It was widely reported that Schiavo died of starvation because her feeding tube was removed. However, the autopsy report from the medical examiner of Pasco and Pinellas Counties, Florida, lists the mechanism of Schiavo's death as "marked dehydration" and rules out starvation as a cause of death.

4. I don't want to presuppose too great a consensus or too large a shared set of beliefs here. Given the way the debate surrounding end-of-life issues is generally framed in social discourse, the question we are supposed to face at the end of life is whether we should stay on life support as long as we can or "let nature take its course." I propose that we should reframe the questions altogether rather than choose one side or the other.

5. Typically, the response again references institutional controls over medications; one simply cannot go to the corner pharmacy and pick up a lethal dose of opiates. This, though, seems to tell doubly against the institution of pharmaceutical prescriptions rather than in favor of maintaining this role for physicians.

6. In Greek mythology, Hygia is the deity associated with health, and Thanatos is the personification of death.

7. "If you ask me what I came into this world to do, I will tell you: I came to live out loud." Quote widely attributed to Emile Zola.

8. See, for example, the BBC's coverage of his suicide and subsequent "burial" (by having his ashes shot out of a cannon).

9. For those who have not seen the film, a "spoiler warning": the real horror of the film is that those who do go to the thanatoria are turned into the human foodstuff that gives the film its name. I will turn to this part of the film in the later sections of this chapter.

10. The problems here are exacerbated in teaching hospitals, where patients are objects of education for young physicians in training. See chapter 12 of this volume for a full discussion of these issues.

11. Charon is the character in Greek mythology that ferries the properly prepared dead to the underworld. My proposal here is that the thanatorium may be a "Charonic" institution for us.

12. I leave open a few questions that are important. Foremost, I leave to the side whether we should endorse or save the traditional model of agency. I also do not address questions about whether the arguments I pursue here break down under more extreme cases of the sort highlighted by the Terri Schiavo tragedy. My goals here are more modest: to show that there are serious incongruities between our accounts of personhood and the institutions that have developed around life and death issues.

13. The version I am quoting from is an online source, so there are no pages to cite beyond the original URL.

14. One should wonder why New York City is envisioned as the place where such things would take root. I imagine the optimistic reading is the sense that New York is a place of social experimentation, a unique civic laboratory; the pessimistic reading is that there is something dehumanizing about living in New York.

15. The point here isn't (or at least isn't just) that the metaphysical account provides a "functional kind"—whereby one knows, in virtue of what kind of thing it is, how well it is functioning. (For example, those who know what a clock is know what makes a clock better or worse.) Functional terms only evaluate instances of their kind in light of their kind. Here, I'm claiming that the metaphysics of the mastery view recommend this sort of agency. To describe someone as an agent on this view is to attribute to them something worthwhile, in the same way that to attribute to someone the characteristic "being a murderer" would be to attribute something bad to them.

16. There might be other grounds for using a thanatorium, but I do not have the space here to provide an exhaustive account of the institution.

17. The role of the pharmacist as gatekeeper has become increasingly worrisome over the last few years, as pharmacists have begun to refuse to fill prescriptions (usually

for emergency contraception) on the grounds of conscience. If this use of conscience becomes legitimated, then it only makes stronger the demands that those facing death acquiesce rather than exercise mastery.

18. The last of these options, an isolated suicide, is the result of not having a thanatorium as an institution in the sense of a "social practice" rather than in the sense of a specific location. If we do not have a social practice that sanctions this manner of choosing death, then the varieties of fear, uncertainty, doubt, and shame that surround suicide now would, *ex hypothesi* govern it in the idealized conditions I'm considering.

19. Obviously, a sense of self is in part determined by the attitudes of others, and the views of others certainly can shape or coerce our own judgments. I don't mean to minimize this point here. The point, though, is that the thanatorium as an institution is a tool, and its uses may be either liberating or repressive.

REFERENCES

Bone, J. 2005. "Gonzo" Said Goodbye to Games, Bombs, Walking and Fun with Suicide Note in Doldrums of February. *The Times (London).* September 10, Section 5.

Chambers, R.W. 1895. *The King in Yellow.* www.gutenberg.org/etext/8492.

Fleischer, R. 1973. *Soylent Green* [motion picture]. Los Angeles: Metro-Goldwyn-Mayer.

Groening, M. 1999–2003. *Futurama* [television series]. Los Angeles: 20th Century Fox Television.

Medical Examiner's Office, District Six (Pasco and Pinellas Counties, Florida). 2005. Death Investigation of Theresa Marie Schiavo (ME case #5050439). June 13.

PART FIVE

The Role of Theory and Culture in Bioethics

EIGHTEEN

"If You Could Cure Cancer by Killing One Person, Wouldn't You Have to Do That?"

Utilitarianism and Deontology in *Extreme Measures*

Jason T. Eberl

Two naked men burst out a door and run down a dark alley. We don't know why they're running, but it's evident they're not healthy. One of them, Claude Minkins, ends up wrapped in a plastic sheet, clearly disoriented, in the middle of a busy street. As in the famous case of Kitty Genovese, no one in this busy city seems inclined to stop and help this obviously distressed person. Instead, passing drivers, who must think he's just another psychotic, probably high, perhaps dangerous, homeless man, honk and curse at him. Not until much later do we learn that Claude, while homeless, is not psychotic and was not ill until he became a "patient" at Triphase—a medical research company.

Dr. Lawrence Myrick (played by Gene Hackman), head of Triphase, has been conducting radical experiments in neural regeneration geared, specifically, to helping persons with cervical fractures walk again. To accomplish his goal by the most expedient means, he needs human subjects and thus "recruits" homeless men like Claude by deceiving them into thinking that they were found ill and are being helped at the Triphase "hospital." In his experiments, Dr. Myrick severs each subject's spinal cord and then applies his experimental treatment to regenerate the neural connection in a macabre, and overly dramatized, example of medical trial-and-error.

What does Myrick believe justifies his experiments? What motivates him and those who support him in carrying out this research program?

What ethical principles should guide medical researchers in risking the health and lives of human research participants? While it may be difficult to identify the correct ethical theory or set of principles to apply in medicine—or in any aspect of life, for that matter—it's pragmatically beneficial to attempt to define and apply such theories or principles to these difficult moral cases. Consider the alternatives: perhaps the judgment of what to do in such moral dilemmas should be left to the individuals involved, appealing to their own values or emotional reactions to the situation, or perhaps society should simply legislate what's to be done based on majority or expert opinion. The problem with both of these alternatives is that individuals, the majority, and even experts may make clearly erroneous judgments or fail to adhere to the basic mandate of justice to "treat like cases alike." There's also little hope of consensus if moral judgments are made on a "to each her own" basis.

In this chapter I use the film *Extreme Measures* (Apted 1996) to address this basic dilemma: is it ever ethical to exploit some persons to benefit others? I do so by examining ethical theories and principles that purport to offer objective normative judgments concerning what should be done and what one's moral attitude should be regarding such cases.

"You Made a Moral Choice . . . Not a Medical One"

Dr. Guy Luthan (played by Hugh Grant) is working in the emergency room at Gramercy Hospital, although he'll soon depart for a neurology fellowship at New York University. In come two trauma patients: a wounded police officer and his assailant, who were both shot in an exchange of gunfire. With only one operating room available, Guy selects the cop for it even though the criminal who shot him is in worse condition. Although Guy attempts to justify his choice as being forced by having only one operating room available, nurse Jodie Trammel (played by Sarah Jessica Parker) doesn't let him off the hook so easily and accuses him of making "a moral choice . . . not a medical one." [1]

What is the "moral choice" Guy made? In this situation, three main moral considerations might be motivating this choice. The first is a *utilitarian* calculation of what would produce "the greatest good for the greatest number." Utilitarians hold that the sole moral imperative is to seek the best consequences—the greatest net amount of happiness—for the majority of persons affected by one's decision. Guy states, "On my right I see a cop with his wife in the corridor and pictures of his kids in his wallet, and on my left some guy who's taken a gun out on a city bus." Because the police officer serves the public good in a greater way than his assailant, not only is the cop's and his family's happiness served by saving him but also society in general is better with him on the streets as opposed to the other patient.

The second possible rationale is a *sympathetic* response to the cop's wife standing in the trauma room's doorway with his fellow brothers in blue; whereas the assailant has no family present to emotionally pressure Guy to save their loved one. Some philosophers, such as Jean-Jacques Rousseau (1712–1778), argue that one's emotional response to a moral dilemma is an excellent guide, if not the sole means, to arrive at a resolution (Rousseau 1762/1979). Utilitarians, on the other hand, take no account of such "sentimentalism." But a utilitarian would recognize the fact that the cop has a family whose happiness (both emotional and material) would be negatively affected by his death; while the assailant may have no family at all as far as is known.

The final means of justifying Guy's decision is by appealing to the concept of *retributive justice*: punishment may be justly administered to those who cause unwarranted harm to others in society. This would be the weakest form of justification insofar as physicians are not agents of justice, but healers whose primary duty is to the patient in front of them. Proper retribution will be administered by the state assuming the assailant survives his wounds.

Rather than retributive justice, the operative concept that should have been at play in this case is that of *distributive justice*: the fair distribution of benefits and burdens in society. In this case, the benefit of optimal medical care must be distributed between the two patients. Jodie points out to Guy that he knew the other patient was in worse condition. The practice of medical triage, in which "you take care of the ones you think you can save," requires that the proper distribution of optimal care is to the worse-off patient assuming that both patients have a relatively equal chance of survival. The preference for the cop would be justified only if the assailant's condition were so bad that his chances of survival even with the benefit of an operating room were slim to none.

"Great Doctors Have the Guts to Do the Right Thing"

The counterpoint to utilitarianism, which mandates fair treatment under both distributive and retributive justice, is *deontology*, the study of moral obligations. In his writings, Immanuel Kant (1724–1804) argues what's known as the principle of respect for persons: "So act that you use humanity, whether in your own person or in the person of any other, always at the same time as an end, never merely as a means" (Kant 1785/1997, p. 38). This principle, based on Kant's recognition of the intrinsic dignity of human persons as rational beings, requires that we don't reduce a person to merely a "thing"—an object of use. Rather, while we can and do use other persons all the time (e.g., a patient uses a physician to be healed; a physician uses a nurse to assist her), we must always respect the fundamental value of persons as we interact with them.

Utilitarianism holds a similar principle of fair treatment. John Stuart Mill (1806–1873), in works such as *Utilitarianism* (1861/2001), argues that, when calculating to whom benefits and burdens will be distributed in a given moral situation, one must be "strictly impartial as a disinterested and benevolent spectator" (p. 17). This is why a utilitarian would object to Guy's being motivated by sympathy for the cop's family and thereby giving more weight to the cop's well-being than to that of the other patient; although, more weight can be given to the cop's well-being insofar as more people may be negatively affected by this death.

The major difference between utilitarianism and deontology is that the former allows a person to be used merely as a means to achieve the best overall consequences. Think of the following example:

> Consider the story (well known to philosophers) of the fat man stuck in the mouth of a cave on a coast. He was leading a group of people out of the cave when he got stuck in the mouth of the cave and in a very short time high tide will be upon them, and unless he is promptly unstuck, they all will be drowned except the fat man, whose head is out of the cave. But, fortunately or unfortunately,

> someone has with him a stick of dynamite. The short of the matter is, either they use the dynamite and blast the poor innocent fat man out of the mouth of the cave or everyone else drowns. Either one life or many lives. (NIELSEN 1972, P. 222)

Kai Nielsen uses this case to illustrate that we must call into question our deontological moral intuitions—namely, the intuition that we can't blow up the innocent fat man because it would constitute using him merely as a means. The gravity of the consequences if we don't blow him up, Nielsen argues, trumps this deontological concern.

Now consider Myrick's experiments and his justification:

> To do the work, we need human subjects, and most of them will die. These men, they're not victims. These men are heroes, Guy. Because of them, millions of people will walk again. We see them every night. They're lost, or cold, or stoned, or worse. And they have nothing, no future, no family, nothing. But here, with us, here they're performing miracles.

Guy responds that those men didn't choose to be heroes, "You chose for them." Tom Beauchamp and James Childress describe four fundamental principles of bioethics: beneficence, nonmaleficence, justice, and respect for autonomy (Beauchamp and Childress 2001). Although Myrick is beneficently attempting to develop a cure for cervical fractures and other neurological impairments, the manner in which he does so violates the other three principles. First, he violates the principle of nonmaleficence by "playing with healthy spines." It would be one thing if Myrick's experimental subjects already had suffered a debilitating spinal cord injury—for example, his assistants Ellen and Billy, or Jodie's brother. For such persons, there is at least a direct benefit to them if Myrick succeeds; although it would still be unjustified without previous animal trials. But the homeless subjects were healthy before Myrick severed their spinal cords.

Second, Myrick violates the principle of justice by targeting a particular socioeconomic group that does not stand out in a medically relevant way that would render them more appropriate subjects than others—this is known as "overrepresentation" (Childress, Meslin, and Shapiro 2005, pp. 151–54). As Guy points out, "You didn't choose your wife or your granddaughter. You didn't ask for volunteers."

In this, Myrick's research echoes nonfictional cases in which medical researchers have targeted racial minorities, prisoners, children, and developmentally disabled persons as research subjects because they were in controlled environments where they could be easily monitored, and consent was not considered a relevant issue. For example, in the infamous Tuskegee syphilis experiments (1932–1972), conducted by the national Public Health Service, researchers targeted poor, African-American men to enroll in a study aimed at understanding how the disease was spread and how it progressed. Four hundred mostly illiterate African-American men in the late stages of syphilis were never informed that they had the disease and were never given treatment for it, though reliable treatment became available in the 1940s.

Another historical example of this phenomenon was the Willowbrook experiments. Beginning in 1956, researchers purposefully infected mentally disabled children with hepatitis at the Willowbrook State School for the Retarded on Staten Island. Parents did give consent for the injections (after 1964 it was a condition for admission), but it's not clear whether they were advised of the hazards. Yet another case of targeting certain, vulnerable populations for research trials happened in 1963, when Cornell Medical School began cancer research on twenty-two patients with dementia at Brooklyn Jewish Chronic Disease Hospital. They were injected with live cancer cells to serve as a control to see if they lived longer than patients with cancer.

Finally, perhaps most importantly, Myrick violates the principle of respect for autonomy insofar as he didn't ask for volunteers or seek informed consent for the experimental treatment. Autonomy, in fact, is the key facet of human nature which, Kant argues, identifies human beings as persons with an inherent dignity that precludes their being used merely as a means. Myrick, in contrast, takes no account of his subjects' autonomy precisely because he doesn't see them as persons with inherent dignity. When two detectives visit a homeless shelter looking for Claude Minkins and Teddy Dolson, the manager reveals to them a virtually nameless, faceless multitude. Even among the homeless, some—the "worms, track rats, mole people"—are dehumanized to a greater degree in the eyes of the surface dwellers. When Guy realizes what's going on, that someone is looking for healthy research subjects, one of the "moles" asks, "Why us?" Guy responds, "Because they think you won't be missed." Myrick subscribes to a view of dignity in which it isn't inherent to a human person but rather is bestowed by others: "Dignity is a relational concept that begins first with the external conferral of dignity before it is claimed by a person as something intrinsic" (Peters 2001, p. 128). If others don't grant value to your existence, then it has none.

While it's clear that a deontologist, following Kant, would abhor Myrick's experiments, would a utilitarian necessarily justify what he does? Utilitarians are open to persons' being used as a means to obtain the greatest overall benefit, and Myrick makes a compelling case for his research on this basis. But Nielsen raises another example in which a magistrate, to quell a violent mob demanding justice for an unpunished crime, frames "a disreputable, thoroughly disliked, and useless man" (Nielsen 1972, p. 223; cf. McCloskey 1957) who is nonetheless innocent; after a brief mock trial, the man is found guilty and executed. While it seems, on first glance, that the magistrate acted in proper utilitarian fashion, Nielsen finds the magistrate's decision short-sighted insofar as worse consequences will result in the long run if word of what he did was leaked to the public: "This would encourage mob action in other circumstances, would lead to an increased skepticism about the incorruptibility or even the reliability of the judicial process, and would set a dangerous precedent for less clear-headed or less scrupulously humane magistrates" (Nielsen 1972, p. 224).

The same conclusion could be applied to Myrick's experiments. Surely, in this age of twenty-four-hour news cycles, an intrepid reporter (or *The Daily Show's* Jon Stewart) would blow the lid off Triphase. The resulting increased cynicism and lack of trust in the medical community would be disastrous for clinicians trying to give patients proper care or researchers attempting to enroll subjects in clinical trials. An increase in distrust of the medical community among African Americans followed the revelation of the unethical Tuskegee syphilis experiments (Gamble 1997). Myrick may have convinced himself that he's acting for the "greater good" and justified his actions by the utilitarian maxim, "The needs of the many outweigh the needs of the few."[2] A more nuanced analysis of the long-term consequences, however, shows his short-sightedness so that he's not justified on either deontological or utilitarian grounds.

Myrick's moral motivation exemplifies the selfless attitude a utilitarian ought to have: "for [the utilitarian] standard is not the agent's own greatest happiness, but the greatest amount of happiness altogether" (Mill 1861/2001, p. 11). After receiving the Wainwright Medal, Myrick receives a telegram from the White House that recognizes his tireless work with "so little regard for personal gain." It's worth noting that, at the celebration in Myrick's house, none of his friends or family shows evident neurological disability. Myrick's not working for his own benefit or that of his loved ones; in fact, the risk he's taking in the event his experiments are uncovered demonstrates his selfless courage, even if it's misplaced.

Other characters, though, appear to have less principled motivations. The two detectives who assist Myrick both have family members who are paralyzed and could be helped by Myrick's research.[3] Just before leaving to frame Guy by planting cocaine in his apartment, one of them turns down a picture of Jesus, evidencing his awareness that he's about to do something wrong; but then we see him kiss his quadriplegic wife—self-interest, extended to a loved one, overcomes moral awareness. We later discover that the reason Jodie is part of the Triphase research team is because she has a paralyzed brother. Guy confronts her asking, "How can you be a part of this?" She responds, "For my brother, because I was driving the car when he was hurt, because I was drunk." Guilt is Jodie's primary motive.

Guy, too, is at first motivated by self-interest when trying to discover the truth about Triphase. Having been framed for cocaine possession, which cost him his job, his fellowship, and his visa, Guy searches out the "mole people" with whom Claude Minkins lived before his death. Why? Because whoever killed Claude has ruined his life to cover it up. He even goes so far as to trade prescriptions for narcotics in exchange for information leading him to the underground dwellers. Although enabling a couple homeless men's drug habit may be a small price to pay to uncover the Triphase conspiracy, Guy's still operating on the motivation of self-interest at this point. This illustrates how easily one's ethical parameters—the lines that one isn't normally willing to cross—may shift if there are sufficiently powerful motivating factors.

We see Guy's ethical parameters shift again after he is deceived into believing that he has a "severe cervical fracture of the sixth vertebra" and is thereby "paralyzed from the neck down" (it's actually just an epidural drip simulating paralysis). When Myrick visits him, Guy immediately asks to be euthanized: "If you want to help me, let me die . . . Please, 400 of potassium chloride in my IV." This is a reversal of Guy's earlier attitude when discussing his father with Jodie. He's clearly disgraced that his father had his medical license revoked for assisting the suicide of a close friend who was dying of terminal cancer.

Some contend that one ought to pursue the maximization of one's own happiness, so long as a person is rationally cognizant of what is in her long-term, best self-interest (Rand 1961). Such people are known as *ethical egoists* and would not begrudge the motivations of Ellen and Billy, who are both paralyzed, of the two detectives whose happiness is obviously affected by that of their loved ones, of Jodie because she is trying to alleviate her guilt, or of Guy, who is initially just trying to clear his name. Kant, however, argues that the only proper moral motivation is to act in accordance with one's duty for the sake of the duty itself, and not for any other purpose, such as happiness or sympathy (Kant 1785/1997, pp. 10–13).

Myrick, although he misunderstands what his moral duty is in this situation, nonetheless appears to be motivated solely by his concept of what is his duty as a medical researcher and not for any profit, recognition, or other self-interest. Although Guy begins his investigation into Triphase for self-interested reasons, he appeals to deontological principles of respect for persons and their autonomy when offered a chance to work with Myrick to "change medicine forever":

> Maybe you're right. Those men upstairs, maybe there isn't much point to their lives. Maybe they are doing a great thing for the world. Maybe they are heroes. But they didn't choose to be . . . You chose for them, and you can't do that, because you're a doctor and you took an oath, and you're not God. So I don't care, I don't care if you can do what you say you can. I don't care if you can find a cure for every disease on this planet. You tortured and murdered those men upstairs, and that makes you a disgrace to your profession, and I hope you go to jail for the rest of your life.

While Myrick's experiments may violate the guiding principles of bioethics governing research with human subjects, it's undeniable that he made great strides in advancing neurological treatment. Myrick boasts of his results: "I can grow nerves. I can grow nerves, and I can control their patterns. Thirty hours before he came to you, Claude Minkins had his spine surgically severed at the fourth vertebra. Teddy Dolson lived for twelve days. I can show you their charts: complete neural regeneration."

After Myrick is accidentally killed in the film's climax, his wife offers Guy his research data. Handing Guy an unrealistically small package of data tapes and log books, she tells him, "I believe there's hope in this package . . . I believe my husband was trying to do a good thing, but in the wrong way. Perhaps you can do it the right way." The film ends with Guy running back into his New York University lab, data in hand, to fulfill Myrick's dream in an ethically appropriate manner. But is his project damned from the start? Is it wrong for Guy and other researchers to develop neurological treatments, and for patients to benefit from such treatments, given the data's ethically "tainted" source?

A deontologist, such as Kant, would be concerned that the use of such data involves continuing to merely use the victims from whom the data were derived without respecting them as persons. On the other hand, a deontologist might argue that we are in fact respecting the victims by making some good come out of their unwilling sacrifice. This argument is more in line with a utilitarian perspective, in which the use of the data is justified so long as a greater amount of net benefit is produced than if it weren't used. A relevant concern for a utilitarian, however, would be if using this data would encourage additional unethical experiments on unwilling subjects—assuming a utilitarian would negatively judge such experiments in the first place.

This last point raises the concern of whether any use of Myrick's data might scandalize future researchers by apparently legitimizing what he did. How should we understand the concept of scandal and apply it to this case? Thomas Aquinas (c. 1225–1274) defines "scandal" as "something said or done less rightly, causing another's [moral] ruin" and occurs when "someone by his admonition, inducement, or example leads another to sin" (Aquinas, *Summa Theologiae* [*ST*; Aquinas 1948] IIa–IIae.43.1).[4] He further specifies two types of scandal. *Active scandal* occurs "when someone by his evil word or deed intends to induce another to sin; or, if he does not so intend, when the deed is such that by its nature it is an inducement to sin; for example, someone publicly commits a sin or something that has a resemblance to sin" (Aquinas *ST*, IIa-IIae.43.1 *ad* 4).

Passive scandal occurs "when it is outside of the agent's intention, and outside the nature of the action, and yet someone who is disposed toward evil is induced to sin" (Aquinas *ST*, IIa-IIae.43.1 *ad* 4). Aquinas contends that active scandal is always an occasion of moral wrongdoing on the part of the agent who scandalizes another, while passive scandal may not entail moral wrongdoing on the agent's part so long as the word or action that led to the other's moral downfall was good in itself (Aquinas *ST*, IIa-IIae.43.2).

Does Guy's willingness to use Myrick's data lead in some fashion to the moral downfall of another researcher who may also use involuntary subjects to perform dangerous medical experiments? To count as a case of active scandal, Guy would have to either (1) perform an immoral action with the intention of leading the other researcher to engage in unethical experimentation or (2) perform an action that is of such a nature that it leads the researcher to perform such experiments—even if Guy didn't intend to induce the researcher to perform such an act—by (a) publicly performing an immoral action or (b) giving the appearance of performing an immoral action that leads the researcher to do wrongful experiments. If Guy supported or explicitly approved of Myrick's use of homeless men as involuntary subjects, then he'd be involved in active scandal under condition 1. Because, though, Guy hadn't supported or approved of what Myrick did, but only uses the resulting data, it's not apparent that he's guilty of active scandal. For condition 2—in the form of either a or b—requires one to commit an immoral action or give the appearance of doing so. Seeking to develop new effective treatments for neurological injury and illness isn't itself an immoral action.

If any scandal occurs merely because Guy uses Myrick's data, it can be at most passive scandal. It constitutes such scandal if a researcher who intends to engage in unethical experimentation is already disposed toward doing so whether or not there's another researcher, such as Guy, who would be willing to use the resulting data. Any moral downfall on the part of another researcher as a result of Guy's action (e.g., using Guy's willingness to use the resulting data as an excuse, a perceived moral "escape route," to conduct further unethical experiments) does not rest on Guy's shoulders. There are limits to the degree to which one can be held responsible for the actions of another moral agent.

Conclusion

Both Guy and Myrick have the same goal as physicians: to help patients to the best of their ability. The difference between them is that Myrick will use any means necessary to fulfill this duty of beneficence in the quickest way possible: "Three years with a rat to get to a dog, then after five years, if I'm lucky, maybe I can work on a chimp. We have to move faster than that." Guy, on the other hand, recognizes that there are certain moral limits, such as the deontological principle of respect for persons, which must not be crossed. The issue at hand is determining what those moral limits are and applying them to specific dilemmas.

For example, the disagreement between Myrick and Guy reflects that between those who support human embryonic stem cell research and those who oppose using human embryos in harmful or destructive research. For proponents, the potential benefits require pursuing this line of research instead of taking the arguably less efficient route of working solely with adult stem cells that are not as pluripotent. Opponents argue that human embryos, with the inherent potential to develop into self-conscious rational beings given the opportunity to develop, fall into the moral category of persons and thus merit respect according to the Kantian imperative. This and a host of other issues within bioethics will continue to highlight the significant difference in moral outlook between utilitarians, deontologists, and other moral theorists. Of course, it would be helpful if we could settle the question of which theory or set of ethical principles is preferable in adjudicating these dilemmas. One problem, however, is that many theories, taken to their logical extremes, lead to counterintuitive conclusions. In the case of utilitarianism, it doesn't match most people's moral intuitions, say, to enslave a minority population to benefit the majority. Deontology, conversely, implies a moral rigidity that intuitively fails in some cases. For example, in addition to not using persons as mere means to an end, deontologists hold other objective moral principles, such as telling the truth. Most people would agree, however, that there are certain situations in which it is appropriate or even morally required to tell a lie—say, to save someone's life or protect them from severe emotional hardship. For this reason, many people, in their everyday lives, combine two or more theories; so, for example, an individual might reason in a utilitarian fashion for the most part but not cross the Kantian line of using another person merely as a means to produce the greatest net benefit. This approach, however, runs the risk of ethical inconsistency or of collapsing into a subjective—"to each her own"—theory of morality. Perhaps the optimal position, which I advocate, is to define an ethical theory that includes a set of objective principles to be adhered to in most cases, but which is sufficiently flexible to allow a variety of circumstances to dictate precisely how these principles are to be applied and to adjudicate situations in which two or more of these principles come into conflict.[5]

QUESTIONS FOR CONSIDERATION

1. *Are there some situations in which "the end justifies the means"? Is it ever morally permissible to sacrifice one, or a few, lives so that a greater number may be benefited?*

2. *How difficult is it to hold onto one's moral ideals in the face of personal tragedy? Is self-interest the foundation on which certain acts, such as euthanasia or the treatment of research subjects, should be morally evaluated?*

3. *Is it permissible to use data that result from unethical medical research? How do we avoid the move from merely using such data to approving or engaging in further unethical research?*

NOTES

1. All quotations, unless otherwise noted, are from the film *Extreme Measures*.

2. This quotation is from a fictional utilitarian, *Star Trek*'s Mr. Spock, who appealed to this principle as his motivation for sacrificing himself to save his shipmates

in *Star Trek II: The Wrath of Khan* (Meyer 1982). Note, though, that Spock uses this principle to justify *self*-sacrifice as opposed to sacrificing the lives of others against their will.

3. From IMDb.com: "In the movie, security for the illegal medical experiments is provided by two supposed police officers named Hare and Burke. In reality, William Hare and William Burke were two men in the business of supplying human cadavers to medical schools in 1820s Edinburgh—until it was learned that the ones they hadn't stolen from graveyards, they had murdered themselves." www.imdb.com/title/tt0116259/trivia.

4. What follows is drawn from Eberl 2006, chapter 4. All translations are mine. For a published English translation of the cited text, see Aquinas 1948.

5. Examples of such theories include W. D. Ross's *prima facie* deontology (Ross 1930) and Thomas Aquinas's theory of "natural law" (Aquinas 1993).

REFERENCES

Apted, M. 1996. *Extreme Measures* [motion picture]. Beverly Hills, CA: Castle Rock Entertainment.

Aquinas, T. 1948. *Summa Theologiae*, trans. English Dominican Fathers. New York: Benziger Bros.

———. 1993. *The Treatise on Law*, ed. R. J. Henle. South Bend, IN: University of Notre Dame Press.

Beauchamp, T., and Childress, J. 2001. *Principles of Biomedical Ethics*, 5th ed. New York and Oxford: Oxford University Press.

Childress, J., Meslin, E., and Shapiro, H., eds. 2005. *Belmont Revisited: Ethical Principles for Research with Human Subjects*. Washington, DC: Georgetown University Press.

Eberl, J. T. 2006. *Thomistic Principles and Bioethics*. New York: Routledge.

Gamble, V. 1997. Under the Shadow of Tuskegee: African Americans and Health Care. *American Journal of Public Health* 87:1773–78.

Kant, I. 1997. *Groundwork of the Metaphysics of Morals,* trans. M. Gregor. New York and Cambridge: Cambridge University Press. (Originally published 1785)

McCloskey, H. J. 1957. An Examination of Restricted Utilitarianism. *Philosophical Review* 66:466–85.

Meyer, N. 1982. *Star Trek II: The Wrath of Khan* [motion picture]. Hollywood, CA: Paramount Pictures.

Mill, J. S. 2001. *Utilitarianism*, 2nd ed., ed. G. Sher. Indianapolis, IN: Hackett. (Originally published 1861)

Nielsen, K. 1972. Against Moral Conservatism. *Ethics* 82:113–24.

Peters, T. 2001. Embryonic Stem Cells and the Theology of Dignity. In *The Human Embryonic Stem Cell Debate: Science, Ethics, and Public Policy,* ed. S. Holland, K. Lebacqz, and L. Zoloth, 127–139. Cambridge: MIT Press.

Rand, A. 1961. *The Virtue of Selfishness.* New York: Penguin Books.

Ross, W. D. 1930. *The Right and the Good.* Oxford: Oxford University Press.

Rousseau, J-J. 1979. *Émile*, trans. A. Bloom. New York: Basic Books. (Originally published 1762)

NINETEEN

Talk to Whom?

Redefining Autonomy in *Talk to Her*

Daniel Sperling

Respect for the patient's autonomy is one of the major guiding principles in medical ethics. In the medical context, autonomy generally has been construed as the patient's ability to prescribe for herself the proper treatment and to make as free and authentic a decision as possible in relation to it (Sherwin 1998, p. 26). However, there are some situations in which the capacity for autonomy is lacking. One such situation is when the patient is in a coma and cannot express for herself the care she would have wanted. Under this situation, it is more helpful to conceptualize the principle of autonomy in a relational context focusing on the patient's complex interrelations and interdependencies with others. In this chapter, I illustrate and defend the relational view of autonomy through a discussion of one of the most fascinating films of the Spanish director Pedro Almodóvar, *Hable con Ella* (which went by the title *Talk to Her* in English-speaking countries; Almodóvar 2002).

The film tells the "love story" between a dancer, who falls into a deep coma following a car accident, and the male nurse who cares for her. The complex web of relations between these two individuals provides a fruitful way of rethinking our understanding of the autonomy of patients and of health care providers and of the proper contours of the therapeutic relationship.

The Value of Autonomy

Philosophers give two main justifications for respecting a person's autonomy. First, an evidentiary account holds that we should respect autonomy for utilitarian reasons even when we regard autonomous decisions as imprudent, because each person usually knows what is best for her better than anyone else does. Nevertheless, this first justification may be problematic, for, as Ronald Dworkin points out, by respecting a person's autonomy we may be required to accept people's choices even when they are manifestly irrational or against their own interests (Dworkin 1993, p. 223).

A more plausible account for why we should respect others' autonomy hinges on the intrinsic value of personal integrity and self-creation. On this account, the value of autonomy consists in the capacity to express one's own character and values. Autonomy allows us to "be responsible for shaping our lives according to our own coherent or incoherent—but, in any case, distinctive personality. It allows us to lead our own lives rather than be led along them, so that each of us can be, to the extent a scheme of rights can make this possible, what we have made of ourselves" (Dworkin 1993, p. 224).

The injunction to respect patient autonomy relies on an idealized image of the rational patient who calculates from a list of social goods and freely chooses among them (Donchin 2001, p. 368). The view of the self here is of an independent, rationally controlling, fixed person, isolated from and inattentive to emotions, communal life, familial and other intimate relationships, and making choices wholly for herself. As such, it ignores the social circumstances and power relations affecting choice making. Moreover, it assumes that all patients are alike and does not take into consideration the fact that some patients are not solely independent, nor do they strictly follow reason (Sherwin 1992, p. 137).[1]

Relational Accounts of Autonomy

In its most common version,[2] the relational feminist critique of the traditional autonomy model holds that human experience is better characterized as involving networks of relationships and interdependencies.[3] Rather than abandoning the traditional notion of autonomy, some feminists opt for redefining autonomy based on a more elaborate understanding of human nature as interconnected and interdependent.[4] Under this new meaning of autonomy, it does not replace the idea of only freedom from interference but also requires that one's relationships with individuals and institutions be constituted in such a way that one will have sincere opportunities to make choices. A relational approach thus attends the ways in which health care practices can contribute to the development and shaping of people's capacity for autonomy and to the role medicine plays in the development and continued exercise of autonomy.

The theory of relational feminism has contributed to the autonomy debate in medical ethics in two interrelated ways: it provides new ways to regard the patient as an autonomous agent and has enriched our perspectives on the medical profession and the physician-patient relationship.

The Patient as Autonomous

Relational feminism centers on the patient as embedded in social relations with others. It asks us to take into account the impact of social and political structures, especially sexism and other forms of oppression, on the lives and opportunities of others (McLeod and Sherwin 2000, p. 260). While in the traditional view, individuals are treated as interchangeable in that no attention is paid to the details of their personal experience, under the relational theory, selfhood is regarded as an ongoing process and relational selves are inherently social beings shaped and modified within a web of interconnected relationships (Sherwin 1998, p. 35).

Moreover, the relational autonomy viewpoint seeks to highlight the relational nature of the autonomy of the oppressed as part of a larger attempt to describe inequalities and exploitation of oppressed groups in the society.[5] As such, it emphasizes the political dimensions of the multiple relationships structuring an individual's self rather than seeking to protect a sphere of purely private relationships that may appear to be free from political influence (Sherwin 1998, pp. 19–20). A feminist approach holds that given the effects of patriarchy, the kinds of medical choices women are asked to make and the cultural association between "femininity" and "irrationality," women's options in health care are frequently construed in ways that limit their autonomy (Dodds 2000, p. 217). Feminists thus invite us to observe the varied circumstances under which health care decisions are made.

Applying the feminist critique of autonomy in the medical context is especially relevant, because by its very nature illness tends to make patients dependent on the care and good will of others, thereby reducing the power of the ill to make free choices. Incompetent patients are, obviously, in an even more dependent position and can be oppressed by their health care providers. Further exacerbating the threats to these patients' autonomy is the physician's tendency to privilege his or her own knowledge over that of the patients and to ignore patients' expressed or implicit values to attain the greater presumed benefit for patients when prescribing treatment. Often, the physician and patient will have different social, educational, and cultural backgrounds. This difference threatens patients' autonomy and free choices pertaining their own health and care.

Professional Autonomy

Although the main focus of relational feminism in health care has been on the autonomy of moral agents, recent suggestions in the literature have called to extend the analysis of relational feminism to apply to the autonomy of health care providers not only as moral agents but also in their capacities as professionals (MacDonald 2002a, 2002b). Chris MacDonald, for example, argues that professional autonomy is explicitly, concretely relational. By professional autonomy MacDonald means the responsibility of a member of a given profession to act according to the shared standards of that profession "in the face of countervailing pressures from institutional authorities, disagreement with members of other professions, or inappropriate demands on the part of patients or clients, or more generally, the public" (MacDonald 2002b, p. 284). Professional autonomy is thus rooted the socially legislated powers of professional societies and in the social status bestowed on professionals by cultural and social institutions. The degree of authority given to physicians over health care and their freedom to shape the health care system stem not just from their skill and knowledge but also from the privileges granted to them by the public. Because of this authority, professionals have substantial control over health care practice including the ability to exercise their judgment in situations in which decisions must be made (MacDonald 2002a, pp. 195–96).

MacDonald pays special attention to professional autonomy of nurses, which in that context means that nursing expertise is independent of, rather than subordinate to, medical expertise. On an individual level, the notion of professional autonomy implies the power of particular nurses to make some decisions that are not subject to authoritative review by those outside of their profession. It implies that nurses have the responsibility to act according to the shared standards of their profession and that, even when nurses carry out physicians' orders, they should retain a sphere of independent judgments concerning the way these orders should be fulfilled. On a more general level, a relational understanding of nursing autonomy helps us understand situations in which nurses themselves are seen as having inadequate autonomy, for example female or gay nurses who are also "oppressed" by physicians or other powerful groups within the medical profession (MacDonald 2002a, pp. 196–97, 201).

Overall, the advantage of regarding professional autonomy as relational is double. It both clarifies the nature of professional ethics and helps us understand how the various professions are at different levels in power hierarchies in health care settings and within society more generally.

Autonomy in the Physician-Patient Relationship

A relational feminist critique of the autonomy model has direct effects on the physician-patient relationship. Under the traditional autonomy model the therapeutic relationship is regarded as a contract between two separate persons, depriving both patients and physicians of virtually all particularity and any possible social interrelations. Feminists illuminate how under this traditional model, the therapeutic relationship is viewed merely as a service provided for the patient usually for the financial benefit of her treating doctor. If there are any social ties between the patient and her physician, they are viewed instrumentally and pursued for their utility and positive consequences. Hence, when dealing with patients with reduced levels of autonomy the typical response of health care team is to exercise paternalism, namely, to make decisions for their patients in the assumption that the health team knows best, definitely better than the patient, what is good for her.

In addition, a feminist perspective invites us to reconsider the physician-patient relationship so that providers can better organize their relational capacities to enhance, and not just protect, the autonomy interests of their patients. There are three models for the reconstruction of such a relationship: mothering, friendship, and sistering (Donchin 2001, pp. 378–82). The first model focuses on the mother-child relation as an idealized metaphor for human relations, arguing for the integration of relational skills such as listening and recognizing others' needs and vulnerability. This model seeks to extend to the whole of society the ethics of care, generalizing maternal relationships in the public sphere (Held 1990).

The second model emphasizes a conception of thoughtfulness and the importance of multiple friendships offering a wide array of perspectives through which one can assess another's choices, values, preferences, and so on. According to this view, our familiarity with others helps us understand the particular needs and capabilities of those around us, thereby enabling us to better care for them (Friedman 1993, pp. 57–58).

Finally, the third model regards relations among actual sisters as structured by a common family history and shared expectations that generate future obligations and suggests applying them to the therapeutic context (Donchin 2001, p. 380). Common to all three models is the view that the physician-patient relationship aims to foster the patient's well-being (beneficence) through shared activity as an expression of a particular relationship. The physician and patient share a common goal particularized to the circumstances and choices of each individual patient. In contrast to a paternalistic approach perpetuating patient dependency on the power and authority of physicians, these models foster development of capacities for self-care advancing one's capabilities to sustain relationships among equal parties.

Hable con Ella

The many issues highlighted by the relational feminist approach to bioethics are nicely explored in the film *Hable con Ella* (*Talk to Her*). The film revolves around two love stories, between the comatose Alicia (played by Leonor Watling) and her nurse, Benigno (played by Javier Cámara), and between Marco (played by Darío Grandinetti), a travel writer in his forties, and Lydia (played by Rosario Flores), a bullfighter who also falls into a coma after she is severely gored by a bull. Throughout the film we also witness an erotic tension between Benigno and Marco, which is mediated by Alicia's body, and toward the end of the film after Alicia awakens and Benigno takes his life, we are aware of a new loving relationship that is being woven between Marco and Alicia.[6]

Although some regard *Talk to Her* as part of a brain-death trilogy,[7] this is a film about love and interconnections between people. As put by Kyndrup, "On the one hand, this film uncompromisingly insists on the presented space's authentic references: to loneliness, to disability, to melancholy, to lack of love—and to beauty, to music, to the good, to the passion. And on the other hand, it constantly makes explicit its own constructional set-up to such an extent that throughout the film, at no single point do you lose the feeling of being led through something and on to something which you cannot (yet) identify" (Kyndrup 2004, p. 24).

Like many of Almodóvar's films, *Talk to Her* is interesting for its dealing with gender roles. As illuminated by Andrew Holleran, "The matador is a woman who's terrified of snakes. The man who rescues her is a macho Argentinean who weeps at concerts. His new friend is a spaced-out Momma's boy we'd say is gay except he is obsessed with a beautiful woman who's comatose" (Holleran 2003, p. 49). In the film, women are represented as immensely powerful and mysterious bodies that intimidate men.[8] While Lydia's physical strength is expressly demonstrated in her battles, Alicia's powerfulness is implicitly present in her ability to stay connected to the outside world, to be an object of love and esteem, and eventually to overcome her tragic situation and return to full competence. The camera focuses on Alicia's white and smooth skin, emphasizing not only its beauty and purity but also the means through which her connections to and from the world are made possible.[9]

But *Talk to Her* can also be viewed as the parallel story of two sets of therapeutic relationships that are each represented by a different love story. The traditional physician-patient bond corresponds to Marco's relationship with Lydia. This relationship is initiated by a contract (to interview Lydia) between a masculine bourgeois man who is always on the run with no home of his own and a depressed woman who has just ended an intimate relationship with a man, admitting in a television interview that it is generally good to talk but who cannot actually do the talking. Their relationship is characterized by rationality, egotism, and permanent movement from one place to another with no real attachment and sense of belonging. It is a relationship in which no talk or communication is genuinely possible and desired, a relationship of solitude and alienation in which emotions are missing or, if they exist, are regarded with shame.

In such a relationship, the patient's body is rarely shown to the viewer, Marco, and others. This body expresses no desires, provokes no reactions, and refuses to return to life (unlike Alicia, Lydia no longer has her period), deteriorating alone until its final decay and ultimate death.

In contrast, the relationship between Benigno and Alicia presents an alternative understanding of the therapeutic model. Such relationship takes place also *outside* the clinic (Benigno holds Alicia's hair clip and a picture of her in his home; he also goes to watch silent movies through which he communicates with Alicia). Prior to her hospitalization Benigno, looking from his window, falls in love with Alicia, having seen her dancing in the studio. Even when he is in jail, Benigno tells Marco he needs information about Alicia. In this relationship, the manifestation of the health providers' talents and skills is not restricted to their working place (Benigno spends most of his life taking care of his mother); their being compassionate and loving is a general attribute exercised not only in relation to their patients but also with regard to peers and close relatives of patients. In such a scenario, the health provider is part of a web of interactions between people and institutions that are both complex and unique. Consequently, reciprocity and mutual reliance exist between parties communicating within this relationship. Benigno talks to Alicia, and the viewer knows she is listening and responding back in her own special ways.[10] This is a relationship of warmth, intimacy, and solidarity in which the body of the patient not only is exceptionally beautiful but also is preserved in the same condition as it was before.

The two different therapeutic models reflect the traditional and relational approaches to autonomy discussed above. The standard autonomy model represents a contractual meeting of two independent agents whose common purpose is to "beat" the disease. Under such model, the physician's role is to supply her patient with the necessary information needed to make a health-related decision, and in return the patient's obligation is to provide some fee for this service. Like Marco and Lydia who meet for an interview, the parties involved in the traditional therapeutic model have a common purpose, a plan. Once the plan is realized each party must go his or her own way. The patient's personal background, her history, and future plans as well as the special role of her close friends and family are irrelevant for ensuring her autonomy in its traditional sense. Thus, when Lydia tells Marco that they will have to talk after the bullfight, Marco replies that they have already been talking for almost an hour. Lydia, who wants to tell Marco she started seeing her ex-partner, Niño, disappointedly replies, "*You* talked for an hour. *I* did not talk at all." In the traditional autonomy model it is indeed the physician who does the talking, and the patient is required to approve (give her consent) or refuse. It is clear from this dialogue that Marco and Lydia do not refer to the same "talk" although they use the same language to express it.

The idea that medicine and cure cannot be effective without a broader understanding and knowledge of particular selves, argued for under the relational feminist view, is successfully represented as successful in the story of Benigno and Alicia, though Benigno's acts may represent an extreme case of it. Unlike most films in the medical-movie genre, the story valorizes the contributions of those for whom care is a central concern, long-term care nurses, rather than, say, emergency medicine physicians or high-powered surgeons.

To use Virginia Warren's distinction, Almodóvar presents two different sets of medical conduct: that involving ongoing relationships, which fades into invisible "housekeeping issues" and that involving crisis issues, which focuses on the decision of whether to continue or discontinue treatment of the patient (Warren 1992). Only in the sphere of the mere "housekeeping issues," however, in the clinic where the women are being cared for—called El Bosque, "the forest"—can miracles come true, and can—as Katerina, Alicia's dance mentor holds—life evolve out of death and enhancement and healing take place. This may also be the reason why Almodóvar bathes the clinic in tones of warm mustard and ochre, eschewing the cold blues and grays stereotypically associated with such a setting (Smith 2002, p. 26).

As a nurse, Benigno is part of a profession that not only is stereotypically "female" but also has an essential component of caring and helping, both of which are associated with the feminine gender role. Through his love for Alicia, Benigno exercises his professional autonomy. His autonomy comes to an end as soon as it reaches its climax, that is when Benigno violates the ethical and legal rules governing his profession and those controlling and shaping his biological nature as a gay person, by impregnating Alicia. In a remarkable way this disgusting act does not result in the viewer's repulsion. As argued by Novoa, "He [Benigno] is part of a reality that is plural and complex, that is difficult to grasp by the standards of law and contemporary reality" (Novoa 2005, p. 236). Moreover, when Benigno's act is regarded as inspired by the *Shrinking Lover*—a silent movie that the director intersperses with the action during Benigno's rape of Alicia—Almodóvar wants us to believe that the rape violates a fictitious body, the body of Aurora and not that of real Alicia. This message is intensified as we watch Aurora experience orgasm when Alfredo crawls inside her.

Indeed, in the film the violation of Alicia's body creates a miracle, namely, saving her and curing her of her previous condition, and eventually brings her life and real love (Marco). From a psychological perspective, Benigno's desire becomes progressively removed from symbolic love as his fantasy is realized in Alicia, namely through merger with her body, a return-to-the-womb fantasy in which he is a "presubject." At this point, according to Kirshner, Benigno sacrifices his life to realize his desire to go "beyond the pleasure principle" of ordinary sexuality (Kirshner 2005, p. 91). Adriana Novoa puts it nicely when she writes, "the emphasis has been placed not on the violation of the autonomy of a person incapable of exercising her will but rather on men's need for female bodies, which both save them and damn them at the same time. By his action, Benigno resolves his persistent conflicts with both masculinity and femininity. On the one hand, the contact with Alicia brings him into the world of men; on the other hand, it is also the first of the labor pains that eventually lead to Alicia's salvation, as his pregnancy finally concludes with her triumphant birth" (Novoa 2005, p. 238).

Benigno's actions highlight the importance of care in the medical context as emphasized by feminists. The act of caring involves a person's responding to another's needs and desires. As put by Daniel Engster, "caring makes the development and basic well being of another its direct end" (Engster 2005, p. 51). After Alicia awakens, Benigno realizes he cannot care for her anymore. Thus, he sees no reason to live in a world where care is absent, and so he takes his own life.

Benigno's relationship with Alicia nicely exemplifies all three care models discussed above. Benigno treats Alicia as if he were her mother.[11] Benigno gets an autograph from a diva inscribed for Alicia, he relates to her detailed descriptions of performances he sees in the theater and silent movies, he grooms and massages her, bathes her, dresses her, makes her up to look pretty, plays music for her, and above all talks to her about daily events.[12] Not only does he treat Alicia as would a mother, but eventually, when Benigno impregnates her, he in a way gives her new life, thereby fulfilling a quasi-maternal function. Benigno acts not only as Alicia's mother but also as her thoughtful friend, perhaps her best friend. He takes care of her and promotes her fundamental interests. A relationship of mutual reliance exists between the two. As much as Benigno gives life to Alicia, she offers him a resolution of his sexual anxieties resulting from his being a confused gay man who is in trauma of the loss of the female body, his mother's body that he knew so well (Novoa 2005, p. 234).[13] Finally and at least symbolically, the sistering model also applies to Benigno's care for Alicia as he belongs to a profession that historically included many women in religious orders, referred to as sisters.

Conclusion

This chapter confronted the traditional understanding of autonomy with the more appealing idea of relational autonomy as it is manifested in the medical context. While according to the first view autonomy is perceived as the ability to deliberate and act on one's own choices and preferences, the latter approach emphasizes the social circumstances and relational powers affecting one's actual but also potential choices, thereby better introducing the ways in which health care practices shape and contribute to one's exercise of autonomy. The article invited the reader to take a feminist perspective to autonomy, highlighting a person's complex and constituting interrelations and interdependencies with others, and to rethink altogether the therapeutic relationship, the medical profession, and the special place of the patient within the physician-patient relationship.

In this chapter the idea of relational autonomy and the feminist critique of traditional autonomy were explored through the discussion of the film *Hable con Ella*. The film enables its viewers to take the perspective of and identify with an individual patient who is incapable of deliberating health-related choices due to her medical condition. Yet this patient is surrounded by a complex net of interconnections with others, which in turn shape her medical condition, the health-related decisions relevant to her, and our understanding of the care she receives under such conditions. The social framework in which care is administered to the patient and the exceptional treatment she receives in that movie cannot leave us unmoved by her capacity for autonomy. The film successfully challenges the medicalization of the therapeutic relationship in general, and the traditional autonomy model specifically.

Reflecting on films that discuss the right to die, James Gordon admits, "to make clinical decisions easier, we sometimes reduce ethics to a utilitarian exercise or an application of laws or principles, when what's needed most is to appreciate the experiences that create ethical conflict." The significance of films such as *Talk to Her* is that they make us listen for the sake of understanding not action. "We get to witness the lives of their characters in all their chaotic complexity—their selfishness, their generosity, their confusion, even their mistaken understanding of the options available to them—without any attendant obligation to correct what's wrong . . . they are didactic in that they teach us that things are more complicated than we might otherwise have thought" (Gordon 2005, p. 8). By highlighting a new perspective of autonomy, both the individual autonomy of a nonsentient patient and the professional autonomy of a gay nurse caring for and communicating to that patient, *Talk to Her* not only makes us rethink our major theories of medical ethics and the most fundamental questions we raise in our daily life but also is a ravishing piece of art that touches us in such a powerful way from which we cannot keep aloof.

QUESTIONS FOR CONSIDERATION

1. *What are the main differences between the traditional view of patient autonomy and the relational feminist view of patient autonomy? Does it seem that the relational feminist view provides a supplement to the traditional view or does it call for a radical rethinking of it?*

2. *Before Alicia's accident, Benigno's obsession with her leads him to violate her privacy and to act in what might be called an oppressive manner toward her. Is Benigno's style of care for Alicia continuous or discontinuous, in your view, with respect to violating her basic rights?*

3. *The type of care Benigno shows Alicia could be said to be both*

more therapeutic and more respectful of the real autonomy of the patient than is the traditional medicalized version of care. Imagine (Heaven forbid!) you were to fall into Alicia's situation, would you want to be cared for by a nurse like Benigno? Why or why not?

NOTES

1. The most famous expression of the traditional autonomy model in the medical context is seen in Beauchamp and Childress's *Principles of Biomedical Ethics,* where the authors contend that "personal autonomy is, at minimum, self-rule that is free from both controlling interference by others and from limitations, such as inadequate understanding, that prevent meaningful choice." According to this view, the autonomous individual "acts freely in accordance with a self-chosen plan, analogous to the way an independent government manages its territories and sets its policies." Therefore, Beauchamp and Childress hold that "to respect an autonomous agent is, at a minimum, to acknowledge that person's right to hold views, to make choices, and to take actions based on personal values and beliefs" (Beauchamp and Childress 2001, pp. 58– 63). However, in their recent edition the authors do not deny that communal life and human relationships help develop one's self and contribute to one's choices, but their acknowledgment of the relation between social connections and one's self is only partial. This is why Anne Donchin regards their revised theory as weak as opposed to strong relational autonomy, which holds that a subject's activities of reflecting, planning, choosing, and deciding are ineluctably social activities (Donchin 2000, pp. 238–39; see also Ellis 2001).

2. Within the feminist critique there exist three major approaches: liberal feminism, focusing on autonomous choices; radical feminism, illuminating women's limited control over the institutions of health care, reproduction, and sexuality; and cultural feminism, identified with a feminine ethic of care (Tong 1996).

3. This argument can be understood either as making a metaphysical claim so that relations with other persons, institutions, and so on, are seen as essentially part of the person, or as making a contingent psychological claim about a person's self-concept, value structure, emotional states, and the like, holding that while personal interactions are dynamic and shifting, they are constitutive elements of a person's psychological states (Christman 2004).

4. Relational feminists articulate such an idea through the discussion of other concepts than autonomy (e.g., field, boundary, the human body, privacy, and property). I explored these concepts in chapter 6 of my *Management of Post-Mortem Pregnancy: Legal and Philosophical Aspects* (2006).

5. But compare Dodds, who argues that the factors identified by relational feminists as limiting health care decision-making affect most patients, not just those who are members of oppressed groups (Dodds 2000, pp. 224–25).

6. The names of all main characters appear to testify for their major traits. "Marco" may be a reference to Marco Polo, the traveler; "Lydia" plays off of "lidiar" or "to fight"; "Alicia" or "Alice" may stand for a storybook standard (Alice in Wonderland), and Benigno may imply his being benign, harmless (Novoa 2005, p. 231).

7. Marsha Kinder, for example, argues that Almodóvar unintentionally created this trilogy in *La Flor de mi Secreto*, *Todo Sobre Mi Madre*, and *Hable con Ella*. In the first film, behind the opening titles a training video shows two young doctors informing a grieving mother that her sixteen-year-old son is brain-dead, a concept she is unable to grasp and refuses to accept. The young doctors aim not to comfort the woman for her loss but to convince her to donate the organs of her loved one. In *Todo Sobre Mi Madre* a fictional training video shows Manuela playing a grieving woman who is told by two doctors that her husband is brain-dead. In this film, Esteban is run down by a car and rendered brain-dead when running to get Huma Rojo's autograph in the rain. Manuela signs away Esteban's heart. Finally in *Hable con Ella*, brain-death takes over the entire film in which the emphasis is put on resuscitation, requiring an interplay between the expressive powers of words and of body language. In Kinder's view, "the image of the comatose youth becomes a new way of refiguring the crucial link between intertexuality and changing subjectivity particularly when these processes are linked to loss, growth and recovery." Although Kinder confuses brain-death with coma, she highlights an interesting motive in Almodóvar's recent films (Kinder 2005, p. 18).

8. Adriana Novoa articulates this view when she writes, "This movie is a set in that mysterious universe to which women may go (the place of lacking) but to which men have no access (the place of prohibition)" (Novoa 2005, p. 227).

9. Compare Catherine Keller's idea of the skin as explored by Jennifer Nedelsky (1990). Along with this line, when Benigno sees Lydia for the first time he remarks to Marco: "This woman is not healthy. Her skin is very dry. Did you talk to her?"

10. In a dialogue with Marco, Benigno urges Marco to talk to Lydia. Marco replies that Lydia's brain is dead and Benigno introduces his philosophy: "One should pay them attention, caress them; they exist; they live; and they are important to us."

11. Indeed, Almodóvar admits, "The idea of motherhood is very important in Spain. It's as if the mother represents the law, the police . . . when you kill the mother, you kill precisely everything you hate. It's like killing the power" (interview with Pedro Almodóvar, mentioned in Kinder 2005, p. 17).

12. The importance of language and communication and their immense contribution to healing is greatly emphasized in the film as is most evidenced from its title. Kinder admits, "In *Hable con Ella*, the nurturing interplay between physical gestures and words proves to have a transformative effect not only on the body of the dancer

who is impregnated and revived, and on the writer who becomes bonded to the male nurse through identification and desire, but also on those of us in the audience whom this film manages to convince that every physical act (no matter how transgressive) can potentially be re-narrativized as an act of love" (Kinder 2005, p. 22).

13. Benigno's most manifested sexual anxiety is conveyed through the *Shrinking Lover*, a silent movie he watches before impregnating Alicia. In that movie, Alfredo, Benigno's alter ego, is rescued by his lover, Aurora, who due to scientific mistake made him shrink almost to the point of vanishing. When the two rest in a hotel, Alfredo elects to disappear into his lover's vagina (Backstein 2003, p. 42).

REFERENCES

Almodóvar, P. 2002. *Hable con ella* [English title, *Talk to Her*; motion picture]. Madrid: El Deseo, S.A.

Backstein, K. 2003. *Talk to Her. Cineaste* Spring: 41–42.

Beauchamp, T. L., and Childress, J. F. 2001. *Principles of Biomedical Ethics*, 5th ed. Oxford and New York: Oxford University Press.

Christman, J. 2004. Relational Autonomy, Liberal Individualism, and the Social Constitution of Selves. *Philosophical Studies* 117:143–64.

Clouser, K. D., and Gert, B. 1990. A Critique of Principlism. *Journal of Medicine and Philosophy* 15 (2): 219–37.

Dodds, S. 2000. Choice and Control in Feminist Bioethics. In *Relational Autonomy: Feminist Perspectives on Autonomy, Agency, and the Social Self*, ed. C. Mackenzie and N. Stoljar, 213–35. Oxford and New York: Oxford University Press.

Donchin, A. 2000. Autonomy and Interdependence: Quandaries in Genetic Decision Making. In *Relational Autonomy: Feminist Perspectives on Autonomy, Agency, and the Social Self*, ed. C. Mackenzie and N. Stoljar, 236–58. Oxford and New York: Oxford University Press.

———. 2001. Understanding Autonomy Relationally: Toward a Reconfiguration of Bioethical Principles. *Journal of Medicine and Philosophy* 26(4): 365–86.

Dworkin, R. 1993. *Life's Dominion*. New York: Alfred Knopf.

Ells, C. 2001. Shifting the Autonomy Debate to Theory as Ideology. *Journal of Medicine and Philosophy* 26(4): 417–30.

Engster, D. 2005. Rethinking Care Theory: The Practice of Caring and the Obligation to Care. *Hypatia* 20(3): 50–74.

Friedman, M. 1993. *What Are Friends For? Feminist Perspectives on Personal Relationships and Moral Theory*. Ithaca, NY: Cornell University Press.

Gordon, J. M. 2005. On Physician-Assisted Suicide: What We Learn from the Movies. *Neurology Today* 5 (4): 8.

Held, V. 1990. Mothering versus Contract. In *Beyond Self-Interest,* ed. J. Masbridge, 287–304. Chicago: University of Chicago Press.

Holleran, A. 2003. Weepers. *Gay and Lesbian Review* May–June: 48–49.

Kinder, M. 2005. Reinventing the Motherland: Almodóvar's Brain-Dead Trilogy. *Film Quarterly* 58 (2): 9–25.

Kirshner, L. A. 2005. Rethinking Desire: The *Object Petit A* in Lacanian Theory. *Journal of the American Psychoanalytic Association* 53 (1): 83–102.

Kyndrup, M. 2004. To Be Shown How to Be Talked To: Narration and Parabasis in Contemporary Film and Almodóvar's *Hable con Ella. P.O.V.: A Danish Journal of Film Studies* 18: 18–27.

MacDonald, C. 2002a. Nurse Autonomy as Relational. *Nursing Ethics* 9 (2): 194–201.

———. 2002b. Relational Professional Autonomy. *Cambridge Quarterly of Healthcare Ethics* 11: 282–89.

McLeod, C., and Sherwin, S. 2000. Relational Autonomy, Self-Trust, and Health Care for Patients Who Are Oppressed. In *Relational Autonomy: Feminist Perspectives on Autonomy, Agency, and the Social Self,* ed. C. Mackenzie and N. Stoljar, 259–79. Oxford and New York: Oxford University Press.

Nedelsky, J. 1990. Law, Boundaries and the Bounded Self. *Representations* 30: 162–89.

Novoa, A. 2005. Whose Talk Is It? Almodóvar and the Fairy Tale in *Talk to Her. Marvels and Tales: Journal of Fairy-Tale Studies* 19 (2): 224–48.

Sherwin, S. 1992. *No Longer Patient: Feminist Ethics and Health Care.* Philadelphia: Temple University Press.

———. 1998. A Relational Approach to Autonomy in Health Care. In *The Politics of Women's Health: Exploring Agency and Autonomy,* ed. S. Sherwin, 19–47. Philadelphia: Temple University Press.

Smith, P. J. 2002. Only Connect. *Sight and Sound* 7: 24–27.

Sperling, D. 2006. *Management of Post-Mortem Pregnancy: Legal and Philosophical Aspects.* Aldershot and Burlington, VT: Ashgate.

Tong, R. 1996. Feminine and Feminist Approaches to Bioethics. In *Feminism and Bioethics: Beyond Reproduction,* ed. S. M. Wolf, 67–94. New York and Oxford: Oxford University Press.

Warren, V. L. 1992. Feminist Directions in Medical Ethics. In *Feminist Perspectives in Medical Ethics,* ed. H. B. Holmes and L. M. Purdy, 32–45. Bloomington and Indianapolis: Indiana University Press.

TWENTY

Stars and Triangles

Controversial Bioethics in Contemporary Spanish Film

Antonio Casado da Rocha

The stars are the apexes of what wonderful triangles!

HENRY DAVID THOREAU

Spain has changed enormously in the last thirty years and at a greater speed than other countries have. The Spanish health care ethos is also changing, even if at a slower pace, from the older paternalist model to one based more on patient autonomy. These changes have been reflected in the way medicine is dramatized by the film industry, providing the viewing public with a new arena in which difficult issues about the end of life can be discussed without the pressures of a real-life scenario.

This trend has been especially visible in recent times. In May 30, 2005, two critics chose the nine best films in the history of *Time* magazine (Corliss and Schickel 2005). Their choice for the first decade of the twenty-first century was a film made in Spain, Pedro Almodóvar's *Hable con ella* (distributed in English as *Talk to Her;* Almodóvar 2002), a disturbing story about patients and their caregivers that won the Academy Award for best screenplay in 2002. On February 27, 2005, the big winner of the Oscar ceremony was *Million Dollar Baby* (Eastwood 2005), and the Spanish *Mar adentro* (distributed in English as *The Sea Inside;* Amenábar 2004) won the Academy Award for best foreign film; both are relevant to bioethics, specifically to issues dealing with euthanasia. Directed and cowritten by Alejandro Amenábar, *The Sea Inside* is based on a real-life case that engrossed Catholic Spain in the 1990s, that of Ramón Sampedro, a fifty-five-year-old former sailor who broke his neck and spent more than twenty-five years as a quadriplegic. On several occasions the Spanish courts denied his petitions for the legalization of assisted suicide, and he died on January 12, 1998, by sipping a solution of cyanide through a straw.

In 2003 the Vancouver Critics gave their Best Canadian Film Award to another film dealing with euthanasia, *Les Invasions Barbares* (*The Barbarian Invasions;* Arcand 2003), and Sarah Polley won the Best Actress Award for her role in Isabel Coixet's *Mi vida sin mí* (*My Life without Me;* Coixet 2003). Polley's character is a young mother whose modest life takes a dramatic turn when her doctor tells her that she has only two months left to live.

Talk to Her, *The Sea Inside*, and *My Life without Me* have much in common. They explore dependence, disability, and vulnerability in subtle ways. They portray emotive end-of-life scenarios in a postmodern context of technological medicine and moral complexity. They are highly original works of art, directed and written by creative filmmakers who manage to transcend the disease-of-the-week genre. Most important, these three films are focused on the patient-professional relationship, raising issues of truth-telling, privacy, confidentiality, and fidelity that are central to bioethics (Beauchamp and Childress 2001, pp. 283–319). The main conflict in *Talk to Her* has to do with the responsibility of a health professional, while *My Life without Me* explores truth-telling from the perspective of the patient, and *The Sea Inside* has more to do with the private and public options regarding assisted suicide. Thus, each of the films is focused on one of the apexes of the health care relationship: the professional, the patient, and "the others," as shown in Figure 20.1, which I will often use in this chapter.

The Four Principles in the Spanish Context

According to Diego Gracia, who has been described by *El País,* the most widely read Spanish newspaper, as the foremost representative of bioethics in Spain (Pérez Oliva 2006), our present situation is a changing one. We are in the midst of a process in which the old paternalistic relationship between health care professional and patient is being challenged by a new one based on the conflicting demands of patient autonomy and professional beneficence (Gracia 1999, p. 25).

The first edition of *The Principles of Biomedical Ethics* (Beauchamp

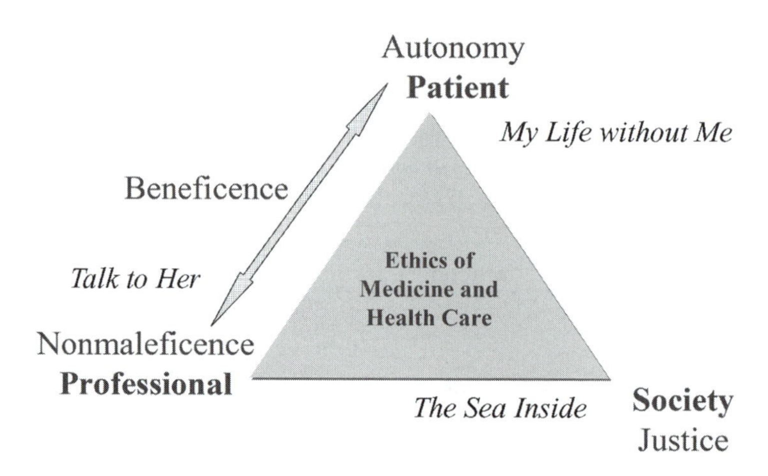

FIGURE 20.1 Proposed correlation of studied films, main principles, and agents in the ethics of medicine and health care. *Source:* Antonio Casado de Rocha.

and Childress 1979) unleashed the four principles of respect for autonomy, nonmaleficence, beneficence, and justice on the newly emerging field of bioethics. These principles were characterized as "midlevel norms" mediating between high-level moral theory and low-level common sense morality, and they immediately became very popular. Now the book is in its sixth edition, and it remains a standard text in the field.

Ten years after Beauchamp and Childress published their book, Gracia published his own *Fundamentals of Bioethics* (*Fundamentos de bioética;* 1989), a book that brought the four-principle approach to Spanish bioethics. Gracia read *The Principles of Biomedical Ethics* in the light of Aristotle, Kant, and Spanish philosophers such as Xavier Zubiri, and he agreed with Beauchamp and Childress that the content of traditional ethical theories is too abstract to explore practical ethical problems within medicine and the life sciences. To establish an agent's actual duty in the face of conflicting obligations, a process of moral deliberation is required. With a theory recalling John Rawls's concept of "reflective equilibrium," Gracia proposed that moral deliberation is a tool by which we examine our considered judgments in the light of principles that are central to bioethics across cultures, as well as with the anticipated outcomes that they might bring about. Of course, there are many amoral persons who do not care about moral obligations, but Beauchamp and Childress believe that all persons in all cultures who are serious about moral conduct do at least accept the norms of commonsense morality (2001, pp. 4–5, 404); Gracia, who in the *El País* interview described himself as a moderate optimist, would surely agree.

The bioethical doctrine proposed by Gracia, which has become very influential in the majority of Spanish and Latin American public health institutions (Guerra 2005), includes a principle of *autonomy* that requires respectful treatment of patients in disclosing information and fostering decision-making free from constraints imposed by others. It also includes a principle of *nonmaleficence*, which asserts an obligation not to inflict harm on others. In addition, the principle of *beneficence* requires that agents take positive steps to help others, balancing an action's possible goods against its costs and possible harms. As for the principle of *justice*, it requires equality of access to medical treatment, research, and the distribution of resources in healthcare services. There is considerable debate about these requirements of justice, but it is clear at least that Spain has been evolving towards a welfare system, one in which universal access to health care is considered by the population to be one of its most cherished rights.

In this sense, Spanish bioethics works in an egalitarian vein, one in which justice is increasingly considered to be of paramount importance (especially by authors such as M. J. Guerra). It is illustrative that Beauchamp and Childress originally presented their principles as "prima facie duties," without prioritization or hierarchical ranking, but Gracia separated the four into two levels: the *private morality* level of autonomy and beneficence, and the hierarchically higher *public morality* level of nonmaleficence and justice. In cases of conflict between a principle on the private level and one of the public, the public one will usually have priority in Spanish bioethics.

Talk to Her, or Silent Movie Paternalism

Almodóvar's previous film, *All about My Mother*, ended with a theater curtain opening to reveal a darkened stage. *Talk to Her* begins with the same opening curtain, but now we see two men who are watching three people: two suffering, sleepwalking women and one man rather frantically attempting to protect them from falling over dangerous wooden chairs.

Those two spectators are, at the same time, narrators. According to Alasdair MacIntyre, human beings are "storytelling animal[s]" (MacIntyre 1981, p. 216), as we need narratives to make sense of our own lives. This point has been applied to bioethics by those who think that the principles of biomedical ethics must be supplemented by an understanding of the narrative structure of human action. These thinkers highlight that narrative elements are pervasive in all forms of ethical reasoning and that our responses to stories are the ground out of which moral theories and principles grow (Nelson 1997). The processes of getting ill, being ill, getting better (or not), and coping with illness (or not), can all be thought of as enacted narratives within the wider stories of people's lives (Greenhalgh and Hurwitz 1999). Notwithstanding growing interest in bioethics in narrative, film as a storytelling medium has received comparatively little attention from bioethicists, and only recently this subject has begun to be discussed in the Spanish context (Marzabal 2004; Muñoz and Gracia 2006).

One of the dance spectators is Benigno (played by Javier Cámara), a nurse who sits patiently at the side of Alicia (played by Leonor Watling), who is in a coma. Benigno teaches the other spectator Marco (played by Darío Grandinetti) to take care of Lydia (played by Rosario Flores), his girlfriend, who is also unconscious. In Almodóvar's films no name is neutral; Benigno is indeed a benign, soft talking, "strangely assured stuffed animal of a man" (Mitchell 2002); Alicia is beautiful and fast asleep, a new "Alice in Wonderland." Eventually, Benigno manages to wake her up, but to do so he transgresses the most basic norms of his profession. In the meantime, Marco learns how to say good-bye both to Lydia and to Benigno, and, as the film ends, he is able to take care of both himself and someone else—Alicia.

What model of interaction between patients and health care professionals can we find here? Partially because Alicia and Lydia are both in a persistent vegetative state, the patient-professional relationship portrayed in this film is a paternalistic one, in which decision-making lies solely within the province of the professional. The patient's needs are cared for, but patient-professional communication becomes a sort of monologue, bringing about dangers of distrust and abandonment.

Beneficence: Why Caring Is an Art

Giving particular attention and personalized care is a difficult and even consuming activity. This is very well illustrated in *Talk to Her*, in which the main characters are not the ill women but rather their caregivers. These two men, according to the script, are "unable to do any harm," but live fundamentally isolated lives and have problems communicating; they both talk too much, or too little, or to the wrong person. When Marco tells Benigno that he cannot take care of Lydia, the latter answers: "Talk to her. Tell her about it." "I wish I could," Marco says, "but she can't hear me." "You never know," replies Benigno. "To caress them, to remember that they exist and that we care for them. That's the only therapy." Initially, Marco lacks this ability to engage in authentic conversations, both to express himself and to listen to others compassionately.

Benigno does know how to "talk to her," but eventually fails to do so in an appropriately professional, detached way. From his perspective, he makes love to her; from ours, he takes advantage of her vulnerability in order to possess her. It is highly ironic that only after Benigno rapes and impregnates Alicia does she actually recover. In a way, the film suggests that the best therapy is to become the ultimate object of an obsessive caretaker's attention, a disturbing theme that appears also in other films by Almodóvar (such as *Tie Me Up! Tie Me Down!*). But here lies Benigno's confusion between beneficent-professional care and consuming-romantic love. He is unable to separate his job and his private life—Benigno became a nurse at home when he had to take care of his mother for fifteen years, and after her death he sought refuge from his loneliness in his professional career as a nurse.

Talk to Her illustrates the centrality of patient autonomy as a concern for contemporary bioethics, showing that beneficence without respect for autonomy becomes paternalism (for a more sympathetic discussion of Benigno's actions and type of care, see chapter 19 of this volume). Actually, the whole film is about the art of respectfully "talking to her." Most of it takes place in a comfortable health institution, a private clinic that looks, according to Almodóvar, "more like a hotel than anything else." But even in the best circumstances there are ethical problems, emerging as they inevitably do from the relationships and conversations that occur in health care organizations. This "art of talking" plays an important role in the deliberation among health care professionals. First, because only the effective exchange of information between the various professionals that participate in the patient's treatment can provide her with the best possible care. Second, communication between hospital staff members can also have an indirectly therapeutic effect for patients, because the treatment can be emotionally draining on caregivers, and one of the best ways to deal with such difficulties is to share one's experience in conversations. This requires an ability on the part of health care professionals that might be called "dialogical competence" (Árnason 2000).

My Life without Me, or Secret Patient Autonomy

Ann is twenty-four years old and has not had much time to think about her life; now she is told that in a few weeks she will die. To avoid bringing suffering to her family and to be able to realize a few plans, she decides not to tell her family the truth about her condition. The patient-professional relationship in this film could be rightly placed inside what has been called the "patient autonomy model" (Árnason 2004). Here we find the primacy of the patient's wishes and at the same time a risk of evasion of professional responsibility, because Ann makes all the choices. The situation is the reverse of that in *Talk to Her*, but with a similarity: once again, only one agent in our triangle does all the talking. The film is based on Ann's monologues, so its design is more "monological" than "dialogical."

This film is entirely based on Ann's perspective—she appears in all the scenes. Before the opening credits, Ann speaks to herself in a soft yet commanding voice that says, "this is you." But this second person addressed, "you," from whose perspective the narrator exercises her autonomy, is divided: something new has happened. Before, she was never "one of those kinds of people who like looking up at the moon." But her imminent death has introduced new demands—or rather it has changed her priorities—and her old self has become a "you" who has to be redirected.

This dialogue with herself constitutes an illustration that a real exercise of autonomy is not common because it requires this kind of deliberation; Ann is simply not used to thinking this way, because she has never had much leisure or spare time in which to do so.

Autonomy: Why Ann Chooses to Lie

My Life without Me contains an extreme argument for the priority of patient autonomy, but how realistic is it? Let us remember that, in opposition to the main message of this film, Gracia's theory gives less normative force to the principles of autonomy and beneficence than to the principles of nonmaleficence and justice, as the latter couple belong to a minimal ethics that is publicly compulsory ("the right," in John Rawls's terminology), while compliance with the former is a matter of private excellence ("the good"). But this position has been challenged in Spain by Simón (1999), who understands the primacy of autonomy as the most important feature of modern morality and argues that respect for autonomy is not a principle like the other three but rather a new perspective on them, one in which nonmaleficence, justice, and benevolence are all understood as autonomy promoting.

This film suggests something similar: in the new list of priorities, respect for autonomy is paramount—at least in palliative care, in which the aim of healing has been replaced by the aim of providing a good death—and consequently many of the other traditional principles lose most of their normative force (conversely, autonomy loses this privileged position in other situations; for instance, in emergency medicine). In the difficult moment occasioned by a terminal diagnosis, the patient needs above all to maintain a certain self-respect, a sense of her own worth as a human being, and the feeling that she has some control over the process of dying. Ann chooses to lie because, as she sees it, that is the only way to satisfy those needs. This exercise of her autonomy is not devoid of a concern with beneficence towards others, as the message she leaves for her daughters is one of self-confidence, but one could ask whether they do not have a moral right to see their mom off.

Some have warned against a person's attempting to control every aspect of his or her life, insofar as doing so may exclude the needs or wishes of others. But self-control is part and parcel of our Western culture, and health care authorities, in both America and Europe, encourage people to take control over end-of-life decisions by completing advance directives. Ann wants to be remembered in a certain way and to control the content of that memory by means of the "advance directives" she gives to Dr. Thompson. In a deleted scene, she makes love with a stranger she has just met in a bar. When he asks her name, she answers, "I'm not going to tell you. I don't want you to forget it." This determination to control how others will remember her is the reason why she forces Dr. Thompson to give up any therapeutic goal, sticking to only the palliative ends of medicine. "I don't want any more tests if they're not going to save me," she tells him at the hospital. "I don't want to be here and I don't want to die here . . . I'm going to do it my way." The physician agrees to the deal as "part of (her) therapy," provided Ann accepts "something to ease the pain."

"No one thinks about death in a supermarket," says Ann. Indeed, mortality is largely invisible in public, though there are certainly significant differences in cultural attitudes toward the end of life and toward communication in this stage. A recent ethnographic study has shown that European Americans and African Americans are likely to view truth-telling as empowering in end-of-life medical contexts, in that it enables the terminal patient to make choices, while Korean-American and Mexican-American respondents are more likely to see truth-telling in this context as cruel, and even harmful, to the patients (Blackhall, Frank, Murphy, and Michel 2001).

For Ann, her only way to overcome death is by facing it on her own: "I don't want people to start treating me like I'm dying." This is why she refuses to bring her husband with her to the hospital and refuses also a second opinion. It has been noted that sometimes the physician's preoccupation with technical activity represents a futile attempt to overcome death (Casado 2003). Terminally ill patients look for clinicians with whom they can build a "therapeutic alliance"—a person who can act as a sounding board or guide them through the dying process (Back 2004). Initially, Dr. Thompson is not very good at that. When Ann tells him she will be twenty-four in December, she adds that she is an Aquarius. Of course, she is not; she is just speaking nonsense because Dr. Thompson is not being helpful as a sounding board. What she really wants to say is: "How about you? What star sign are you? What the hell is happening to me?" After that, Ann refuses to take part in more tests ("they're trying out a new machine, they're like little kids"). She wants to be free of death talk so that she can live the end of her life autonomously, not to evade death (as in the supermarket), but to deal with it, and, to use Thoreau's words in *Walden*, "to live deep and suck out all the marrow of life."

The Sea Inside, or Bioethics at the Courts

Our third story follows Ramón Sampedro's case as he tries to persuade those who love him and the high court that he should be given the right to die. Although the authorities reject this wish, his friends ultimately help him prepare this last journey. One of those friends, Julia (played by Belén Rueda), is also ill, and plans to end her life in the same way as Ramón (played by Javier Bardem), but eventually she takes a different path. (A few scenes dealing with the development of Julia's character, actually a collage of several real persons, were deleted in the final cut to make the film shorter. This obscures her reasons for choosing a different path from Ramón and makes the final cut somewhat unbalanced in its point of view, which is dominated by the impressive presence of Ramón.)

This film lacks patient-professional relationships, in the sense that no health care personnel are involved. But it is clearly about relationships of care and advice, and there are also issues of professional ethics, as Julia and Gené are lawyers who actively assist Ramón in his plea. The model of interaction is dominated by relationships between the patient and society, the legal system, and even institutionalized religion. In this sense, the film has to do with the role of power and the law throughout the world of health care—what some would call the "judicialization of bioethics."

Let's go back to our assessment of the current Spanish bioethical scenario. It is time to recall that this situation is not only characterized by the conflict between paternalism and the new patient autonomy model. There is a third part: society and the state, which are always present in the patient-professional relationship, often through the law and the economy. The standards of care have never been better or more universal in Spain, but the expectations of the citizenry have also increased, and the triangle is more problematic than ever (Gracia 1999, p. 25). Beauchamp and Childress maintain that the principles of justice foster questions about "what the people of a nation should expect from their health care system and how the nation can address citizens' needs" (2001, pp. 64, 113, 165–66, 272). However, can a nation help someone if he asks to die?

Justice and Nonmaleficence: Why Ramón Chooses to Die

The Sea Inside has been the most viewed and acclaimed film in Spain in recent history, as Sampedro's case has caused a great public controversy (Guerra 1999). Newspapers have published a wide range of articles and letters to the editor, both "for" and "against" euthanasia, forgetting that Ramón was not terminally ill, and therefore that his case was not one of "euthanasia" in the usual sense of the word. Moreover, on September 22, 2004, the *Diario de Navarra* published a piece suggesting that the debate over Ramón Sampedro had the intent of making it easier for doctors to kill patients to save the rising costs of health care in an aging society. The Catholic Church published leaflets against the film, and some bioethicists complained that it was misleading because it ignored the influence that Ramón's example could have in medical practice (Simón 2004).

Some critics (de Prada 2004) ridiculed the presumed use of autonomy as a moral justification for assisted suicide by pointing out that anyone choosing this option thereby terminates his or her capacity for autonomous choice. But there is nothing about the principle of respect for autonomy as such that precludes one's choosing options that rule out one's own future autonomous choices (Preston, Gunderson, and Mayo 2004). Others mentioned the risk of a slippery slope in reference to the much-debated Dutch experience (Hendin, Rutenfrans, and Zylicz 1997) with legal, physician-assisted suicide, and many remarked that, since euthanasia and physician-assisted suicide play no part in the dying process of 90 percent of terminally ill patients, the objective must be to improve the quality of care at the end of life and not to win the battle over legalizing euthanasia, which is "an emotionally charged irrelevance" (Emanuel 2001).

However, these films are emotionally charged because they are made to be moving, to appeal to the senses and the emotions by means of image and sound—that is, after all, the aim of cinema, and it would be silly to consider this characteristic a fault of the film. In addition, *The Sea Inside* is not an apology for pure, irrational emotion. Quite the contrary: Ramón is an unflinchingly Socratic figure, who for instance says to his nephew, "Look, if you want to persuade me you've got to rationally justify your point." He is aware that the topic of death raises powerful emotions, but he wants to face them and think them through. "At the end of the day," he acknowledges, "this is just about fear."

"What is the future for you?" Julia asks. "Death," he replies, "for me as well as for you." Other critics condemned Ramón's obsession with death, as if his position was that the life of a quadriplegic was not worth living. But, as he says in the film, "who is talking about quadriplegics here? I'm talking about myself. About Ramón Sampedro." We might agree with this basic existentialist claim that we determine our values through our choices, that is, through the course of our actions. In this sense, by choosing to die, Ramón somehow values death. But he does not value any type of death, or death in general; what he values is rather the result of *his* specific circumstances, *his* deliberation, and *his* choice. And he agrees that others may choose differently. As his friend Gené says, "what we support is freedom: that of those who want to live, and that of those who prefer to get out of the way."

Not everyone who asks for an assisted suicide is depressed or unloved. From the fact that a person in a certain situation decides not to go on living, we cannot infer a negative judgment regarding those in similar circumstances who decide otherwise. Ramón is choosing for himself, not for others. Although by setting a precedent he may inevitably be paving the way for others in a comparable position. Western societies are characterized by an attitude of reasonable pluralism, meaning that they are not dominated by a belief in a single moral code but rather that there are several conceptions of the good life, each of them with its own conception of the good death. What was a good death for Ramón Sampedro might not be as good for another quadriplegic person, and it is reasonable that this be so.

Human beings are moral because they can choose, even if they choose to die. In this sense, the argument between Father Francisco ("Life-denying freedom is not freedom!") and Ramón ("A life without freedom is not a life either!") is a false dichotomy. Battin and Quill (2004) show how the argument over physician-assisted dying has often been based on similar statements: "What would you have, access to hospice and palliative care or access to physician-assisted death?" Put it this way, most people would choose the former option, not the latter. But that is not a genuine choice, they argue, as the state of Oregon and Holland's institutions of legal physician-assisted suicide show that good palliative care, including that provided by hospice, is compatible with physician-assisted death. The film strongly suggests the possibility of a model that integrates assisted dying with excellent end-of-life care, and also its moral necessity, because suffering may be more tolerable when it is endured voluntarily.

In *The Barbarian Invasions*, it seems that no one who helped in the suicide of the main character was convinced that it was morally wrong. *Mar Adentro* (and *Million Dollar Baby*) depicts a more complex situation, one in which family and friends are divided about it, but also one suggesting that suicide—whether or not it is, generally speaking, "wrong"—is not a wrong that should be forbidden by the law. There are, of course, other wrongs that should be legally prevented—Alicia's rape, for instance. Thus one who would assist another in a rape should be prevented from doing so, but one who would assist another in a genuine suicide should not.

Conclusion

Bioethics is an attempt to bring together moral theory and health care practice, and film provides us with an excellent laboratory for this task. Here we have explored the contribution of three recent Spanish films to the philosophical debate about issues surrounding disability and the end of life. These films have attracted great attention in Spain and abroad, but their underlying bioethics had not yet been systematically studied.

Underlying the emergence of the moral questions introduced by these films is the greatly increased medical capacity to keep people alive beyond a point that would have been hardly imaginable in Spain (or anywhere else) in the nineteenth or early twentieth centuries. The films provide nuanced treatments of the three sides of the triangle. We have seen that the main conflict in *Talk to Her* has to do with the principle of beneficence, whereas *My Life without Me* represents the principle of autonomy at its fullest expression, and *The Sea Inside* has to do with the justice of an act of assisted suicide. But each film also shows the risks of putting too much emphasis on one moral principle and forgetting the others. Benigno's beneficence becomes a controlling domination and violation of Alicia's autonomy, Ann's autonomy alienates her from family and friends, and Ramón's plea is rejected by church and courts of justice in the name of nonmaleficence. In all three cases what we have is a value model based on the preeminence of a single principle, a relationship centered on just one of the apexes of the relationship, a monologue.

Without authentic conversations, the patient-professional relationship becomes a silent movie where good health care is absent. At the end of his *Fundamentos de bioética*, Gracia approvingly quotes Adela Cortina, a contemporary philosopher who claimed that such a dialogical competence was absent from the Spanish public sphere. Indeed, the absence of a "civil morality" brings about a number of ills afflicting contemporary societies, such as "a lack of tolerance, little willingness to take part in dialogue and to accept its outcome, the pretension of having a monopoly over truth, etc." (Gracia 1989, p. 574). These films show how standard bioethics, as it is taught today in Spain, is still characterized by an unresolved tension between the older paternalistic outlook and the newer autonomy-centered models, which combine multiple principles. Only authentic conversations and deliberation between the three main agents in our triangle—patients, professionals, and "the others"—can address such a tension in a comprehensive, cooperative way. Otherwise—as we have seen in the cases of Ramón, Ann, Lydia, or Alicia—the primacy of autonomy in modern ethical *theory* will be hard to put into practice. In real *practice*, however, the key is often to attend to the particularities of the cases, and to allow the guiding principles to emerge from a respectful and informed dialogue among all parties in these tangled, yet sometimes wonderful, triangles.

As in ancient times, stars help us navigate.

QUESTIONS FOR CONSIDERATION

1. *Is Lydia better treated than Alicia? Where is the line that separates beneficence from maleficence in both cases?*

2. *On what basis is Ramón's plea justifiable? Is the battle over legalizing euthanasia an emotionally charged irrelevance?*

3. *Is Ann's decision right? Is it based on particular considerations about how a culture understands autonomy?*

ACKNOWLEDGMENTS

I am indebted to Vilhjálmur Árnason, Garrett Barden, Arantza Etxeberria, and Koldo Martínez for their valuable comments and insights on the subject of this chapter.

REFERENCES

Almodóvar, P. 2002. *Hable con ella* [English title, *Talk to Her*; motion picture]. Madrid: El Deseo, S.A.

Amenábar, A. 2004. *Mar adentro* [English title, *The Sea Inside*; motion picture]. Madrid: Sogepaq Productions.

Arcand, D. 2003. *Les Invasions Barbares* [English title, *The Barbarian Invasions*; motion picture]. Quebec: Astral Films.

Árnason, V. 2000. Gadamerian Dialogue in the Patient-Professional Interaction. *Medicine, Health Care and Philosophy* 3 (1): 17–23.

———. 2004. Ética y sanidad: Dignidad y diálogo en la relación asistencial [Ethics and Health: Dignity and Dialogue in the Patient-Professional Relationship]. *Laguna. Revista de filosofía* 14:23–35.

Back, A. L. 2004. Doctor-Patient Communication about Physician-Assisted Suicide. In *Physician-Assisted Dying: The Case for Palliative Care and Patient Choice,* ed. T. E. Quill and M. P. Battin, 102–117. Baltimore: Johns Hopkins University Press.

Battin, M. P., and Quill, T. E. 2004. False Dichotomy versus Genuine Choice: The Argument over Physician-Assisted Dying. In *Physician-Assisted Dying: The Case for Palliative Care and Patient Choice,* ed. T. E. Quill and M. P. Battin, 1–12. Baltimore: Johns Hopkins University Press.

Beauchamp, T. L., and Childress, J. F. 1979. *Principles of Biomedical Ethics*, 1st ed. Oxford and New York: Oxford University Press.

———. 2001. *Principles of Biomedical Ethics*, 5th ed. Oxford and New York: Oxford University Press.

Blackhall, L., Frank, G., Murphy, S., and Michel, V. 2001. Bioethics in a Different Tongue: The Case of Truth-Telling. *Journal of Urban Health: Bulletin of the New York Academy of Medicine* 78 (1): 59–71.

Casado, A. 2003. Ética al final de la vida [Ethics at the End of Life]. In *Cuidados paliativos en enfermería* [Palliative Care in Nursing], ed. W. Astudillo, A. Orbegozo, A. Latiegui, and E. Urdaneta, 323–350. San Sebastián: Sociedad Vasca de Cuidados Paliativos.

Coixet, I. 2003. *Mi vida sin mí* [English title, *My Life without Me*; motion picture]. Madrid: El Deseo, S. A.

Corliss, R., and Schickel, R. 2005. 9 Great Movies from Nine Decades. *Time* 165 (22): 78–79.

de Prada, J. M. 2004. Eutanasia, *El Seminal*, October 31, 12.

Eastwood, C. 2004. *Million Dollar Baby* [motion picture]. Burbank, CA: Warner Bros. Pictures.

Emanuel, E. J. 2001. Euthanasia: Where the Netherlands Leads Will the World Follow? *British Medical Journal* 322: 1377.

Gracia, D. 1999. Planteamiento general de la bioética. In *Bioética para clínicos,* ed. A. Couceiro, 19–35. Madrid: Triacastela.

———. 2007. *Fundamentos de bioética* [Fundamentals of Bioethics], 2nd ed. Madrid: Triacastela.

Greenhalgh, T., and Hurwitz, B. 1999. Why Study Narrative? *British Medical Journal* 318: 48–50.

Guerra, M. J. 1999. Euthanasia in Spain: The Public Debate after Ramon Sampedro's Case. *Bioethics* 13: 426–32.

———. 2005. Bioética en España: Treinta años de interdisciplinariedad y controversias [Bioethics in Spain: Thirty Interdisciplanary and Controversial Years]. In *Bioética: Entre la medicina y la ética* [Bioethics: Between Medicine and Ethics], ed. M. T. López de la Vieja, 1730190. Salamanca: University of Salamanca Press.

Hendin, H., Rutenfrans, C., and Zylicz, Z. 1997. Physician-Assisted Suicide and Euthanasia in the Netherlands: Lessons from the Dutch. *Journal of the American Medical Association* 277, 21:1720–22.

MacIntyre, A. 1981. *After Virtue.* South Bend, IN: University of Notre Dame Press.

Marzabal, I. 2004. *Deliberaciones poéticas: Cine y ética narrativa* [Poetic Deliberations: Film and Narrative Ethics]. Bilbao: University of the Basque Country Press.

Mitchell, E. 2002. A Time When Loyalty Overrides Love. *New York Times,* October 12, Section B, p. 9.

Muñoz, S., and Gracia, D. 2006. *Médicos en el cine. Dilemas bioéticos: sentimientos, razones y deberes* [Medical Doctors at the Movies. Bioethical Dilemmas: Feelings, Reasons, and Duties], Madrid: Complutense University Press.

Nelson, H. L., ed. 1997. *Stories and their Limits: Narrative Approaches to Bioethics.* New York: Routledge.

Pérez Oliva, M. 2006. Diego Garcia, El maestro deliberador [Diego Garcia, the Master Deliberator]. *El País,* January 29, Section EPS, 12–17.

Preston, T., Gunderson, M., and Mayo, D. J. 2004. The Role of Autonomy in Choosing Physician Aid in Dying. In *Physician-Assisted Dying: The Case for Palliative Care and Patient Choice,* ed. T. E. Quill and M. P. Battin, 39–54. Baltimore: Johns Hopkins University Press.

Simón, P. 1999. La fundamentación del consentimiento informado [The Grounding of Informed Consent]. *Revista de calidad asistencial* 14: 100–109.

———. 2004. Mar adentro: Las otras orillas [The Sea Inside: The Other Shores], *El País,* October 12, 33.

TWENTY-ONE

Ikiru and Net-Casting in Intercultural Bioethics

Michael C. Brannigan

Life is so short,
Fall in love, dear maiden,
While your lips are still red,
And before you are old,
For there will be no tomorrow.

Life is so short,
Fall in love, dear maiden,
While your hair is still black,
And before your heart withers,
For today will not come again.

FROM THE MUSICAL THEME IN *Ikiru*

Intercultural studies are not immune from the hazard of exaggerating distinctions and differences in ways that cast monolithic nets over other traditions and perspectives. Akira Kurosawa's classic 1952 film *Ikiru* can easily convey an impression to many Western viewers that Japanese clinical practice tends (or, at least, tended in the early twentieth century) to be impersonal, bureaucratic, and paternalistic in ways that differ from European and American health care encounters, which seem more compassionate and respectful of patients' rights. However, although the film's protagonist undergoes an encounter that appears to reflect a vastly different clinical style, it remains unfair to typecast Japanese clinical ethics on its basis. In a particularly poignant scene, the main character, Kanji Watanabe, visits the clinic and discovers that he has stomach cancer with only months left to live. In considering aspects of Watanabe's clinical encounter, we explore whether and to what degree alleged differences in the Japanese clinical encounter are real.

On an anecdotal basis of disclosure styles in Japanese clinical practice, we may infer that Japanese physicians generally lie to their patients concerning a diagnosis of terminal illness. This cultural net-casting, as I dub it, also occurs when we inflate alleged similarities among cultures. Because Japanese health care professionals are increasingly more familiar with the idea of informed consent in clinical practice, we may suppose that they have uncritically adopted Western views of informed consent, even though the Japanese term for informed consent, *setsumei to doi* ("explanation and consent") does not quite mean the same for Japanese as it does for us. In this chapter, I will examine perceived differences more closely than similarities.

Though my chapter's title seems enigmatic, the theme is straightforward. Casting nets over Japanese health care is wrongheaded in that it unfairly homogenizes the complexity of institutional, professional, interpersonal, and cultural dramas. Cultural net-casting also pays less attention to different cultures' common ground by suggesting artificial incompatibilities among cultural and societal practices within the arena of health care and health care ethics. I do not diminish the importance of generalization as a tool for understanding cultures, subcultures, and their various patterns of beliefs, values, and behaviors. We generalize through noting patterns of similarities and discrepancies. This naturally descriptive methodology helps cultivate proper understanding of the whole picture. We've succumbed to net-casting, however, when we exaggerate similarities or differences as representing a given culture.

Background

Ikiru was sandwiched between Kurosawa's typical period films (*jidaigekei*) *Rashomon* and *Seven Samurai*. Unlike his rendering of medieval Japan and its warring factions of samurai, loyal and disloyal to their daimyos and ruling dynasties, *Ikiru* is contemporary, restrained, and without the scope and force of violence depicted in his samurai scenes. *Ikiru*'s violence takes another form—the inner quake that occurs when one unexpectedly stumbles on the truth of impending death as the ultimate interruption in one's securely inconsequential life.

The film slowly unveils the extraordinary transformation of an ordinary midlevel bureaucrat, Kanji Watanabe, who rises from his lifeless everyday paperwork to help create a community playground for children. He inspires the makeover from a wasteland and cesspool of mosquitoes and drudge to a pristine park. This is especially remarkable in postwar Japan, where the rule of thumb for *sarariman* (Japanese adaptation for "a salaryman" or "a company man") is to live one's life in predictable duty to one's organization in acquiescence to its bureaucratic foibles. In the second half of the film, the deceased Watanabe is remembered by his coworkers for his unexpected labor against the wheels of civil service. Yet, even though one colleague seems stirred personally by Watanabe's example, the others return to business as usual.

Often a single defining moment can lift one out of the ashes of ordinariness. For Watanabe (who embodies "all the attributes of insignificance" as Albert Camus describes the municipal clerk Joseph Grand in *The Plague*), this decisive event begins with his clinical encounter and his confrontation with the indelible truth of his approaching death from stomach cancer. It is not the fact of death in itself that transforms him, but the awakening to various profoundly personal, naked truths that the acknowledgment of death's interruption can generate.

The film's existential current permeates some archetypal questions in bioethics. How does one genuinely "live"? What is quality of life? Who determines it? How important is the acceptance of death? What does it mean to face the truths we often choose to ignore or deny? What is the purpose of medicine? Is there a distinction between curing and healing? What should be the proper relationship between health professionals and patients? Should truth always be disclosed to patients? How does our confrontation with death define who we may become?

Watanabe's metamorphosis comes about only after facing his death sentence head on. After bouts of depression and hanging on to straws of false hope, pleasure, and remorse, his final response is his redemption. The film's title, *Ikiru*, literally means "to live." Watanabe emerges from his melancholy, transcends the thoroughgoing blackness of his dreaded death sentence, and shows us that "to live" means "to act."[1] How? By freeing himself from the prison of self-interest and acting totally and tirelessly on behalf of others, including present and future children, Watanabe helps to give life to a clean, wholesome park where there was once a breeding ground for disease. Peeling away these existential layers, let us return to our more pragmatic theme. In view of the scene below, what can we learn regarding the danger of net-casting in intercultural bioethics?

Intercultural Bioethics

As a prelude, my use of "intercultural bioethics" in the title is deliberate. In my work on the subject (Brannigan and Boss 2001; Brannigan 2004, 2005), though I have resorted to other designations such as "cross-cultural bioethics," I'm now more inclined to prefer intercultural bioethics. Bioethics has evolved as a field that is both conceptually and practically interdisciplinary. As a field committed to examining ethical issues in the biosciences, medicine, and health care, bioethics requires the discerning engagement of various disciplines. Given the normative aims of the field, the relevant disciplines have predominantly been philosophical, theological, medical, legal, and biological; neither sufficient attention nor respect were attributed to other areas like social science, anthropology, and ethnology, yet these latter disciplines are surely crucial when it comes to looking at bioethics through an intercultural lens.

In view of bioethics' interdisciplinary basis, "intercultural" therefore makes sense. The prefix "inter-" implies an active engagement that "multi-" and "cross-" do not evidently convey. "Multicultural" clearly indicates awareness of and proper respect for plurality, but sans dialogue. Recognition of pluralistic worldviews and values is critically important. Yet without engagement, an effort at genuine discourse and dialogue among these worldviews, mere awareness and respect do not preclude net-casting. "Cross-cultural" denotes awareness of and respect for plurality, but the idea of "crossing over" cultures suggests a privileged point of reference and comparison—crossing over from where and from what perspective? To illustrate, we can compare and contrast the conventional Western mainstream approach to bioethics with certain viewpoints in Japan. Despite an earnest effort to explore these "other" perspectives, these perspectives can be "flattened" and viewed as "other," without the struggle involved in self-examination and reassessment in the light of these worldviews, values, and beliefs. Indeed, when it comes to studies of other cultures, the ubiquitous challenge will always be whether or not and to what degree we can avoid a privileged position. In any case, assuming a privileged viewpoint is conducive to unfair cultural net-casting.

Looking outward is at the same time a looking inward. The term *intercultural* at least conveys the ideal aim of more actively and genuinely engaging with another culture and thereby with our own cultures and sets of biases in open and honest discourse and dialogue to enable the possibility of self-understanding, growth, and renewal. This sort of change cannot take place through net-casting. "Intercultural" underscores the need to avoid the fallacy of cultural net-casting that inflates either differences or similarities. Given this, after we examine the following scene from *Ikiru*, we will scout out a few of its "red flags" or more hazardous areas that may lend themselves to cultural net-casting. My caution to colleagues is to beware of showing the film to students and others, pointing out how "Japanese practice health care in this way," whereas "we do it this way."

From Waiting Room to Office

Just before he meets with his doctor, Watanabe, who has been experiencing ongoing abdominal symptoms for some time, encounters another patient in the waiting room. This character acts as sort of an unsolicited interpreter, one who will prepare Watanabe and translate for him some of the medical rhetoric he might hear from his physician. This purveyor of the truth, sensing Watanabe's apprehension, alludes to Suzuki, a different patient. Suzuki has just been diagnosed with stomach cancer, but Suzuki himself is not informed of this. The unwelcome interpreter informs Watanabe of specific details of the deceit. When the physician tells the patient that he or she suffers from a "mild ulcer," this actually means stomach cancer and that the victim has less than a year left to live. This dishonesty is reaffirmed with further statements such as "no need to operate" and "eat anything you want."

Our interpreter then ominously describes the signs of stomach cancer (see Figure 21.1). Watanabe becomes increasingly distressed since he has

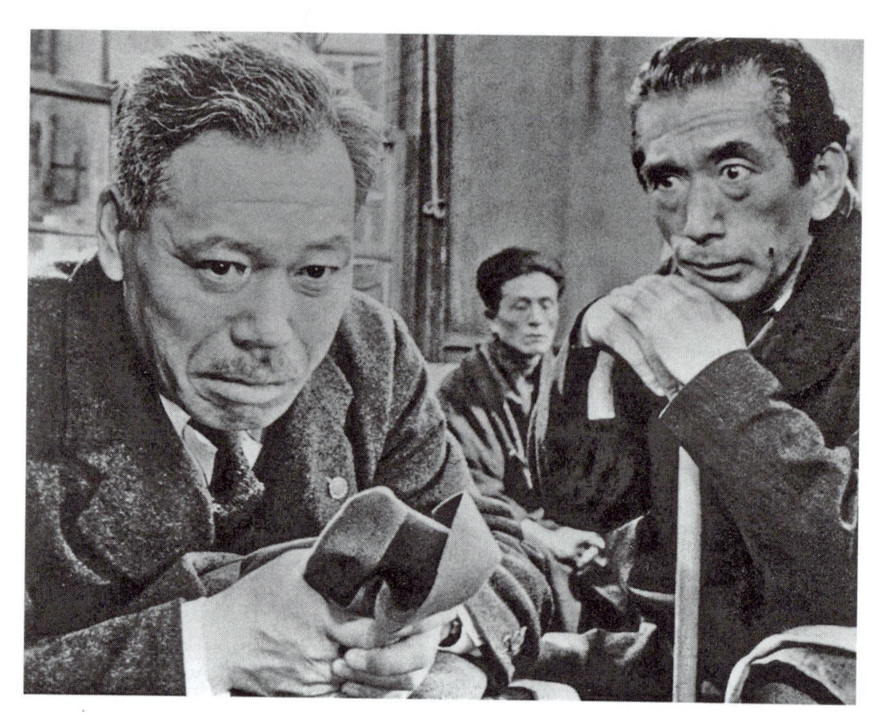

FIGURE 21.1 Kanji Watanabe, played by Takashi Shimura, anxiously awaits the bad news in *Ikiru*. *Source*: Toho Company, The Kobal Collection, provided by The Picture Desk.

been having these same symptoms: a heavy pain in the stomach region, incessant burping, dry tongue, relentless thirst, diarrhea or constipation, black bowel movements, loss of appetite, and constant vomiting. The persistence of these symptoms forces Watanabe to miss his first day of work in nearly thirty years to make this visit to the clinic. The more he hears, the further he moves away, seeking to distance himself from further uninvited truths. All this prepares the viewer for Watanabe's clinical encounter and conversation with his physician.

"Watanabe-san. Watanabe Kanji-san."

As his name is called, Kanji Watanabe sits in another room, isolated, away from his interpreter, the other waiting patient who just spoke with him. Watanabe looks despondent and appears utterly alone.

"Watanabe-san."

Watanabe stands up to go to the doctor's office. When he rises, he drops his overcoat.

"Yes."

Watanabe enters the doctor's office. He is at first barely visible behind the medicine cabinet. Nurses are busy with their paperwork, not one of them acknowledging him as he enters. At the same time, two physicians seem fixed on the x-ray of Watanabe's stomach. Finally the older physician moves away from the film, momentarily glances at Watanabe, and sits first at the desk, gesturing to Watanabe to be seated.

"Sit down."

The doctor looks over some papers, apparently Watanabe's report.

"Um. It looks like you've got a mild ulcer."

Watanabe is still standing, his back now to the physician. On hearing this, he drops his coat again. The film's musical backdrop beats ominously as he stares ahead. Both doctors look at him as if inspecting his reaction. Just when Watanabe turns around to face his physician, the doctor looks down again at his report.

"Honestly . . . please tell me the truth."

Watanabe's voice nearly pleads. Hearing this, the nurse, now sitting at the same desk with the doctor, appears occupied with paperwork and writing. The doctor continues to stare down at his report, while Watanabe gazes at him imploringly, waiting for his response, and asks once more.

"Tell me it's stomach cancer."

After a pause, the doctor briefly looks up at Watanabe.

"I just told you, it's a mild ulcer."

Watanabe lowers his head, nearly touching the desk as if in resignation. The doctor and nurse look at each other. The nurse walks over to the window, picks up Watanabe's coat from the floor, and stares out the window. As she returns to the desk, the camera now moves to the back of the other physician who is listening all this time. Watanabe continues to question.

"What about an operation? Can you operate?"

As Watanabe stares up at the doctor with pleading eyes, both doctor and nurse find escape in their reports.

"Oh, there's no need to operate. It'll heal on its own."

Now, with his hands folded together, the physician's eyes finally meet Watanabe's.

"And my diet?"

Watanabe stares back.

"Well, just use your common sense. As long as it's easy to digest."

The nurse remains immersed in her paperwork. Perhaps out of discomfort or nervousness, she briefly pats the back of her hair to ensure that it's still in place. She then picks up a slip of paper as the doctor repeats himself.

"You can eat whatever you like."

The physician and Watanabe look into each other's eyes. Watanabe then leans forward, still peering straight ahead at the doctor. The doctor goes back to his report, and Watanabe again lowers his head, and here the scene ends.

In the next scene, Watanabe has left the office. The older physician sits and lights a cigar, while the younger physician and the nurse stare ahead, lost in thought. The younger physician asks:

"Does that patient have a year?"
"No. I'd give him six months."
"Six months?"

The younger doctor seems surprised.

"Yeah."

The doctor quickly looks at his younger colleague, looks downward, and poses a question.

"What would you do if you had only six months left to live, like him?"

The nurse stares ahead, and the young physician lowers his head. The doctor turns and looks at the nurse, asking her the same question.

"What about you, Aihara?"

Aihara shrugs her shoulders and answers indifferently.

"The barbiturates are over there."

When the young doctor hears this, he looks down reflectively. He then walks over to Watanabe's x-ray, turns on the screen light, and gazes at the outlined mass of cancer in Watanabe's stomach.

Nothing New

Surely, in the above clinical encounter, the health professionals exhibit little emotion. Yet, we still need to be careful and not make unfair generalizations. This portrayal of aloofness is also situated within an historic, social, and political context. The film's setting takes place during the American occupation of Japan in the postwar period, in its bold attempt to instill the principles of democracy in a defeated society. The film demonstrates that during this turbulent period, Japanese society has become so heavily bureaucratized that any effort to reconstruct in the wake of collapse is monumentally difficult. This context is crucial to understand further aspects of the film.

There is an unambiguous bleakness in Watanabe's brief encounter. As he enters, no one acknowledges him. Physicians and nurses are busy in their paperwork, reminiscent of Watanabe's workplace, where paperwork is also a substitute for human encounter. However, the scene is hardly a sufficient cultural marker to make general claims about the greater impersonality of Japanese health care. The film is set in the decades before the Western emphasis on patients' rights, an idea that only slowly took hold within Japanese health care, and although one can argue that the notion of patients' rights is still relatively foreign in Japan,[2] aloofness in the clinical encounter is inarguably familiar in the West as well. Despite mechanisms in place in U.S. health care institutions to help ensure recognition of patients' rights, honest disclosure, and informed consent, our health system's fragmentation of its health delivery still lends itself to hospitals' inhospitableness. Considering both the time in which the film was made and the currency of impersonality even now in our own health care system, there are no grounds here for net-casting.

The viewer is prepared for this impersonality from the start. *Ikiru's* opening scene shows the x-ray of Watanabe's stomach, a mass of cancer filling a sizable portion of the stomach cavity. This medicalizes the main character as a "cancer," even worse, a "stomach cancer," and again such medicalization is hardly a stranger to U.S. health care. As the narrator tells us, this "stomach belongs to the protagonist." Watanabe *is* in effect his cancer.

The narrator goes on: "He may as well be dead. In fact, this man has been dead for more than twenty years now." He and his coworkers are "worn down by the minutiae of bureaucracy." Thus the clinical encounter's detached objectivity clearly reflects that of Watanabe's workplace. In the doctors' office, the film switches from the sterile medicine cabinet to nurses' and physicians' superfluous attention to paperwork rather than to communicating face-to-face with the patient. Throughout the scene, paperwork offers a safe shield from interpersonal encounter. Both in the workplace and in the doctors' office, immersion in paper represents meaningless activity, an officially sanctioned escape from human engagement.

This is evident in an early scene when mothers visit Watanabe's workplace to complain of a disease-laden swamp in an area that has led to their children's intestinal parasites and skin rashes. Their request is simple—to clean the area and rid it of any pollution. The response is predictable—unconcern and bureaucracy prevail. The mothers are taken on a farcical runaround. The company sidesteps their request, starting with the Health Department, to the Sanitation Department, to Environmental Sanitation, to Department of Prevention, to Infectious Disease, to Pest Control, to City Hall's Sewage Department, to Roads, City Planning, Ward Reorganization, to Fire Department, Education and Child Welfare Committee, to Ward Representative to City Council, Deputy Mayor, to Deputy Director, to Public Affairs, Engineering, and finally to sector chief, Watanabe, who happens to be absent due to a doctor's appointment. Entirely put off by this charade, the mothers are then asked to submit their request in writing. The irony is brutal. Because paper in the first half of the film signifies meaningless activity in a senseless and inefficient bureaucracy, urging the women to put their request in writing so that their written request can occupy the same empty and useless space as all other forms shows inarguable disdain for the mothers.

Can human compassion, responsibility, and accountability take root in this bureaucratic grind? Along similar lines, can Watanabe regain what little is left of his "living"? After being hit hard with the truth that he will soon die, another truth eventually seeps in—that he had been unofficially "dead" and buried in endless piles of paperwork throughout most of his adult life. Is redemption possible? In such dire prognosis, can Watanabe truly *live* out his remaining days?

Medical Paternalism

There are features of Watanabe's clinical visit that, at least on the surface, seem distinct enough to be considered by some as cultural markers specific to the Japanese context, specific not only over fifty years ago when the film was made, but even today. Yet again, tagging these features as uniquely Japanese is risky. Consider first his compliance with his doctor. Watanabe clearly defers to the authority of his physician. From our contemporary lens, his doctor exerts his control in a nearly despotic though benign way and comes across as somewhat insensitive to Watanabe's plight. That, combined with his lack of honesty can churn out an image of a cold-hearted, disinterested physician who lacks both communicative skills as well as any capacity to empathize with his patient.

Moreover, there is the aspect of gender. Just as women appear to customarily fill subordinate roles to men, nurses appear as second-class citizens in Japan's medical hierarchy. The nurses plainly assume a docile role in the doctors' office. The nurse Aihara is not addressed with the honorific suffix of *san*, but is simply called by her family name. Her presence is passive as she plays no active role in the conversation with Watanabe.

Furthermore, the relationship between physician and patient in Japan has had a long-standing historical footing in the Confucian ethos that stressed respect and obedience for those in authority in order to maintain filial piety and to ensure the social order. A strong medical paternalism was the norm in that physicians had a fundamental duty to protect their patients from harm. Patients, likewise, were obliged to follow their physician's orders.

Ikiru takes place in the 1950s. One may rightly point out that Japanese health care still manifests this medical paternalism. In a strong, hierarchical society where rank is all-important, respect continues to be shown to those of higher rank. The more educated continue to be treated with greater respect and deference. Thus, respect for the authority of the physician, a professional trained and licensed to heal, is still paramount. Yet is any of this different in any substantive way from how the clinical team interacts with the patient in U.S. health care? Does the scene's hierarchy reveal a distinct cultural marker about Japanese health care? Again, we need to be cautious about any tendency to cast cultural nets and claim this as a typical Japanese feature. This is clearly the case when we consider the increasing dominance of medical technologies in Japanese health care within a more contextual framework.

Before the Meiji Period (1868–1912), the prevailing health practice was traditional Chinese medicine (*kanpo*). *Kanpo* is the application of herbal (and occasionally animal) medicine, acupuncture, and moxibustion (burning mugwort plant cones on specific parts of the body to infuse heat). For example, ginseng is commonly used to promote blood circulation. Despite earlier efforts to suppress *kanpo*, it still continues to thrive today in Japan to treat chronic conditions and degenerative disorders (Otsuka 1976; Lock 1980).[3] However, toward the end of the Edo Period (1603–1867, preceding the Meiji), medicine was open to other influences, despite a 265-year era of *sakoku*, or closed period. The influences of Dutch medical theory, German medical education, and American medicine, respectively, led to a view of medicine as a specialized science with an increasingly sophisticated application of medical technologies in health practice. Diagnosis in *kanpo* rested on patients' perceptions of illness symptoms and healers' detection of bodily imbalance as well as physiological and environmental factors. This changed in the "new medicine," biomedicine, as diagnosis relied more on medical technologies and laboratory tests to ascertain pathogenic causes of illness. We see this with the fixation on the x-ray of Watanabe's stomach and its menacing mass of cancer. The x-ray in effect demonstrates the "triumph" of medical technology in that it replaces interpersonal intervention.

The end of World War II witnessed the increasing power of modern medicine and medical technology as well as continued deference to physicians. A strict system of licensure enabled physicians to be credentialed in ways that guaranteed social status and economic security. Mandatory licensing of physicians began earlier with the Meiji government when it required all practitioners of medicine, including practitioners of *kanpo*, to obtain officially sanctioned degrees in biomedicine (Long 1987).[4] Just as power and privilege accompanied modern scientific medicine, the same power and privilege was attributed to its ardent practitioners, the modern physicians.[5] Modern medicine thus assumed a dominant role in the Japanese health system, while other more traditional expressions such as *kampo* remained subordinate.

In this context, *Ikiru* illustrates how both hierarchy and medical technology supersede interpersonal interventions. At the same time, understanding the above context should enable us to refrain from net-casting. Clinical encounters in the United States often display a similar dominance of hierarchy and medical technology. Many of the ethical issues in U.S. health care, with its escalating fragmentation of health delivery, are bred by an overreliance on medical technologies, insufficient shared decision-making between patients and their health care providers, and increasing impersonality. And deeper moral questions in health care have to do with determining who or what is in control. In the film, the x-ray's seductive power suggests medical technologies, not physicians, as the wielders of power. The physicians are both interpreters and intermediaries of the medical technologies while remaining under their spell. Clearly, when technique substitutes for human interaction, impersonality is the inevitable consequence, whether this is the case in Japan, the United States, or anywhere else.

Nondisclosure

What about the issue of nondisclosure? Contemporary viewers in the United States can be easily shocked by the physician's degree of deceit. Although nondisclosure has been an established practice in Japan (even Emperor Hirohito was spared the truth about the cancer that went on to kill him in 1989), to us it still seems unpardonable. Could this be reasonable cause for net-casting? May we legitimately claim that Japanese physicians generally lie to their dying patients and that this is a special cultural trait?

Japanese health care in recent decades has undergone a bit of a face lift. First, growing interest and discussion about patients' rights and truth-telling has led to the practice of more open and honest disclosure. Today in Japan, more physicians convey the truth to their patients, and more patients expect to be told the truth. Honest disclosure is now considered the standard of care, as evidenced in the National Cancer Center's 1996 "Manual on Disclosing Cancer Diagnosis" (Steineck 2005). Second, there is more discussion about the need for public health awareness and responsibility for health. Citizens are urged to take more personal responsibility for their health through improved diet and lifestyles. Third, though the incidence of stomach cancer was high in Japan during Watanabe's time, due to earlier screening and improved treatment, the diagnosis of stomach cancer no longer carries the same ring of death and is no longer viewed as essentially hopeless.

Despite this growing awareness and discussion of patients' rights, quite a few physicians are still reluctant to disclose the diagnosis and prognosis of cancer, particularly if the condition is terminal (Bioethical Committee for the Japanese Medical Association 1994). And when family members object to disclosure, some physicians hesitate to disclose the truth to the patient.[6] In view of this apparent ambivalence toward disclosure, it may be the case that moral grounds are not the driving force behind the idea of patients' rights. To illustrate, when the former Ministry of Health and Welfare (now called the Ministry of Health, Labor, and Welfare, or *Kosei-rodo-sho*) set up a council to study the matter of disclosure, they outlined practical reasons rather than moral ones for telling the truth to dying patients: when patients are deceived, they still suspect that something is wrong; due to increased access to medical information, it is unrealistic to hide the truth; because patient cooperation is needed in more specialized interventions, sharing the truth would enable this cooperation (Steineck 2005). In either case, whether the grounds for enhanced disclosure are primarily moral or prudential, nondisclosure is not a cultural marker for net-casting Japanese medical practice. It is simply wrong-headed to assert that Japanese physicians generally do not tell the truth.

Stomach—*Hara*

One cultural marker or distinguishing feature in Japanese health care lies in the dread of stomach cancer. Then and now, their high salt-and-fish diet is directly related to a high incidence of stomach disorders and cancer among Japanese. And for Watanabe, the waiting patient, probably Suzuki, and many Japanese, stomach cancer is feared above all other cancers. What is it about the stomach that induces this fear?

A clue lies imbedded in a complex web of spiritual beliefs and tradition and is reflected in language. Historically, the Japanese have thought of the region of the stomach, *hara*, as the physical locale for the soul. *Hara* harbored a person's spirit. For this reason, foot soldiers in medieval warfare feared injuring their abdominal region. They believed that wearing a *haramaki*, a cloth tightly wrapped around their stomachs, offered special protection to that organ. Centuries later, during World War II, Japanese women sewed one thousand red knots in each *haramaki* to again offer protection, particularly for soldiers about to face possible death from fighting in the front lines (Ohnuki-Tierney 1984).

Hara as a haven for one's spirit is further linked with beliefs regarding "saving face," that is, saving spirit by restoring honor. Samurai were able to "save face," for example after losing honor during battle, by taking their own lives, ripping through their stomachs. *Harakiri* literally means "killing the stomach." The ritual suicide called *seppuku* involves committing *harakiri* while another trusted second (*kaishaku-nin*) swiftly decapitates the person who is performing *harakiri*.[7]

Related to this idea of harboring the person's spirit, *hara* also signified a person's true disposition, or character, in a sense, the individual's being. According to anthropologist Emiko Ohnuki-Tierney, *hara* "represents a combination of the heart and the brain. It is the seat of both thought and feeling, or intellect and affect" (Ohnuki-Tierney 1984, p. 59). We see this combination of heart and mind in linguistic usage. This idea of the stomach's representing an individual's character is evident in common expressions. Someone with a "black stomach" (*hara ga guroi*) is someone of bad character. A person with a "big stomach" (*hara no ookii*) is altruistic and kind (someone whom we would think of as "bighearted"). To "display the stomach" (*hara o miseru*) is to show one's true feelings. When a person reaches a decision, that person "decides the stomach" (*hara o kimeru*). Note the nuance between *harakiri*, "killing the stomach," and *hara o watte hanasu*, "slicing the stomach open in order to speak," in other words speaking openly without holding anything back. We say something similar in "spilling the guts." In both cases, opening the stomach is a sort of emptying of the self.

As we see in the film, the stomach plays an important role in views toward the body in health and illness. Because it is believed that this region houses the person's spirit and character, protecting the stomach is of utmost importance. In view of this, Watanabe's perceived death sentence from stomach cancer and his consequent despondency and deep-rooted existential transformation take on added weight.

The significance of the stomach and, hence, the dreaded decree of stomach cancer are rather unique to Japanese culture and may be the single cultural feature relevant to health care ethics that stands out in the film. Even here, however, we need to exercise caution and not assume that other cultures do not share similar attitudes and beliefs regarding the stomach. Incidentally, with rumors of Hollywood hoping to remake the film in an American version with Tom Hanks in the leading role, if this crystallizes, it would be interesting to see how the remake can redo this symbol of the stomach and the accompanying dread of stomach cancer.

Conclusion

There was no sense of bioethics (later referred to as *seimei rinri*) in Japan in the 1950s and little or no thought given to notions of patients' rights. Indeed, the Japanese language did not have a term signifying "moral rights." Only when the Meiji Restoration introduced ideas regarding civil and legal rights did the closest approximation come about, *kenri*. This term, however, still does not mean the same as Western philosophical constructs of moral rights that embrace a clear distinction between moral and legal, between positive and negative moral rights, and that convey the nonabsoluteness of moral rights.

Even during the Meiji reform in education, law, and government, the pervasive Confucian ethos with its emphases on filial piety and respect for parents, teachers, and others in public authority still held sway in medicine. Physicians naturally acted in the role of parents, looking out for the best interests of their patients. In return, patients showed dutiful respect and obedience to them. This translated into a strong medical paternalism that embraced a fiduciary relationship between physicians and patients in that the mandate to protect patients meant acting in ways that would safeguard them from harm.

Given the meaning of the stomach and the dread associated with diseases of the stomach, Watanabe faces harm. For his physician, honestly disclosing the fact of stomach cancer to his patient could cause further injury in the form of serious depression and isolation. Westerners who do not dig beneath the surface of apparent differences between Japanese and Western clinical encounters might conclude that the Japanese health care setting treats patients immorally. And if one does not take the time and effort to more closely fathom moral grounds for these discrepancies, one overlooks the fact that, within this cultural milieu, deception occurs as a way of protecting the patient from the serious harms of depression and isolation. Given the particular significance of the stomach—as the seat of the soul—in Japanese culture, it would seem that compassion and care for the patient would require nondisclosure, rather than the opposite.

Responsible bioethics must seriously heed the social, cultural, and historical contexts of concerns that permeate its rich interdisciplinary field. The same can be said for intercultural bioethics, indeed even more so in view of the illuminating quality of cultures' situatedness. A well-informed intercultural approach avoids reductionist claims that Japanese physicians are unjustifiably paternalistic or deceitful. Both assertions demonstrate net-casting, the path of least resistance. In the case of Japanese clinical encounters, an intercultural bioethics is trustworthy when it can reasonably weigh and carefully assess the relevant social, cultural, and historical parameters of paternalism and deception. At the same time, with respect to meanings associated with stomach cancer, there are surely grounds for at least cautiously claiming the distinctiveness of the fear and dread among Japanese surrounding stomach cancer.

As to lessons we can learn from *Ikiru*, one is the need to be vigilant against making facile generalizations about cultures. It is all too easy to assert that the United States is essentially "rights-driven" whereas Japan is more "duty-driven," or to allege that the United States promotes independence whereas Japan reinforces interdependence (Kawashima 1967; Doi 1973; Markus 1991; Yamada 2002; Young 2002).[8]

Deeper issues underlie these apparent surface tensions, and, as I see it, these have to do with matters of self-definition and personal identity. That is, there is a vital relationship between one's view of one's "self" and how one believes one ought to act with others. There is an intimate link between ontology and ethics. For instance, the expression of autonomy, self-rule, hinges pretty much on how one defines "self." In mainstream Western philosophical thought, patient autonomy refers to the *individual* patient's self-determination. Yet, because "self" may be perceived differently in other cultural contexts, autonomy is not necessarily abandoned in cultures that view identity in more collective ways. For this reason, I argue for an "ontological shift" in ways of understanding personal identity as a necessary condition for reasoned discourse among cultures. By this, I pose the challenge as to whether we can gradually move from a privatized notion of "self" (as an independent, isolated "I") to a sense of "I" that is more communal (other-oriented).[9] Clearly, there is still a danger in this appeal if based on assumed ontological polarities, that is, private and independent versus collective and interdependent. Thinking in terms of such polarities violates the first commandment in intercultural studies—"Let us not cast unfair nets over cultures."

Responsible intercultural bioethics refuses to typecast a group on the bases of specific narratives such as Watanabe's. At the same time, this intercultural approach cultivates an informed sensitivity to and knowledge of both germane internal discrepancies within the same group and certain shared features with other groups. While admitting that certain traits (such as meanings attached to the stomach) may be unique, an informed intercultural bioethics will make every effort to understand and appreciate such beliefs within their proper contexts and resist the temptation to presume that distinction in itself suggests exclusivity and incompatibility.

QUESTIONS FOR CONSIDERATION

1. *In view of the problematic in intercultural bioethics, are there sufficient grounds to make a reasonable claim for a global bioethics? For a global ethics?*

2. *Considering the natural tendency and need to generalize, when would generalization cross the line into net-casting?*

3. Ikiru *is a Japanese film, and translators may offer various nuances in interpretation to enable audience comprehension. Intercultural dialogue is possible only if there is intercultural discourse. Is intercultural discourse possible? Are some worldviews radically incongruent with others?*

NOTES

1. Here I am reminded of the teachings of the neo-Confucian philosopher Wang Yang-ming (Wang Shou-jen, 1472–1529), whose radical equation of knowledge and action profoundly influenced failed revolutionaries in Japan such as Oshio Heihachiro (1793–1837) and Mishima Yukio (1925–70). On behalf of the impoverished working class, Oshio led an unsuccessful revolt against the ruling dynasty in 1837 in which he and his followers, including his son, lost their lives. So also, Mishima committed ritual suicide, *seppuku*, after failing in his attempt to lead his right-wing Shield Society (*Take no kai*) in a coup against the Japanese army in 1970.

2. During my research fellowship in 1995 at the University of Tokyo to examine Japanese perspectives on organ transplants and brain-death, Japanese faculty and graduate students at the School for International Health desired to learn more about mainstream principles of American bioethics. They were genuinely interested in knowing more about our approaches and values.

3. In contrast, biomedicine's success lies in its effectiveness in dealing with acute illness and disease.

4. Even before the Meiji Restoration, during the last decade of the Edo Period, there was an official government bias in favor of the "new medicine." Until then, there was little emphasis on officially credentialing healers.

5. The Japanese Medical Association (Dai Nippon Ikai), formed in 1893, just a few decades after the start of the Meiji Restoration, remains a powerful voice in Japanese politics as well as health care.

6. This was the case in a study at Fukuoka University School of Medicine (Hattori et al. 1991; Akabayashi et al. 1999; Seo et al. 2000).

7. Ohnuki-Tierney points out that this use of *hara* is used more often by men and underscores a masculine attitude behind ritual suicide (Ohnuki-Tierney 1984, 59).

8. Japanese psychologist Takeo Doi's *Anatomy of Dependence* is a classic account of the notion of *amae*, the "desire to be loved and cared for." According to Doi, *amae* captures the Japanese wish to lean on others' good will and underscores the need for

dependency. More recently, we see this in Haru Yamada's *Different Games, Different Rules*. Even though she warns us of stereotypes, her linguistic analysis of communication styles still points out how Americans value independence and Japanese value mutual dependence. As for the rights-duties polarity, Jerome Young's essay on suicide describes a pervading sense of duty among Japanese stemming from a powerful Confucian ethic of propriety, duty, and ultimately loyalty to the collective. Also, Kawashima Takeyoshi's article on rights offers an insightful discussion of the origins of the idea of "rights" in Japan.

9. I addressed this issue in a Communication, Medicine, and Ethics conference at the University of Cardiff, Wales, sponsored by its Health Communication Research Centre (see www.cardiff.ac.uk/encap/hcrc/comet2006) and more recently at the University of Tokyo, Center for Biomedical Ethics and Law, February 8, 2008.

REFERENCES

Akabayashi, A., Fetters, M., and Elwyn, T. 1999. Family Consent, Communication, and Advance Directives for Cancer Disclosure: A Japanese Case and Discussion. *Journal of Medical Ethics* 25, 4:296–301.

Bioethical Committee for the Japanese Medical Association. 1994. Report Regarding Informed Consent. *Journal of the Japanese Medical Association (Nihon Ishika Zashi)* 103:515–28.

Brannigan, M. C., ed. 2004. *Cross-Cultural Biotechnology: Ethical, Legal, and Social Issues*. Maryland: Rowman & Littlefield.

———. 2005. *Ethics across Cultures*. New York: McGraw-Hill.

Brannigan, M., and Boss, J. 2001. *Healthcare Ethics in a Diverse Society*. New York: McGraw-Hill.

Doi, T. 1973. *Anatomy of Dependence*, trans. J. Bester. Tokyo: Kodansha International.

Hattori, H., Salzberg, S. M., Kiang, W. P., et al. 1991. The Patient's Right to Information in Japan: Legal Rules and Doctor's Opinions. *Social Science and Medicine* 32:1007–16.

Kawashima, T. 1967. The Status of the Individual in the Notion of Law, Right, and Social Order in Japan. In *The Japanese Mind*, ed. C. Moore, 262–87. Honolulu: University of Hawaii Press.

Kurosawa, A. 1952. *Ikiru* [motion picture]. Tokyo: Toho Company.

Lock, M. M. 1980. *East Asian Medicine in Urban Japan*. Berkeley and Los Angeles: University of California Press.

Long, S. O. 1987. Health Care Providers: Technology, Policy, and Professional Dominance. In *Health, Illness, and Medical Care in Japan: Cultural and Social Dimensions,* eds. M. Lock and E. Norbeck, 66–88. Honolulu: University of Hawaii Press.

Markus, H. A., and Kitayama, S. 1991. Culture and the Self: Implications for Cognition, Emotion, and Motivation. *Psychological Review* 98, 2:224–53.

Ohnuki-Tierney, E. 1984. *Illness and Culture in Contemporary Japan: An Anthropological View*. Cambridge: Cambridge University Press.

Otsuka, Y. 1976. Chinese Traditional Medicine in Japan. In *Asian Medical Systems,* ed. C. Leslie, 322–40. Berkeley and Los Angeles: University of California Press.

Seo, M., Tamura, K., Shijo, H., et al. 2000. Telling a Diagnosis to Cancer Patients in Japan: Attitude and Perception of Patients, Physicians and Nurses. *Palliative Medicine* 14:105–10.

Steineck, C. 2005. Handling Cancer: Ethical Discussions about Cancer in Japan. At www.jsps-club.de/staticfiles/Vortrag_Steineck.pdf.

Yamada, H. 2002. *Different Games, Different Rules: Why Americans and Japanese Misunderstand Each Other.* New York: Oxford University Press.

Young, J. 2002. Morals, Suicide, and Psychiatry: A View from Japan. *Bioethics* 16, 5:412–24.

Index